Human sperm acrosome reaction

*Réaction acrosomique
du spermatozoïde humain*

Human sperm acrosome reaction

Réaction acrosomique du spermatozoïde humain

Proceedings of the international symposium on " Human sperm acrosome reaction, physiological and pharmacological induction and transduction pathways", held in Collioure, France, 7-9 September 1995

Actes du symposium international sur "La réaction acrosomique du spermatozoïde humain, mécanismes d'induction physiologique et pharmacologique et voies de transmission du signal" Collioure, France, 7-9 septembre 1995

The symposium was held under the patronage of
Le symposium s'est tenu sous le patronage de

L'Institut National de la Santé et de la Recherche Médicale (INSERM)

Edited by

Patrick Fénichel
Jean Parinaud

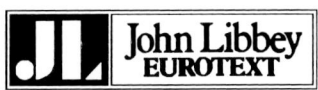

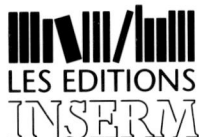

British Library Cataloguing in Publication Data

A catalogue record for this book is available from the British Library

ISBN 2-7420-0094-1
ISSN 0768-3154

First published in 1995 by

Editions John Libbey Eurotext
127, avenue de la République, 92120 Montrouge, France.
(33) (1) 46 73 06 60
ISBN 2-7420-0094-1

John Libbey and Company Ltd
13 Smiths Yard, Summerley Street, London SW18 4HR, England.
(44) (81) 947 27 77

Institut National de la Santé et de la Recherche Médicale
101, rue de Tolbiac, 75654 Paris Cedex 13, France.
(33) (1) 44 23 60 00.
ISBN 2-85598-627-3

ISSN 0768-3154

© 1995 Colloques INSERM / John Libbey Eurotext Ltd,
  All rights reserved
  Unauthorized publication contravenes applicable laws

Préface

Le processus de fécondation implique, aussi bien chez les invertébrés marins que chez les mammifères supérieurs, une phase d'activation du spermatozoïde au contact des enveloppes de l'œuf. Cette étape calcium-dépendante, appelée "réaction acrosomique", met en jeu la libération d'un granule sécrétoire, l'acrosome, situé à la face antérieure de la tête, qui permet la pénétration du spermatozoïde jusqu'à la membrane ovocytaire.
Les dix dernières années ont vu les connaissances de la fonction acrosomique progresser de manière très importante grâce à l'avènement de nouveaux outils d'étude de l'acrosome. C'est ainsi qu'il a pu être montré qu'elle ne peut être réalisée que si le spermatozoïde a subi des modifications membranaires appelées capacitation. Les inducteurs physiologiques ont été identifiés comme étant les stéroïdes du liquide folliculaire et les glycoprotéines de la zone pellucide. Les mécanismes moléculaires mis en jeu lors de la réaction acrosomique ont été partiellement caractérisés. Ils semblent impliquer plusieurs voies de transmission du signal (tyrosine kinases, protéine kinases C et A, canaux ioniques).
Ces connaissances fondamentales ont trouvé des applications cliniques. C'est ainsi que l'exploration de la fonction acrosomique a pris une place importante dans le bilan d'infertilité masculine et que des agents pharmacologiques sont utilisés *in vitro* afin d'augmenter la capacitation. De plus, des applications prometteuses telles que la contraception vaccinale ou le tri des spermatozoïdes ayant effectué leur réaction acrosomique sont en cours de développement.
Depuis quelques années, l'intérêt pour cette fonction du spermatozoïde est allé croissant comme l'atteste le grand nombre de publications sur ce sujet. Il nous a donc paru opportun d'organiser, avec le soutien de l'INSERM, un symposium international sur la réaction acrosomique réunissant les meilleurs spécialistes internationaux, afin de faire le point sur les aspects cliniques et fondamentaux. Cet ouvrage collige les textes des conférences de cette réunion qui s'est tenue à Collioure en septembre 1995. L'année 1995 représente une période charnière en raison du développement rapide de la micro-injection de spermatozoïdes dans le cytoplasme ovocytaire. Cette technique sophistiquée, qui donne des résultats spectaculaires, ne représente néanmoins qu'une solution de remplacement qui ne fait que constater l'échec dans la compréhension des mécanismes physiologiques et dans la thérapeutique. Il reste donc souhaitable de progresser dans le démembrement des différentes étapes de la fécondation et de développer des approches pharmacologiques de l'infertilité masculine.

Les éditeurs

Preface

In marine invertebrates as well as in mammals, the fertilization processes imply an activation phase of the spermatozoa induced by the egg vestments. This calcium-dependent step, called acrosome reaction, is the exocytosis of the acrosome, a secretory granule localized at the anterior part of the sperm head, which allows the spermatozoa to reach the oocyte plasma membrane.

Due to the appearance of new tools for acrosome study, the knowledge of acrosome function has greatly progressed during the past ten years. It has been shown that acrosome reaction is possible only if the spermatozoa has undergone membrane modifications in the course of capacitation. The physiological inducers have been identified as follicular steroids and glycoproteins of the zona pellucida. The molecular mechanisms have been partially characterized and involved several transduction pathways, *i.e* protein kinases A and C, tyrosine kinases, ionic channels.

These basic data have allowed clinical applications and the assessment of acrosome function is now used for checking male fertility. Moreover, high promising applications such as pharmacological enhancement of capacitation, immunocontraceptives and selection of acrosome reacted spermatozoa are in development.

Recently, the interest for this sperm function has been growing as attested by the number of scientific communications in this area. Therefore, we thought opportune to organize, under the high patronage of INSERM, an international symposium on "acrosome reaction" to gather together some of the outstanding experts to report the most recent basic and clinical advances. This book collects the texts of the communications of this meeting held in Collioure in September 1995.

In 1995, the great development of intra-cytoplasmic sperm injection has induced a big change in the clinical aspects of andrology. However, this technique, which gives very good results, is only a palliative and reflects failures in both the understanding of physiological processes and the medical therapy. Therefore, it is still necessary to increase the knowledge of fertilization events in order to develop pharmacological treatments of male infertility.

The editors

International Scientific Committee
Comité Scientifique International

P. Fénichel, Faculté de Médecine de Nice, France
R.A.P. Harrison, AFRC Babraham Institute Cambridge, England
Y. Menezo, INSA Lyon, France
D. Mortimer, Sydney IVF, Pty Ltd, Australia
J. Parinaud, Faculté de Médecine de Toulouse, France

Organizing Committee
Comité d'organisation

P. Fénichel, Faculté de Médecine de Nice, France
J. Parinaud, Faculté de Médecine de Toulouse, France

The symposium has been supported by
Le symposium a reçu le soutien de

L'Institut National de la Santé et de la Recherche Médicale (INSERM)
Les laboratoires Organon Pharmagyne, Serono et Theramex

Acknowledgments
Remerciements

We would like to express our gratitude to the speakers who accepted to come from a long way to present in Collioure their most recent data.
The authors specially thank Hélène Moutaffian (Toulouse) for her great contribution to the symposium organization and to the book edition.

Nous remercions vivement les conférenciers qui ont accepté de se déplacer pour présenter, à Collioure, leurs résultats les plus récents.
Des remerciements particuliers vont à Hélène Moutaffian sans les efforts considérables de laquelle ce symposium n'aurait pu avoir lieu.

List of participants
Liste des participants

AANESEN Arthur,
Karolinska Hospital, Department of Obstetrics and Gynaecology, Box 140, 17176 Stockolm (Sweden)
AITKEN John,
MRC Reproductive Unit, 37 Chalmers Street, Edinburgh EH3 9EW (Scotland)
ARAN Begona,
Institut Dexeus, P Bonanova, 89-91, 08107 Barcelona (Spain)
ARTS Eugène,
University Hospital Groningen, Oostersingel 59, Groningen NL-9713 EZ (The Netherlands)
BAKER Gordon,
University of Melbourne, Department of Obstetrics and Gynaecology, Royal Women Hospital, Melbourne 3053 (Australia)
BALDI Elisabetta,
Andrology Unit, University of Firenze, Viale Pierraccini 6, Florence 50139 (Italy)
BALTES Petra,
Andrological Research Unit, Department of Dermatology and Andrology, Justus Liebig University, Gaffykstrasse 14, D 35392 Gießen (Germany)
BARNABE Renato,
Perreira Leite 341, Sao Paulo 05442-015 (Brazil)
BARNABE Valquiria,
Perreira Leite 341, Sao Paulo 05442-015 (Brazil)
BARRIERE Paul,
Maternité du CHU de Nantes, quai Moncousu 44035 Nantes Cedex 01 (France)
BARTHELEMY Claire,
CECOS, CHU Bretonneau 37044 Tours Cedex (France)
BASTIT Pierre,
CEGOP Saint Antoine, Clinique Saint Antoine, 696 rue Pinchon 76230 Bois Guillaume (France)
BECKER Andreas,
Schering AG, Institute for Cellular and Molecular Biology, Berlin D-13342 (Germany)
BLACKMORE Peter,
Eastern Virginia Medical School, Department of Pharmacology, PO Box 1980, Norfolk Virginia 23501 (USA)

BOUCHER Daniel,
CHU Gabriel Montpied, Laboratoire de BDR, place H. Dunant, 63003 Clermont-Ferrand Cedex 1 (France)
BREITBART Haim,
Bar Ilan University, Department of Life Sciences, Ramat Gan 52900 (Israel)
BREWIS Ian,
Department of Molecular Biology and Technology, University of Sheffield, Sheffield S10 2UH (United Kingdom)
BRINGMANN Peter,
Schering AG, Institute for Cellular and Molecular Biology, Berlin D-13342 (Germany)
BUJAN Louis,
CECOS, CHU la Grave, place Lange, 31052 Toulouse (France)
CHEN John,
CSCG del CMR, via T.Pendola 62, Siena 53100 (Italy)
COHEN-BACRIE Paul,
Laboratoire d'Eylau, 55 rue Saint Didier, 75116 Paris (France)
COHEN-DAYAG Anat,
Weizmann Institute, Rehovot 76100 (Israel)
COZZI Jean,
CHU de Grenoble, Hôpital de la Tronche, 38043 Grenoble Cedex (France)
CZYBA Jean-Claude,
Hôpital Edouard Herriot, place d'Arsonval 69437 Lyon Cedex 03 (France)
DE JONGE Christopher,
University of Nebraska, Medical Center, 600 sth 42nd street, Omaha NE 68198-3255 (USA)
DECAUX Joel,
Hôpital Manchester, Maternité, 08000 Charleville- Mézières,
EA 1719, IRCL Lille, place de Verdun, 59045 Lille Cedex (France)
DEMOULIN André,
Centre de PMA, Hôpital de la Citadelle, boulevard du 12ème de Ligne, Liège (Belgique)
DONZEAU Michèle,
CHU de Nice, 38 avenue de la République, 06300 Nice (France)
EMILLIOZI Clélia,
Centre de PMA, CHU de Nice, 38, avenue de la République, 06300 Nice (France)
FENICHEL Patrick,
CHU de Nice, 38 avenue de la République, 06300 Nice (France)
FERET Christophe,
Aster Biotechnologies, ZA Les Nertières, 06140 La Gaude (France)

FERNANDEZ Pedro,
Andrology-IVF Laboratory, Human Reproduction Unit, Hospital Universitario La Fe, avda. Campanar 21, 46009 Valencia (Spain)
FLORMAN Harvey,
Worcester Foundation for Experimental Biology, 222 Maple Street, Shrewsburry MA 01545 (USA)
FOLIGUET Bernard,
Maternité Antoine Pinard, 10, rue du Docteur Heydenreich, 54042 Nancy Cedex (France)
FRANKEN Daniel,
Department of Obstetrics and Gynaecology, 19063 Tygerberg Hospital, Bellville 7505 (South Africa)
FRASER Lynn,
Biomedical Science Division, King's College London Strand, London WC2R 2LS (United Kingdom)
FRIEDRICH Kai-Jochem,
Department of Dermatology, Andrology, Sigmund Freud str 25, Bonn 53105 (Germany)
GADELLA Bart,
Babraham Institute, Babraham hall, Cambridge CB2 4AT (United Kingdom)
GARCIA Manuel,
University of California, Department of Cell Biology (USA)
GOJALAS Laura,
Weizmann Institute, Rehovot 76100 (Israel)
GOMEZ Martha,
University of Sydney, Department of Animal Sciences, Sydney MSW 2006 (Australia)
GRILLO Jean-Marie,
CHU de la Belle de Mai, 23 rue F.Simon, 13001 Marseille (France)
GRIVEAU Jean-François,
Unité de Biologie de la Reproduction, Hôtel-Dieu, 1bis, rue de la Cochardière Rennes 35000 (France)
GRIZARD Geneviève,
CHU Gabriel Montpied, Laboratoire de BDR, place H. Dunant, 63003 Clermont-Ferrand Cedex 1 (France)
GRUNDY Carolyn,
Department of Applied Biology, University of Hull, Cottingham Road, Hull HU6 7RX (United Kingdom)
GUERIN Jean-François,
Hôpital Edouard Herriot, place d'Arsonval, 69437 Lyon Cedex 03 (France)
GUICHAOUA Marie Roberte,
CHU de la Conception, Bd Baille, 13385 Marseille Cedex 05 (France)

HAMAMAH Samir,
Unité de Biologie de la Reproduction, Département de Gynécologie Obstétrique, Faculté de Médecine, CHU Bretonneau, 37044 Tours Cedex (France)
HARRISON Robin,
Department of Development and Signalling, AFRC Babraham Institute, Cambridge CB2 4AT (United Kingdom)
HENKEL Ralf,
Department of Dermatology / Andrology, Gaffkystr 14, Giessen 35392 (Germany)
HERR John,
University of Virginia Health Sciences, Department of Anatomy and Cell Biology, Box 439, Charlottesville VA 22908 (USA)
HINSCH Klaus-Dieter,
Hautklinik Giessen, Gaffkystr 14, 35392 Giessen (Germany)
HOLT William,
Institute of Zoology, Regents Park, London NW1 4RY (United Kingdom)
HUSZAR Gabor,
Department of Obstetrics and Gynaecology, Yale University School of Medicine, 333 Cedar street FMB 331, New Haven CT 06510 8063 (USA)
KALENTAR SEYED Medhi,
Jessop Hospital for Women, Leavygrave road, Sheffield S3 7RE (United Kingdom)
KEATING Jean,
University of Hull, Applied Biology, Cottingham rd, HU6 7RX (United Kingdom)
KOHN Frank,
Department of Dermatology, Gaffkystrasse, 35385 Gießen (Germany)
KOPF Gregory
University of Pensylvannia Medical Center, DRB, Philadelphia, Pensylvannia 19104-6080 (USA)
LE LANNOU Dominique,
Unité de Biologie de la Reproduction, Hôtel-Dieu, 1bis, rue de la Cochardière, Rennes 35000 (France)
LIU De Yi,
Royal Women Hospital, 132 Grattan st, Carlton Victoria, Melbourne, 3053 (Australia)
LUCAS Hervé,
Unité de Biologie de la Reproduction, CHU Nantes (France)
LUCONI Michaela,
Andrology Unit, University of Firenze, viale Pierraccini 6, Florence 50139 (Italy)

MAC CANN Christine,
University of Sheffield, Firth Hall, Western Bank, Sheffield (United Kingdom)
MARTINEZ Paz,
Instituto de Biologia Fondamental, Universidad Autonoma Barcelona, Bellaterra 98193 (Spain)
MATHIEU Claudine,
Maternité Pellegrin, place Amélie Raba-Léon, 33000 Bordeaux (France)
MAYER Guy,
Maternité Pellegrin , place Amélie Raba-Léon, 33000 Bordeaux (France)
MEIZEL Stanley,
University of California, Department of Cell Biology, Davis California 95618643 (USA)
MENESINI Maria Julia,
CSCG del CNR, via T. Pendola 62, Siena 53100 (Italy)
MENEZO Yves,
IRH Fondation Mérieux, 1 rue Laborde, Bron 69500 (France)
MERCIER Georges,
FIV Marseille-Provence, 77 rue du Docteur Escat, 13006 Marseille (France)
MIEUSSET Roger,
CECOS, CHU La Grave , place Lange 31052 Toulouse Cedex (France)
MILHET Pierrette,
Laboratoire de Fécondation in vitro, CHU La Grave, 31500 Toulouse (France)
MISKA Werner,
Department of Dermatology/ Andrology, Gaffkystr 35392 Giessen (Germany)
MOOBRATEN Larry,
Jackson Laboratory, 600 Main street, Bar Habor, ME 04609 (USA)
MOORE Harry,
University of Sheffield, Department of Cell Biology and Biotechnology, Sheffield (United Kingdom)
MORALES Patricio,
Faculty of Biological Sciences, Catholic University of Chile, Santiago (Chile)
MORTIMER David,
SIVF Sydney, 187 Macquirie Street, Sydney 2000 (Australia)
MOUTAFFIAN Hélène,
CHU La Grave, Laboratoire de FIV, 31052 Toulouse Cedex (France)
NADAV Zamir,
Department of Physiology and Pharmacology, Faculty of Medicine, Tel Aviv University, Tel Aviv 69978 (Israel)

NAOR Zvi,
Tel Aviv University, Faculty of Life Sciences, Ramat Aviv, Tel Aviv 69978 (Israel)
NAZ Rajesh,
Albert Einstein College of Medicine, Department of Obstetrics and Gynaecology, 1300 Moris Park Avenue, New York 10461 (USA)
NUNEZ Rocio,
Ramon y Cajal Hospital, Andrology Laboratory, CTRA Colmenar km 9100, 28034 Madrid (Spain)
O'TOOLE Chris,
King's College, Strand, London WC2R 2LS (United Kingdom).
OSTERHOFF Carolyn,
Institute for Hormones and Fertility Research, Grandweg 164, Hamburg D 22529 (Germany)
PARINAUD Jean,
CHU La Grave, Laboratoire de FIV, 31052 Toulouse Cedex (France)
PARIS Jacques,
Laboratoire Theramex, 6 av du Prince Albert, 98000 Monaco (Monaco)
POSILICO James,
Intermune Life Sciences, BCE place suite 2500, 181 Bay street, Toronto M6J 2T7 (Canada)
REVELLI Alberto,
University of Torino, Department of Obstetrics and Gynaecology, Largo Turati 62, Torino 10128 (Italy)
ROLDAN Eduardo,
Departamento de Reproduccion Animal, CIT-NIA, Ctra de la Coruna Km 5,9 28040 Madrid (Spain)
ROUSSEAUX PREVOST Roselyne,
EA 1719, IRCL Lille, place de Verdun 59045 Lille Cedex (France)
ROUSSEAUX Jean,
EA 1719, IRCL Lille, place de Verdun 59045 Lille Cedex (France)
SALING Patricia,
Box 3648, Duke University Medical Center, Durham NC 27710 (USA)
SELVA Jacqueline,
Hôpital Antoine Béclère, 157 rue de la Porte de Trivaux, 92141 Clamart (France)
SI Yuming,
Tokyo University, Department of Biology, Komaba, Meguro-Ku, Tokyo, 153 Tokyo (Japan)
SIDHU Kuldhip,
Andrology Laboratory, Department of Zoology, Punjab Agricultural University; Ludhiana 141 004 (India)

SION Benoît,
CHU Gabriel Montpied, Laboratoire de BDR, place H. Dunant, 63003 Clermont-Ferrand Cedex 1 (France)
SULLIVAN Robert,
Hôpital Maisonneuve, 5415 l'Assomption, Montréal H1T 2M (Canada)
SWEENEY Antoinette,
Toxicology Unit, Regional College, Athlone (Ireland)
TESARIK Jan,
Hôpital Américain de Paris, Laboratoire de Spermiologie, 92202 Neuilly (France)
THEPOT François,
Centre de PMA, CHU d'Amiens, 124, rue Camille Desmoulins, 80000 Amiens (France)
TOMKINS Paul,
Regional College, Toxicology Unit, Athlone 05442-015 (Ireland)
TOURNAYE Herman,
Centre of Reproductive Medicine, Laarbeeklaan 101, Brussels B-1090 (Belgium)
TROUP Stephen,
Manchester Fertility Services, BUPA Hospital, Russel road, Whalley range, Manchester MIC8AJ (United Kingdom)
VAN DER MERWE Elisabeth,
Medical Research Council, PO box 19070, Tygerberg, Cape Town 7505 (South Africa)
VAN KOUIJ Roelof,
University Hospital, Heidelberglaan 100, Utrecht, PO box 85500 (The Netherlands)
VIEITEZ Gérard,
Laboratoire de Fécondation in vitro, CHU La Grave, 31052 Toulouse (France)
VITTORI Christian,
Aster Biotechnologies, ZA les Nertières, 06140 La Gaude (France)
WHITFORD William,
Life Technologies, 2086 Grandisland Blvd, Grandisland NY, 14072 (USA)
WOLF Jean-Philippe,
Clinique Universitaire de Baudelocque, 123 boulevard de Port-Royal, 75674 Paris Cedex 14 (France)

Contents
Sommaire

Foreword
Préface

Acknowledgments
Remerciements

List of participants
Liste des participants

Chapter I / *Chapitre I*

Capacitation / *Capacitation*

1   The sperm plasma membrane
La membrane plasmique du spermatozoïde
W.V. Holt

17   Mechanisms regulating capacitation and the acrosome reaction
Mécanismes contrôlant la capacitation et la réaction acrosomique
L.R. Fraser

35   Modification of sperm membrane antigens during capacitation
Modification des antigènes membranaires pendant la capacitation
H.D.M. Moore

45   Membrane changes during capacitation with special reference to lipid architecture
Modifications membranaires et particulièrement de l'architecture lipidique pendant la capacitation
R.A.P. Harrison, B.M. Gadella

67   Lipid transfer protein: a natural stimulator of the sperm capacitation process
Les protéines de transfert lipidique: un stimulateur naturel de la capacitation
C.H. Muller, S.E. Ravnik

Chapter II / *Chapitre II*

Physiological induction of acrosome reaction /
Induction physiologique de la réaction acrosomique

85   Sperm interaction with the zona pellucida: the role of ZRK
Les interactions du spermatozoïde avec la zone pellucide: rôle de ZRK
P.M. Saling, D.J. Burks, M.R. Carballada, C.A. Dowds, L. Leyton, S.B. McLeskey, A. Robinson, C.N. Tomes

105   Induction of the human acrosome reaction by rhuZP3
Induction de la réaction acrosomique par la ZP3 recombinante
C.L.R. Barratt, D.P. Hornby

123   The role of proteases in the mammalian sperm acrosome reaction
Rôle des protéases lors de la réaction acrosomique chez les mammifères
J. Tesarik

133   Role of the acrosome reaction in egg vestments and plasma membrane penetration
Rôle de la réaction acrosomique dans la pénétration des enveloppes de l'œuf
P. Morales, M. Llanos

151   Initiation of human sperm acrosome reaction by progesterone
Initiation de la réaction acrosomique par la progestérone
S. Meizel

165   Effect of steroids on calcium fluxes in human sperm
Effets des stéroïdes sur les flux calciques dans le spermatozoïde
P.F. Blackmore, J.F. Fisher, C.H. Spilman, W.B. Im, J.E. Bleasdale

Chapter III / *Chapitre III*

Transduction pathways during acrosome reaction
Les voies de transduction du signal au cours de la réaction acrosomique

179 Exo(cyto)tic ion channels in mammalian sperm
Les canaux ioniques exo(cyto)tiques dans les spermatozoïdes de mammifères
H.M. Florman, J.R. Lemos, C. Arnoult, J.A. Oberdof, Y. Zeng

191 Integration of tyrosine kinase and G protein-mediated signal transduction pathways in the regulation of mammalian sperm function
Place des voies de transmission du signal impliquant les tyrosine kinases et la protéine G dans la régulation de la fonction du spermatozoïde de mammifère
G.S.Kopf, P.E. Visconti, J. Moos, H.L. Galantino-Homer, X.P. Ning

217 Role of protein kinase C in human sperm acrosome reaction
Rôle de la protéine kinase C dans la réaction acrosomique du spermatozoïde humain
Z. Naor, R. Rotem, M. Kalina

225 Role of phosphoinositides in the mammalian sperm acrosome reaction
Rôle des phospho-inositides dans la réaction acrosomique chez les mammifères
E.R.S. Roldan

245 Role of membrane tyrosine kinases in human sperm function
Rôle des tyrosine kinases membranaires dans la fonction spermatique
R.K. Naz

257 Role of cAMP pathways: cross-talk mechanisms for the acrosome reaction
Rôle des voies de l'AMPc: mécanismes de réaction croisée
C. De Jonge

Chapter IV / *Chapitre IV*

Clinical applications /
Applications cliniques

277 Methods for evaluating the acrosomal status of human sperm
Méthodes d'évaluation du statut acrosomique du sperme humain
N.L. Cross

287 Culture media, capacitation and acrosome reaction
Rôle des milieux de culture sur la capacitation et la réaction acrosomique
Y. Ménézo

295 *In vitro* induction of the human sperm acrosome reaction
Induction in vitro *de la réaction acrosomique*
D. Mortimer

315 Acrosomal function and sperm fertilizing ability
La fonction acrosomique et le pouvoir fécondant du sperme
P. Fénichel

327 Physiopathology of acrosome dysfunctions
Physiopathologie des dysfonctionnements de l'acrosome
F.M. Köhn, R. Henkel, K.F. El-Mulla, W.B. Schill

339 Mechanisms and prevention of lipid peroxidation in human spermatozoa
Mécanismes et prévention de la peroxidation lipidique dans les spermatozoïdes
J. Aitken

355 The acrosome and intracytoplasmic sperm injection
Acrosome et injection intracytoplasmique du spermatozoïde
A.Van Steirteghem, Z. Nagy, J. Liu, H. Joris, P. Devroey

363 Selection of acrosome reacted spermatozoa
Sélection des spermatozoïdes réactés
J. Parinaud, H. Moutaffian

373 The use of acrosomal antigens as contraceptive immunogens: studies on the intra-acrosomal antigen SP-10
Utilisation des antigènes acrosomiques dans la contraception vaccinale: étude de l'antigène intra-acrosomique SP-10
J.C.R Herr

Chapter V / *Chapitre V*

Posters / *Posters*

387 Fluidity changes in sperm membranes during capacitation
Morros A., Iborra A., Alsina M., Martinez P.

388 Fluorescence techniques used to study sperm membrane lipid architecture during capacitation
Gadella B.M., Harrison R.A.P.

390 Extracellular calcium inhibits tyrosine kinase activity during capacitation of human spermatozoa
Luconi M., Krausz C., Forti G., Baldi E.

392 Protein phosphorylation on tyrosine during human sperm capacitation
Emiliozzi C., Philip P., Ciapa B., Fénichel P.

393 Fate of two novel human sperm antigens HE4 et HE5 during *in vitro* capacitation
Osterhoff C., Kirchhoff C., Ivell R.

395 Quantification of energetic patterns of human spermatozoa during capacitation process by 31p magnetic resonance spectroscopy (31p-MRS)
Hamamah S., Seguin F., Barthélémy C., Royere D., Perrotin F., Lansac J.

397 Sperm capacitation in human is transient and correlates with chemotactic responsiveness
Cohen-Dayag A., Tur-Kaspa I., Dor J., Mashiach S., Eisenbach M.

399 Stimulation of human sperm during capacitation *in vitro* by an analog of adenosine
Fénichel P., Gharib N., Emilliozzi C., Donzeau M., Ménézo Y.

400 Origin and nature of the acrosome reaction-inducing substance (ARIS) of human follicular fluid (hFF)
Baltes P., Sanchez R., Schalles U.K., Villegas J., Peña P., Henkel R., Turley H., Miska W.

402 Preincubation in peritoneal fluid affects follicular fluid induced acrosomal reactivity *in vitro*
Revelli A., La Sala G.B., Modotti M., Miceli A., Balerna M., Massobrio M.

403 Inhibition of zona binding using solubilized human zona pellucida
Franken D.R., Henkel R., Kaskar K., Habenicht U.F.

404 The production and purification of recombinant human ZP3 from *E. coli*
Chapman N.R., Hornby D.P., Barratt C.L.R., Moore H.D.M.

406 The use of antibodies raised against synthetic peptides to conserved and unconserved regions of human ZP3 for characterization of sperm-egg interactions
Mc Cann C.T., Barratt C.L.R., Moore H.D.M.

408 Calcium/progesterone mediated acrosome response and sperm maturity are not related in human spermatozoa
Huszar G., Vigue L.

410 Effect of lysophospholipids on the human sperm acrosome reaction
Llanos M., Morales P., Salgado A.M., Vigil P.

412 Evidence suggesting that reacted human spermatozoa express a L-selectin
Lucas H., Harb J., Le Pendu J., Mirralie S., Bercegeay S., Jean M., Barrière P.

414 Localization and characterization of protein 4.1 in human spermatozoa
Roussseaux Prevost R., Dalla Venezia N., Saint Pol P., Delaunay J., Rousseaux J.

416 P 34 H: an epididymal protein associated with the acrosome of human spermatozoa
Sullivan R., Balis J., Boué F.

418 Relationship between timing of the acrosome reaction induction and the fusiogenic capacity of human spermatozoa
Cozzi J., Chevret E., Rousseaux S., Pelletier R., Sele B.

419 Induction of human sperm capacitation and acrosome reaction in the reproductive tract of hamster cultured *in vitro*
Dhindsa J.S., Sidhu K.S., Guraya S.S.

420 Mechanisms underlying ANP- induced acrosomal exocytosis in bovine sperm
Zamir N., Barkan D., Keynan N., Naor Z., Breibart H.

421 Role of reactive oxygen species (ROS) on human sperm acrosome reaction
Fernandez P.J., Doncel G.F., Acosta A.A., Romeu A.

422 Superoxide anion production by human spermatozoa as a part of the ionophore induced acrosome reaction process
Griveau J.F., Renard P., Le Lannou D.

423 Participation of protein kinases in calcium ionophore induced human acrosome reaction
Asin S., Doncel G.F., Acosta A.A.

425 Progesterone induces Ca^{2+} dependent cAMP increase in human spermatozoa
Milhet P., Parinaud J.

426   The signal transduction pathway of the acrosome reaction in human spermatozoa in response to purified recombinant human ZP3
Brewis I.A., Chapman N.R., Barratt C.L.R., Hornby D.P., Moore H.D.M.

428   Comparison of two cryopreservative media on acrosomal status
Barthelemy C., Saussereau M.H., Fricot G., Hamamah S., Royère D., Tharanne M.J.

430   Effect of caffeine citrate and heparin on post-thawed motility and on acrosomal cap of buffalo bull spermatozoa frozen in different diluents: assay for *in vitro* fertilization technique
Barnabe V.H., Barnabe R.C.

431   Effects of lipids in cryoprotective diluants on motility and fertilization potential of post-thaw human spermatozoa
Grizard G., Sion B., Renard P., Artonne C., Boucher D.

432   A simple method for assessment of the human acrosome reaction (AR) of spermatozoa bound to the zona pellucida (ZP): lack of relationship with ionophore A23187 induced AR
Liu D.Y., Baker H.G.W.

434   Clinical characteristics of disordered zona pellucida induced acrosome reaction: a newly described cause of infertility
Baker H.W.G., Liu D.Y., Bourne H.

436   Correlation between clinical diagnosis and acrosomal protease assay for the evaluation of male infertility
Chen J.S., Ma J., Chang H.S., Chang T.S., Sensini C., Collodel G., Piombini P., Baccetti B., Menesini Chen M.G.

438   Detection of patients defective in acrosome reaction
Arts E.G.J.M., Van Kooij R.J., Kastrop P.M.M., Hobo A.C.

439   Sperm function tests and fertilization failure following IVF
Kalantar S.M., Lenton E.A., Barratt C.L.R.

441 The effect of testosterone enanthate administration on the acrosome reaction to ionophore challenge (ARIC) test
Troup S.A., Bellis A., Wu F.C.W., Lieberman B.A.

442 Use of acrosome reaction for predicting *in vitro* fertilization results
Richoilley G., Moutaffian H., Vieitez G., Milhet P., Labal B., Parinaud J.

444 Effect of four sperm capacitation treatments on fertilization *in vitro* and after intracytoplasmic injection of *in vitro* matured sheep oocytes
Gomez M.C., Catt J.M., Maxwell W.M.C., Evans G.

446 Prognostic value of hamster test with calcium ionophore A 23187
Van Kooy R.J, Arts E.G.J.M, Kastrop P.M.M, Velde E.R

447 A novel method for evaluating the acrosomal status of mammalian spermatozoa
Margalit I., Rubinstein S., Breitbart H.

448 Changes in lectin receptors in ejaculated, capacitated and acrosome reacted rhesus monkey spermatozoa
Sivashanmugam P., Navaeetham D., Rajalakshmi M.

449 Expression of sperm binding-receptors in different groups of human spermatozoa
Friedrich KJ., Haidl G., Deiss B., Kreysel H.W.

450 Modifications of lectin binding sites on the surface of human sperm during acrosome reaction
Fierro R.C., Daniel M., Foliguet B., Bene M.C., Barbarino P., Faure G., Grignon G.

452 Response of human spermatozoa to five different acrosome reaction inducers
Kohn F.M., El-Mulla K.F., El-Beheiry A.H., Schill W.B.

454 Studies on the kinetics of human sperm acrosome reaction; a mathematical model for assessment
Henkel R., Franken D.R., Maritz. J.S., Schill W.B., Habenicht U.F.

456 The application of scanning probe microscopy to the visualization of the human sperm acrosome reaction
Sweeney A., Tomkins P.T.

458 Using flow cytometry for acrosome status evaluation in human sperm
Nikoaleva M.A., Gougassian I.A., Philippova R.D., Sukhikh G.T.

460 The extrusion of doublet ODF-s (outer dense fibers) 5-6 associating with fibrous sheath sliding in mouse sperm flagella
Si Y., Okuno M.

Chapter I
Chapitre I

Capacitation
Capacitation

The sperm plasma membrane

W.V. Holt

Institute of Zoology, Zoological Society of London, Regent's Park, London NW1 4R, United Kingdom

ABSTRACT

Changes to the lateral organization of the membrane begin during spermiogenesis, continue during epididymal maturation, and after a period of stability during storage in the cauda epididymidis, must reorganize yet again in preparation for fertilization. The mechanisms which control the initial establishment of sperm membrane domains, and their subsequent reorganization may involve selfassembling lipid and protein interactions, and the actions of endoproteases. Capacitation is accompanied by significant changes in membrane architecture, possibly to facilitate membrane fusion and signalling events during fertilization. The equatorial segment is a prime target for much of the reorganization, and contains an array of proteins and lipids with fusogenic, structural and cell binding activity. This review highlights some relevant recent findings, but also evaluates the possible relationships between separate lines of evidence which can sometimes appear conflicting.

Les modifications de structure de la membrane débutent au cours de la spermiogénèse et se poursuivent durant la maturation épididymaire, puis après une période de stabilité au cours de leur stockage dans la queue de l'épididyme, doivent se réorganiser de nouveau en vue de la fécondation. Les mécanismes contrôlant la mise en place initiale des domaines membranaires ainsi que leurs réorganisations consécutives semblent impliquer l'autoassemblage des lipides et les interactions protéiques ainsi que l'action des endoprotéases. La capacitation s'accompagne de changements importants de l'architecture membranaire, probablement afin de faciliter la fusion des membranes et la transmission de signaux lors de la fécondation. La plaque équatoriale est le lieu de prédilection de la plupart des réorganisations et contient une multitude de protéines et de lipides ayant des propriétés fusogéniques, structurales et de liaison. Cette revue souligne quelques-unes des découvertes récentes, mais également évalue les relations probables entre différentes données pouvant parfois paraître contradictoires.

The ultrastructural differentiation of the sperm plasma membrane into domains is now well known (for reviews, see (1, 2)) and for several species, including the human, the changes in membrane structure during epididymal maturation and prior to fertilization have also been recorded (for example, (3-6)). The criteria for distinguishing membrane domains include morphology, antibody specificity, lectin binding, membrane-sterol content, lipid asymmetry and lipid phase state. The challenge now facing gamete biologists is to elucidate the functional significance of the heterogeneity during the events prior to fertilization. The wealth of recent research in this area has identified a potentially confusing richness of processes upon which sperm membrane function reportedly depends.

ORGANIZATION, ORIGIN AND MAINTENANCE OF SPERM PLASMA MEMBRANE DOMAINS.

Domain formation begins during the post-meiotic period when the haploid spermatid undergoes elongation (1, 7-9). This stage is important for subsequent sperm development as subsequent membrane modifications cumulatively build upon pre-existing membrane components. In keeping with current models of membrane protein targeting, it is generally believed that sperm membrane components are synthesized within the endoplasmic reticulum and processed by the Golgi apparatus. There are, however, indications that mechanisms which bypass the Golgi apparatus may also operate (10). Targeting of membrane components to specific regions of the spermatid plasma membrane may occur during spermiogenesis. For example, domain formation during spermiogenesis has been deduced in the guinea pig (11) from observations that two related integral membrane proteins (PM52 and PM35) are detected only in the periacrosomal region of the sperm head prior to entry into the epididymis. Earlier cytochemical studies (12) demonstrated redistribution of acrosomal components within elongating spermatids from the guinea pig and other mammals, leading to domain formation in the outer acrosomal membrane. The disposition of acrosomal contents could govern the architecture of the overlying plasma membrane through intermembrane contacts (13).

Studies of sperm antigen PH-20, initially detected in the guinea pig (9, 14, 15) then in mouse, cynomolgous monkey and human (16-17), showed that although its final distribution in spermatozoa was confined to specific surface and internal sites on the head, it first appeared within the Golgi apparatus of round spermatids and was later distributed over the entire cell surface of testicular spermatozoa. This antigen was regionalized late in epididymal transit, disappearing from the flagellum, and (in the guinea pig at least) being concentrated into the post-acrosomal domain. Species differences are evident here as mouse and monkey PH-20 is localized over the acrosomal region. The mechanism of regionalization is obscure. Although PH-20 is phosphatidylinositol linked and potentially free to diffuse laterally like a lipid, Phelps et al (15) failed to show that its mobility depended upon the lipid phase state of the membrane and suggested that restriction was imposed by interactions of its ectodomain. If this particular antigen is regionalized in response to the reorganization of others, how do they in turn become organized?

The ultrastructure of the annulus suggests that this ring-like array of tightly packed intramembranous particles situated at the posterior end of the middle-piece would prevent the lateral diffusion of integral membrane proteins. Supporting evidence was provided by Myles et al (18), who showed that a guinea pig antigen, PT-l, was freely diffusible within the confines of the posterior sperm tail region but could not traverse the annulus. Studies of a rat sperm integral membrane protein, CE-9, (19-20) provided similar evidence that an antigen can be freely diffusible within a barrier-limited membrane domain, the posterior region of the sperm tail. However, these studies also showed that whilst CE-9 was restricted to the posterior tail region in testicular and caput epididymal spermatozoa, it was redistributed anteriorly during epididymal transit, thereby inevitably bypassing the annulus. Correlative studies carried out in vitro showed that before redistribution this antigen, originally a 251 amino acid protein, underwent endoproteolytic cleavage with the removal of 75 extracellular amino acids. Significantly, redistribution was temperature- sensitive and energy (ATP) dependent. By analogy, proteolytic processing of extracellular peptide sequences may stimulate the redistribution of several antigens, such as the PH20 mentioned above (21). The difficulty with this view is that the required proteases are insensitive to high concentrations of protease inhibitors, and with particular relevance to CE-9, treatment with exogenous protease neither proteolyses it nor stimulates redistribution. However, a specific protease of appropriate function cannot be ruled out.

Critical judgment about the validity of data must be exercised when considering this evidence. Phillips et al (22) evaluated changes in staining patterns of rat spermatozoa from different epididymal regions and discussed the technical artefacts which could confound immunocytochemical evidence. They showed that some apparent redistribution could be caused by epitope exchange between different parts of the membrane. The evidence cited above for domain formation and the behavior of membrane antigens does not invoke the need for stabilization by underlying cytoskeletal elements. Early experiments in cell fusion showed that some membrane antigens are freely and laterally miscible (23) a finding confirmed in numerous subsequent studies.

However, spermatozoa clearly possess mechanisms which confine some protein populations, and indeed lipids (24, 25), to particular membrane domains. The potential involvement of a regulated cytoskeletal network in controlling the diffusibility of membrane components is attractive. Lateral diffusion of membrane components may be retarded by three independent factors,; viscous drag, steric effects and transient binding to relatively immobile structures (for review, see (26)). Evidence is accumulating that candidate components of a sperm cytoskeletal network are indeed present in the membrane. While remaining independent these could act together to control the formation and maintenance of membrane domains. Evidence of extensive cytoskeletal linkages between the plasma membrane and underlying structures has been derived from ultrastructural studies (13), and immunocytochemical studies have identified some of the proteins involved. Some main findings are reviewed below.

CYTOSKELETAL PROTEINS AND SPERM MEMBRANE ORGANIZATION.

G-actin is present in spermatozoa from a variety of species but although its distribution appears to be consistent during spermiogenesis (27) inter-species differences have emerged for mature spermatozoa. Human spermatozoa show actin localization in the acrosomal cap (28) neck and principal piece (29) whilst rabbit, boar and ram spermatozoa exhibit equatorial segment or postacrosomal localization (27, 30). It is therefore difficult to interpret such differences in functional terms.

Virtanen (28) localized an immunoanalogue of erythrocyte α-spectrin over the acrosomal cap and principal-piece of rabbit and human spermatozoa, and moreover identified this antigen as a calmodulin-binding protein. In somatic cells this polypeptide is typically located beneath the plasma membrane, and by binding to F-actin filaments forms a framework for plasma membrane organization. Currently there is no evidence for F-actin in ejaculated spermatozoa, although its transient formation from G-actin cannot be excluded. Virtanen (28) reported that the localization of actin, spectrin and vimentin in human spermatozoa coincided with distinct surface specializations. For example, vimentin, an intermediate filament protein, was localized to the equatorial segment, the initial site of sperm egg fusion. This finding was subsequently confirmed and extended (31); vimentin was localized in permeabilized (28) and non-permeabilized cells (31). This protein, which is partly exposed on the cell surface, thus potentially provides anchor sites between the plasma membrane and underlying structures. It may be significant for sperm regulation that vimentin in other situations has phosphorylation sites for protein kinase C and cAMP dependent kinase (32, 33), which control assembly and disassembly of its structure, and that protein kinase C has also been localized to the equatorial segment of human spermatozoa (34). Although no direct connection has so far been made, numerous reports point to the involvement of phosphorylation mechanisms in sperm capacitation (e.g. (35, 36). Annexins, a class of proteins which may be involved in the membrane attachment of cytoskeletal elements, have also been detected in the equatorial segment of human spermatozoa (37) and would be worthy of further investigation for a potential role in sperm-egg fusion.

    The equatorial segment of human and rat spermatozoa contains band-3 related proteins (38). These are members of the anion exchange protein family (for review, see (39)) responsible for bicarbonate-chloride exchange and regulation of intracellular pH, which have also been implicated in the flipping of anionic phospholipids (40, 41). Given current evidence that bicarbonate is essential for capacitation (36, 42) and can also induce rapid (i.e. <90 sec) fluidization of membrane lipids (43), the possible involvement of band-3 proteins in capacitation is of interest. Fibronectin, a high molecular weight (250 kd) glycoprotein was recently localized to the equatorial segment of human spermatozoa (44). It was detected on the surface of both acrosome intact and acrosome-reacted cells, and since the sperm-egg interaction was inhibited by antifibronectin antibodies it was proposed that fibronectin acted to promote the initial binding of the sperm head to the egg plasma membrane surface.

LIPIDS AND MEMBRANE ORGANIZATION

The organization of membranes into domains requires either interaction between integral membrane components and underlying cytoplasmic structures, or a range of self-assembly mechanisms. Cytoskeletal protein activity is therefore likely to be mediated through protein-lipid interactions. There is increasing evidence that physiological events involve these interactions, and that lipids may be the primary targets of physiological agonists during the prefertilization period.

The sperm plasma membrane contains an unusual array of lipids. The phospholipids typically adopt unusual configurations in mammals; there is a relatively high proportion of plasmalogens, which contain ether-linked fatty acids instead of the more common ester linkages. No satisfactory explanation for this idiosyncrasy currently exists, although a role in protection against oxidative stress is one possibility (45). Phospholipids account for 65 - 75% of the total, but a large proportion of these comprises docosahexaenoic acid, a component which confers membrane fluidity and instability. Possibly to counteract this destabilizing effect the membrane also contains sterols such as cholesterol, cholesterol-sulphate and desmosterol (46).

The finely balanced biophysical status of the mammalian sperm plasma membrane has been demonstrated in several studies (e.g. (47-51)), and at physiological temperatures the sperm membrane contains coexistent regions of fluid and gel phases. During capacitation the sterols appear to be removed by lipid-transfer proteins (52) and albumin (53-55) in preparation for fertilization. It is important to note that the increase in temperature which the spermatozoa experience as they enter the female tract would act synergistically with such biochemical changes to produce a fusogenic, but unstable, membrane lipid environment.

Studies of guinea pig, boar and human spermatozoa indicate that sterols and acidic phospholipids are concentrated over the acrosomal cap region (2, 56). In human spermatozoa, the cholesterol sulphate can occupy up to 20% of the sperm head surface area. Desulphation of sterol sulphates in the female reproductive tract, and their subsequent removal, would dramatically change the biophysical properties of the sperm plasma membrane towards a more fusogenic state. A model for capacitation based around this mechanism was proposed by Langlais and Roberts (55). Cheetham et al (57) proposed an alternative model of capacitation which was similarly based, but allowed for the observation that not all sterol sulphate was removed during capacitation. Deriving their data mainly from in vitro studies of liposomes, these authors suggested that cholesterol sulphate could interact with Ca^{2+} to cause membrane destabilization in preparation for membrane fusions during the acrosome reaction.

The potential involvement of lipid-protein and lipid-lipid interactions in the maintenance of membrane domains has recently seen a resurgence of interest. Liposomes, containing a fluorescent lipid analogue to indicate fusion and acidic phospholipids to promote fusogenicity, fused with the equatorial segment of acrosome-reacted bovine and human spermatozoa (58). Interestingly they did not fuse with acrosome-intact spermatozoa nor with other membrane domains of acrosome-reacted cells, but could fuse with frozen-thawed cells. Further studies of this system (59) in human spermatozoa suggested that the fluorescent label was restricted within the equatorial segment domain by barriers to lateral diffusion which existed in both the inner and outer membrane leaflets. The diffusion barriers could not be abolished by external protease treatment; however, 10 mM EDTA treatment allowed the fluorescent label to spread over the sperm head and even over the flagellum. The authors were certain that this was not a facilitation of liposome-membrane fusion occurring after preliminary labeling of the equatorial segment membrane, but a real promotion of lateral random diffusion. One explanation for these results was that EDTA treatment, which would bind calcium and other divalent cations, might perturb plasma membrane proteins. This might modify the properties of cytoskeletal or lipid-binding proteins (60). Calcium is also known to interact directly with a number of lipid groups modifying their phase separation behavior. The importance of glycolipids in this process has recently been highlighted by the observation that mammalian spermatozoa contain sulphogalactosylceramide (seminolipid) which becomes redistributed from the apical segment into the equatorial segment during capacitation (61). It was proposed that desulphation of this lipid by aryl sulphatase in seminal plasma could promote its redistribution towards the equatorial segment. The formation of the hexagonal IT phase of phospholipids within the membrane might then follow, thus facilitating fusion. There is some similarity between this proposal and Cheetham's model (57) where the formation of the hexagonal II phase was invoked as a role of sterol sulphates in membrane destabilization. The capacity to form fusogenic intermediates seems to be correlated with the ability to form hexagonal phase structures although this does not mean that the hexagonal structures are actually required for fusion (62).

The uniquely fusogenic ability of the equatorial segment was underlined when ram spermatozoa were experimentally induced to fuse with avian erythrocytes (63). In this instance the fusogenicity was augmented by adding microdispersed glyceryl mono-oleate to a mixture of cells. Similarly, lysolipids have been used to provoke the acrosome reaction (64). The possibility that such fusogenic derivatives are active in vivo has recently been highlighted by the detection and localization of lysophospholipase over on the plasma membrane overlying the acrosome of human spermatozoa (65), as well as on the inner acrosomal membrane. This would provide a mechanism for deactivating lysolipids formed through the action of phospholipases.

These results are not wholly in agreement with recent studies in the guinea pig, where evidence exists for the role of a sperm integral membrane protein (PH-30) in mediating fusion between the oocyte and sperm plasma membranes. This protein consists of two subunits, one of which resembles a viral fusion protein and the other contains a peptide related to a family of soluble integrin ligands (66). In this instance the PH-30 is localized over the post-acrosomal region of the sperm head (67), a position which does not entirely accord with the role of the equatorial segment as the initial site of sperm-oolemma interaction.

INITIATION OF CAPACITATION AND THE ACROSOME REACTION

Conceptual disagreement between various hypothetical mechanisms for the membrane fusion process itself are also relevant here. Some models for membrane fusion (68, 69) propose that the perturbation of the membrane lipid bilayer by fusogens increases the proportion of hydrocarbon chains in the liquid state. When such bilayers are apposed, components become intermingled with the resultant formation of unstable intermediates and membrane fusion. This model accommodates the relocation of intramembranous proteins as seen in freeze-fracture images of capacitating and acrosome-reacting spermatozoa (70), with the appearance of particle-free, and presumably fusogenic, membrane regions. Recent opinion has favored an active role for integral membrane proteins in fusion, and suggests that membrane fusion is accompanied by protein aggregation (for reviews, see (71, 72)). Freeze-fracture studies of acrosome reacting boar spermatozoa (73) lent support to this view by showing that fusion (the acrosome reaction) was initiated in areas rich in transmembrane glycoproteins which had become clustered over the apical region. This model is more consistent with the hypothesis that a viral fusion protein is involved in sperm-egg fusion, but both models are compatible with the possibility that extensive lateral relocation of plasma membrane components is a prerequisite to fertilization. Like the relocation of seminolipid discussed above, it is clear that a number of membrane components undergo redistribution during the period prior to fertilization, and conversely that membrane destabilization can result from the artificial induction of redistribution. For example, cross-linking a variety of sperm membrane antigens with antibodies induces the acrosome reaction in different species (mouse (74, 75); sheep (76); human (77)). The zona pellucida component ZP3 is also thought to induce the acrosome reaction by aggregating sperm surface receptors (78).

Although somewhat speculative, a capacitation mechanism can be envisaged which is initiated by a fluidization of membrane lipid components through exogenous influences such as lipid-transfer proteins, albumin and sterol sulphatases, and which leads to lipid phase changes and the relocation of membrane proteins. Such a mechanism was elaborated by Visconti et al (36), who suggested that changes in membrane fluidity would provoke a pre-programmed series of membrane and intracellular events. Their model linked the initial fluidization of the plasma membrane to increased calcium permeability, the activation of adenylyl cyclase and protein kinase A, and a cascade of events involving the tyrosine-phosphorylation of several proteins. Physiological changes not involving membrane fusion, such as hyperactivation, can be accommodated within such a model and it is a useful basis for further investigation.

The view that capacitation and the acrosome-reaction involves intra-membranous modification and redistribution of membrane lipids and proteins has been strengthened recently by the realization that progesterone can initiate the acrosome reaction in a variety of species (see (79) and references therein). Several lines of evidence suggested that progesterone binds to specific receptors in the plasma membrane, which then aggregate over the equatorial segment and elicit rapid calcium uptake at the same time. The mechanisms involved in the progesterone-induced acrosome reaction are discussed at length within this volume and a comprehensive consideration of the topic would be inappropriate. However, it is important to note that recent work in the mouse suggests that the progesterone response involves the activation of a γ-aminobutyric acid receptor (GABA) receptor which in turn leads to the opening of calcium channels (80). These findings indicate that progesterone is not merely acting through its intrinsic ability to modify membrane lipid fluidity.

CONCLUSIONS

Recent evidence about specific lipid and protein interactions of the sperm plasma membrane underlines the view that its complex architecture constantly changes throughout the developmental process, from spermiogenesis to fertilization. Intrinsic localized factors, such as highly specific proteases, may be essential in this process, preparing the membrane for signal transduction and fusion. Many potential signal transduction pathways are apparently activated during capacitation and the possibility of some redundancy within this system must be considered. While variability in characteristics such as sperm shape or length is obvious, signaling pathways may also have undergone subtle biochemical evolution. Such cryptic differences may be contributing to current difficulties in the interpretation of sperm membrane function. The human spermatozoon appears to conform in many respects with what is known about other mammalian species, and the case for extrapolation between species seems reasonably strong. However, spermatologists may have to consider the species differences more seriously when judging the respective merits of particular cell mechanisms.

REFERENCES

1. Holt WV. Membrane heterogeneity in the mammalian spermatozoon. Int Rev Cytol 1984: 159-194.
2. Friend DS. Membrane organization and differentiation in the guinea pig spermatozoa., In: Van Blerkom J, Motta PM eds. Ultrastructure of Reproduction. Boston: Martinus Nijhoff, 1984: 75-85.
3. Singer SL, Lambert H, Cross NL, Overstreet JW. Alteration of the human sperm surface during in vitro capacitation as assessed by lectin-induced agglutination. Gamete Res 1985; 12: 291-299.
4. Cross NL, Overstreet JW. Glycoconjugates of the human sperm surface: distribution and alterations that accompany capacitation in vitro. Gamete Res 1987; 16: 23-25.
5. Cerezo JMS, Beuno MI, Skowronski B, Cerezo AS. Immunohistochemical localization of concanavalin A and wheat germ lectin receptors in the normal human spermatozoa. Am J Reprod Immunol 1982; 2: 246-249.
6. Kallojoki M, Malmi R, Virtanen I, Suominen J. Glycoconjugates of human sperm surface. A study with fluorescent lectins and Lens culinaris agglutination affinity chromatography. Cell Biology Int Reports 1985; 9: 151-164.
7. Holt WV. Functional development of the mammalian sperm plasma membrane. In: Firm CA ed. Oxford Rev Reprod Biol, Oxford: Clarendon Press, 1982: 195-240.
8. Pelletier RM, Friend DS. Development of membrane differentiations in the guinea pig spermatid during spermiogenesis. Am JAnat 1983; 167: 119-141.
9. Phelps BM, Myles DG. The guinea pig sperm plasma membrane protein, PH-20, reaches the surface via two transport pathways and becomes localized to a domain after an initial uniform distribution. Dev Biol 1987; 123: 63-72.
10. Tanii I, Toshimori K, Araki S, Oura C. Extra-Golgi pathway of an acrosomal antigen during spermiogenesis in the rat. Cell Tiss Res 1992; 270: 451-457.
11. Westbrook-Case VA, Winfrey VP, Olson GE. Characterization of two antigenically related integral membrane proteins of the guinea pig sperm periacrosomal plasma membrane. Mol Reprod Dev 1994; 39: 309-321.
12. Holt WV. Development and maturation of the mammalian acrosome. J Ultrastruct Res 1979; 68: 58-71.
13. Escalier D. The cytoplasmic matrix of the human spermatozoon: cross-filaments link the various cell components. Biol Cellulaire 1984; 51: 347-364.

14. Primakoff P, Hyatt H, Myles DG. A role for the migrating sperm surface antigen PH-20 in guinea pig sperm binding to the egg zona pellucida. J Cell Biol 1985; 101: 2239-2244.
15. Phelps BM, Primakoff P, Koppel DE, Low MG, Myles DG. Restricted lateral diffusion of PH-20, a PI-anchored sperm membrane protein. Science 1988; 240: 1780-1782.
16. Lin Y, Mahan K, Lathrop WF, Myles DG, Primakoff P. A hyaluronidase activity of the sperm plasma membrane protein PH-20 enables sperm to penetrate the cumulus layer surrounding the egg. J Cell Biol 1994; 125: 1157-1163.
17. Gmachi M, Sagan S, Ketter S, Kreil G. The human sperm protein PH-20 has hyaluronidase activity. FEBSLetts 1993; 336: 545-548.
18. Myles DG, Primakoff P, Koppel DE. A localized surface protein of guinea pig sperm exhibits free diffusion in its domain. J Cell Biol 1984; 98: 1905-1909.
19. Petruszak JAM, Nehme CL, Bartles JR. Endoproteolytic cleavage in the extracellular domain of the integral plasma membrane protein CE9 precedes its redistribution from the posterior to the anterior tail of the rat spermatozoon during epidydimal maturation. J Cell Biol 1991; 114: 917-927.
20. Nehme CL, Cesario MM, Myles DG, Koppel DE, Bartles JR. Breaching the diffusion barrier that compartmentalizes the transmembrane glycoprotein CE9 to the posterior-tail plasma-membrane domain of the rat spermatozoon. J Cell Biol 1993; 120: 687-694.
21. Phelps BM, Koppel DE, Primakoff P, Myles DG. Evidence that proteolysis of the surface is an initial step in the mechanism of formation of sperm cell surface domains. J Cell Biol 1990; 111: 1839-1847.
22. Phillips DM, Jones R, Shalgi R. Alterations in distribution of surface and intracellular antigens during epididymal maturation of rat spermatozoa. Mol Reprod Dev 1991; 29: 347-356.
23. Frye LD, Edidin M. The rapid intermixing of cell surface antigens after formation of mouse-human heterokaryons. J Cell Sci 1970; 7: 319-335.
24. Wolf DE, Voglmayr JK. Diffusion and regionalization in membranes of maturing ram spermatozoa. J Cell Biol 1984; 98: 1678-1684.
25. Wolf DE, Lipscomb AC, Maynard VM. Causes of nondiffusing lipid in the plasma membrane of mammalian spermatozoa. Biochemistry 1988; 27: 860-865.
26. Zhang F, Lee GH, Jacobson K. Protein lateral mobility as a reflection of membrane microstructure. BioEssays 1993; 15: 579-588.
27. Camatini M, Colombo A, Bonfanti P. Cytoskeletal proteins involved in cell polarity: mammalian spermatozoa and insect enterocytes., In:

Lanzavecchia G, Valvassori R eds. Form and function in Zoology, Modena: 1991: 15-31.
28. Virtanen I, Badley RA, Paasivuo R, Lehto VP. Distinct cytoskeletal domains revealed in sperm cells. J Cell Biol 1984; 99: 1083-1091.
29. Flaherty SP, Winfrey VP, Olson GE. Localization of actin in human, bull, rabbit and hamster sperm by immunoelectron microscopy. Anat Rec 1988; 221: 599-610.
30. Holt WV, North RD. Cryopreservation, actin localization and thermotropic phase transitions in ram spermatozoa. J Reprod Fert 1991; 91: 451-461.
31. Ochs D, Wolf DP, Ochs RL. Intermediate filament proteins in human sperm heads. Exp Cell Res 1986; 167: 495-504.
32. Inagaki M, Nishi Y, Nishizawa K, Matsuyama M, Sato C. Site-specific phosphorylation induces disassembly of vimentin filaments in vitro. Nature 1987; 328: 649-652.
33. Geisler N, Weber K. Phosphorylation of desmin in vitro inhibits formation of intermediate filaments: identification of three kinase A sites in the aminoterminal head domain. EMBO J 1988; 7: 15-20.
34. Rotem R, Paz GF, Homonnai ZT, Kalina M, Naor Z. Protein kinase C is present in human sperm: possible role in flagellar motility. Proc Nat Acad Sci USA 1990; 87: 7305-7308.
35. Visconti PE, Bailey JL, Moore GD, Pan D, Olds-Clarke P, Kopf GS. Capacitation of mouse spermatozoa. 1. Correlation between the capacitation state and protein phosphorylation. Development 1995; 121: 1129-1137.
36. Visconti PE, Moore GD, Bailey JL, Pan D, Leclerc P, Connors SA, Olds-Clarke P, Kopf GS. Capacitation in mouse spermatozoa. II: Capacitation and protein tyrosine phosphorylation are regulated by a cAMP-dependent pathway. Development 1995; 121: 1 139-1 150.
37. Berruti G. Calpactin-like proteins in human spermatozoa. Exp Cell Res 1988; 179: 374-384.
38. Parkkila S, Rajaniemi H, Kellokumpu S. Polarized expression of a band 3-related protein in mammalian sperm cells. Biol Reprod 1993; 49: 326-331.
39. Reithmeier RAF. Mammalian exchangers and co-transporters. Curr Opinion in Cell Biology 1994; 6: 583-594.
40. Ortwein R, Oslender-Kohnen A, Deuticke B. Band 3, the anion exchanger of the erythrocyte membrane, is also a flippase. Biochim Biophys Acta 1994; 1191: 317-323.
41. Vondenhof A, Oslender A, Deuticke B, Haest CWM. Band 3, an accidental flippase for anionic phospholipids. Biochemistry 1994; 33: 4517-4520.

42. Neill JM, Olds-Clarke P. A computer-assisted assay for mouse sperm hyperactivation demonstrates that bicarbonate but not bovine serum albumin is required. Gamete Res 1987; 18: 121-140.
43. Harrison RAP, Ashworth PJC, Miller NGA. Rapid effects of bicarbonate/CO_2 on boar spermatozoa detected by merocyanine, a probe of lipid packing. J Reprod Fert 1993; Abstract Ser. 12: Abstr. 18.
44. Hoshi K, Sasaki H, Yanagida K, Sato A, Tsuiki A. Localization of fibronectin on the surface of human spermatozoa and relation to the sperm-egg interaction. Fert Steril 1994; 61: 542-547.
45. Darin-Bennett A, White IG, Hoskins DO. Phospholipids and phospholipid-bound fatty acids and aldehydes of spermatozoa and seminal plasma of rhesus monkeys. J Reprod Fert 1977; 49: 119-122.
46. Lin DS, Connor WE, Wolf DP, Neuringer M, Hachey DL. Unique lipids of primate spermatozoa - desmosterol and docosahexaenoic acid. JLipidRes 1993; 34: 491-499.
47. Holt WV, North RD. Determination of lipid composition and thermal phase transition. J ReprodFert 1985; 73: 285-294.
48. Holt WV, North RD. Thermotropic phase transitions in the plasma membrane of ram spermatozoa. J Reprod Fert 1986; 78: 445-457.
49. Buhr MM, Canvin AT, Bailey JL. Effects of semen preservation on boar spermatozoa head membranes. Gamete Res 1989; 23: 441-449. 1 0
50. Crowe JH, Hoekstra FA, Crowe LM, Anchordoguy TJ, Drobnis E. Lipid phase transitions measured in intact cells with Fourier transform infrared spectroscopy. Cryobiology 1989; 26: 76-84.
51. Wolf DE, Maynard VM, McKinnon CA, Melchior DL. Lipid domains in the ram sperm plasma membrane demonstrated by differential scanning calorimetry. Proc Natl Acad Sci USA 1990; 87: 6893-6896.
52. Ravnik SE, Zarutskie PW, Muller CH. Purification and characterization of a human follicular-fluid lipid transfer protein that stimulates human sperm capacitation. Biol Reprod 1992; 47: 1126-1133.
53. Davis BK, Byrne R, Bedigian K. Studies on the mechanism of capacitation: albumin-mediated changes in plasma membrane lipids during in vitro incubation of rat sperm cells. Proc Natl Acad Sci USA 1980; 77: 1546-1550.
54. Go KJ, Wolf DP. Albumin-mediated changes in sperm sterol content during capacitation. Biol Reprod 1985; 32: 145-153.
55. Langlais J, Roberts KD. A molecular membrane model of sperm capacitation and the acrosome reaction of mammalian spermatozoa. Gamete Res 1985; 12: 183-224.
56. Peterson RN, Gillott M, Hunt W, Russell LD. Organization of the boar spermatozoan plasma membrane: evidence for separate domains (subdomains) of integral membrane proteins in the plasma membrane

overlying the principal segment of the acrosome. J Cell Biol 1987; 88: 343-349.
57. Cheetham JJ, Chen RJB, Epand RM. Interaction of calcium and cholesterol sulphate induces membrane destabilization and fusion: implications for the acrosome reaction. Biochim Biophys Acta 1990; 1024: 367-372.
58. Arts E, Kuiken J, Jager S, Hoekstra D. Fusion of artificial membranes with mammalian spermatozoa - specific involvement of the equatorial segment after acrosome reaction. Eur J Biochem 1993; 217: 1001-1009.
59. Arts E, Jager S, Hoekstra D. Evidence for the existence of lipid-diffusion barriers in the equatorial segment of human spermatozoa. Biochem J 1994; 304: 211-218.
60. Jones R, Hall L. A 23 kDa protein from rat sperm plasma membranes shows sequence similarity and phospholipid binding properties to a bovine cytosolic protein. Biochim BiophysActa 1991; 1080: 78-82.
61. Gadella BM, Gadella TWJ, Colenbrander B, Van Golde LMG, Lopes-Cardozo M. Visualization and quantification of glycolipid polarity dynamics in the plasma membrane of the mammalian spermatozoon. J Cell Sci 1994; 107: 2151-2163.
62. Ellens H, Bentz J, Szoka FC. H+-induced and Ca2+-induced fusion and destabilization of liposomes. Biochemistry 1985; 13: 3099-3106.
63. Holt WV, Dott HM. Chemically induced fusion between ram spermatozoa and avian. J Ultrastruct Res 1980; 71: 311-320.
64. Fleming AD, Yanagimachi R. Effects of various lipids on the acrosome reaction and fertilizing capacity of guinea pig spermatozoa with special reference to the possible involvement of lysophospholipids in the acrosome reaction. Gamete Res 1981; 4: 253-273.
65. Lepage N, Roberts KD. Purification of lysophospholipase of human spermatozoa and its implication in the acrosome reaction. Biol Reprod 1995; 52: 616-624.
66. Blobel CP, Wolfsberg TG, Turck CW, Myles DG, Primakoff P, White JM. A potential fusion peptide and an integrin ligand domain in a protein active in sperm-egg fusion. Nature 1992; 356: 248-252.
67. Blobel CP, Myles DG, Primakoff P, White JM. Proteolytic processing of a protein involved in sperm egg fusion correlates with acquisition of fertilizing competence. J Cell Biol 1990; 111: 69-78.
68. Ahkong QF, Cramp FC, Fisher D, Howell JI, Tampion W, Verrinder M, Lucy JA. Chemically-induced and thermally-induced cell fusion: lipid-lipid interactions. Nature, New Biol 1973; 242: 215-217.
69. Lucy JA. Mechanisms of chemically induced cell fusion. In: Poste G, Nicolson GL eds. MembraneJusion, Amsterdam: Elsevier / North Holland, 1978: 267-304.

70. Flechon J. Sperm surface changes during the acrosome reaction as observed by freeze-fracture. Am J Anat 1985; 174: 239-248.
71. White JM. Membrane fusion. Science 1992; 258: 917-924.
72. Plattner H, Knoll G, Erxleben C. The mechanics of biological membrane fusion. Merger of aspects from electron microscopy and patch-clamp analysis. J Cell Sci 1992; 103: 613-618.
73. Aguas AP, Pinto da Silva P. Bimodal redistribution of surface transmembrane glycoproteins during Ca2+-dependent secretion (acrosome reaction) in boar spermatozoa. J Cell Sci 1989; 93: 467-479.
74. Aarons D, Boettger-Tong H, Holt G, Poirier GR. Acrosome reaction induced by immunoaggregation of a proteinase inhibitor bound to the murine sperm head. Mol Reprod Dev 1991; 30: 258-264.
75. Macek MB, Lopez LC, Shur BD. Aggregation of 1-, 4-galactosyltransferase on mouse sperm induces the acrosome reaction. Dev Biol 1991; 147: 440-444.
76. McKinnon CA, Weaver FE, Yoder JA, Fairbanks G, Wolf DE. Cross-linking a maturation-dependent ram sperm plasma membrane antigen induces the acrosome reaction. Mol Reprod Dev 1991; 29: 200-207.
77. Tesarik J, Mendoza C, Moos J, Fenichel P, Fehlmann M. Progesterone action through aggregation of a receptor on the sperm plasma membrane. FEBS Letts 1992; 308: 1 16-120.
78. Leyton L, Saling P. Evidence that aggregation of mouse sperm receptors by ZP3 triggers the acrosome reaction. J Cell Biol 1989; 108: 2163-2168.
79. Brucker C, Lipford GB. The human sperm acrosome reaction: physiology and regulatory mechanisms. An update. Human Reprod Update 1995; 1: 51-62.
80. Shi QX, Roldan ERS. Evidence that a $GABA_A$-like receptor is involved in progesterone-induced acrosomal exocytosis in mouse spermatozoa. Biol Reprod 1995; 52: 373-381.

Human sperm acrosome reaction. Eds P. Fénichel, J. Parinaud.
Colloque INSERM/John Libbey Eurotext Ltd © 1995. Vol. 236, pp. 17-33.

Mechanisms regulating capacitation and the acrosome reaction

Lynn R. Fraser

Anatomy and Human Biology, King's College London, Strand, London, WC2R 2LS, United Kingdom

Abstract

Successful mammalian fertilization requires that sperm first undergo capacitation and then the acrosome reaction, an exocytotic event that allows cells to penetrate the zona pellucida and to fuse with the oocyte plasma membrane. These events require a permissive extracellular environment, with the ionic composition playing a major role in the stimulation/inhibition of requisite processes that are needed for successful sperm function. Considerable evidence indicates that this is due to consequent changes in the intracellular ionic composition. This chapter will address some of the mechanisms that may play important roles in controlling ion fluxes, particularly in the sperm head. Regulation of Ca^{2+} fluxes appears to play the pivotal role in capacitation and the acrosome reaction, but other ions clearly participate in the complicated changes that promote/accompany the acquisition of fertilizing ability. Control of Ca^{2+}, as well as other cations and some anions, will therefore be considered.

La réussite de la fécondation chez les mammifères implique que les spermatozoïdes soient préalablement capacités puis qu'ils accomplissent leur réaction acrosomique. La réaction acrosomique est un phénomène d'exocytose permettant aux cellules de pénétrer la zone pellucide et de fusionner avec la membrane plasmique ovocytaire. Ces événements nécessitent un environnement extracellulaire favorable incluant la composition ionique qui joue un rôle primordial dans la stimulation/

inhibition des processus nécessaires aux fonctions du spermatozoïde. De nombreux signes indiquent que cela est dû à des changements importants de la composition ionique intracellulaire. Ce chapitre abordera quelques-uns de mécanismes qui pourraient jouer un rôle important dans le contrôle des flux ioniques, et plus particulièrement dans la tête spermatique. La régulation des flux calciques semble jouer le rôle central dans la capacitation et la réaction acrosomique, mais il est clair que d'autres ions participent aux changements complexes qui initient / accompagnent l'acquisition du pouvoir fécondant. Le contrôle du Ca 2+, ainsi que celui d'autres cations, sera donc considéré.

INTRODUCTION

In all mammals, sperm cells are required to fertilize oocytes, thereby (1) providing a haploid set of chromosomes with a paternal pattern of genomic imprinting needed for normal development and (2) triggering oocyte activation and the consequent initiation of metabolic events needed to support early embryonic development. It has long been known that successful fertilization is dependent on the extracellular ionic environment, in large part because this can modify the intracellular ionic composition of the gametes. The first observations on this were published 80 years ago, when Loeb (1) noted that fertilization in the sea urchin did not occur in the absence of extracellular Ca^{2+}. Later studies revealed that this was due to defective sperm function, namely failure of the acrosome reaction to occur. After the development of successful culture systems for mammalian gametes, it was possible to demonstrate that mammalian sperm fertilizing ability, like that of invertebrate sperm, can be modulated by alterations in the extracellular ionic composition.

Unlike their invertebrate counterparts, mammalian sperm are not immediately fertile upon release from the male reproductive tract, despite their ability to exhibit vigorous motility. They require a species-dependent period of time during which they undergo a series of changes, collectively referred to as 'capacitation' (2), that are needed for cells to become fully competent to fertilize an oocyte. When capacitated, mammalian sperm can (1) express hyperactivated motility, the very vigorous, thrusting pattern of motility that is needed for penetration of the oocyte investments (3) and (2) interact with oocytes (including cumulus cells, follicular fluid and zona pellucida) to undergo the acrosome reaction. The latter is an exocytotic event that promotes interaction with and penetration through the zona pellucida and confers fusogenic properties on the remaining plasma membrane in the sperm head (3). It has been suggested (4) that the importance of capacitation may actually be to prevent sperm from becoming fertile too quickly, given that cells are deposited into the lower regions of the female reproductive tract and must then move some considerable distance to reach the site of fertilization (usually the ampullary region of the oviduct). Indeed, the success of intracytoplasmic sperm injection proves that neither capacitation nor the acrosome reaction is an absolute requirement for the sperm nucleus to participate in normal embryonic and subsequent fetal development. This strengthens the argument that the mechanisms controlling capacitation and the acrosome reaction are designed to promote delivery of the sperm cell's 'payload', i.e. the nucleus, into the oocyte cytoplasm once a sperm has reached the vicinity of its target.

Although it is clear that, under normal assay conditions in vitro, uncapacitated sperm are not fertile while capacitated cells are, it has proved difficult to identify capacitated cells other than by demonstrable fertilizing ability. Thus, microscopic observation of uncapacitated and capacitated suspensions reveals no obvious morphological changes that accompany the acquisition of fertilizing potential. It is possible to detect and quantify changes in two sperm parameters that do reflect the acquisition of fertilizing ability, namely the ability to undergo the acrosome reaction and the ability to express hyperactivated motility. However, these do not necessarily provide information on the relative proportions of uncapacitated and capacitated cells in a population.

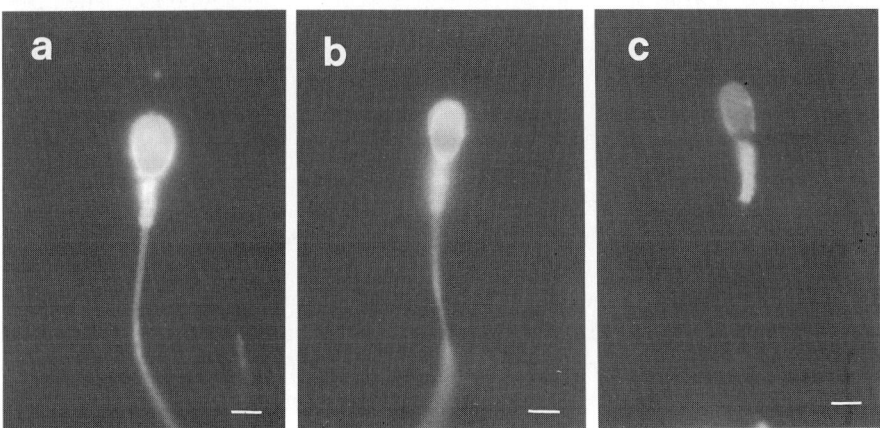

Figure 1: **Chlortetracycline fluorescence patterns observed in human sperm cells:** *(a) F, with fluorescence over the entire head (characteristic of uncapacitated, acrosome-intact cells); (b) B, with a fluorescence-free band in the postacrosomal region (characteristic of capacitated, acrosome-intact cells); (c) AR, with dull fluorescence over the entire head (characteristic of capacitated, acrosome-reacted cells). The bar represents 2.5 µm (from (7) with permission).*

During the past decade, numerous studies have indicated that the fluorescent antibiotic chlortetracycline (CTC) provides a useful tool for monitoring capacitation-related changes in sperm populations. CTC binds to membrane-associated cations, especially Ca^{2+} (5). When incubated briefly with mammalian sperm suspensions, CTC interacts with cells to give different binding patterns on the sperm head. Three main patterns were originally described for mouse sperm (6) and similar patterns of fluorescence have been observed in human (7), bull (8) and boar sperm (9). The main patterns are: F, with bright fluorescence over the entire head (characteristic of uncapacitated, acrosome-intact cells); B, with a fluorescence-free band in the postacrosomal region (characteristic of capacitated, acrosome-intact cells); AR, with dull fluorescence over the head (characteristic of capacitated, acrosome-reacted cells). In all cells, the midpiece is brightly fluorescent, whatever the distribution of fluorescence on the head. Typical examples of CTC patterns observed with human sperm are shown in Fig. 1. In general, temporal changes in relative proportions of the patterns reflect changes in the fertilizing ability of the whole population. When used on cells either selected for motility or stained with a vital dye (e.g. Hoechst bis-benzimide 33258), CTC provides information not available with conventional techniques used to assess occurrence of the acrosome reaction. By allowing assessment of the relative proportions of uncapacitated and capacitated sperm within the acrosome-intact group of cells, CTC analysis provides unique information relating to functional potential.

The value of the CTC technique was demonstrated recently during investigation of a possible physiological role for pyroglutamyl-glutamylprolineamide, a TRH-related peptide produced by the prostate gland and secreted into the seminal plasma of a number of mammals, including man (10). At concentrations of ≥ 25 nM, the tripeptide significantly stimulated capacitation (promoted more rapid transition from the F to the B pattern of CTC fluorescence) but had no stimulatory effect on the acrosome reaction. These results suggested that the peptide would stimulate fertility and in vitro fertilization experiments confirmed this, the peptide-treated cells being significantly more fertile than untreated counter parts. For this reason, it has been proposed that the peptide be called fertilization-promoting peptide (FPP) (10). The important point is that a conventional technique would only have revealed the lack of a stimulatory effect on the acrosome reaction and there would have been no obvious reason to study the peptide further. It should be emphasized that CTC analysis clearly focuses attention on changes in the sperm head. However, since successful fertilization requires coordinated alterations in both head and tail compartments, it is plausible that FPP also promotes requisite changes in motility. More recently, we have used CTC analysis to demonstrate that FPP at concentrations of ≥ 25 nM also stimulates human sperm capacitation, but not acrosomal exocytosis (11). Since FPP is found in human seminal plasma at a mean of ~ 50 nM (12), it may well play a positive role in promoting human sperm fertilizing ability. Impaired fertility in some men may reflect insufficient FPP or defective FPP-sperm interaction.

While the acrosome reaction, which involves fusion, vesiculation and eventual loss of membranes in the anterior portion of the sperm head, is clearly irreversible, current evidence indicates that capacitation itself is reversible. This reversibility appears to reflect the time-dependent dissociation from the sperm surface of proteins that inhibit fertilizing ability. At least some of these molecules, termed 'decapacitation factors' or DFs, can reassociate with sperm cells when they are added back to suspensions of capacitated cells and inhibit fertility, thereby reversibly altering sperm functional ability. These DFs may be either of epididymal or seminal plasma origin (13). In species that fall into the latter category, it is sometimes the case that epididymal sperm may actually be more fertile than ejaculated sperm since no time is needed to allow for dissociation of DF molecules and the consequent physiological 'switching on' of sperm. Therefore, the acquisition of DFs inhibits, at least temporarily, the fertilizing ability of cells. In vivo, the time required for dissociation of DF molecules may well coincide with the amount of time required for ejaculated sperm to reach the site of fertilization, thereby maximizing the possibility that potentially fertilizing sperm cells will be present when the oocyte(s) arrives. The fact that in some instances human sperm aspirated from various regions of the epididymis and even the testis have been able to fertilize oocytes successfully, leading to normal embryonic development and the establishment of full-term pregnancies, indicates that complete transit through the male reproductive tract is not required for acquisition of fertilizing potential.

In the mouse, at least one DF is of epididymal origin. Comparison of capacitation times in vitro required by epididymal and ejaculated mouse sperm to become highly fertile revealed no detectable differences, suggesting that contact with seminal plasma does not markedly alter capacitation kinetics in the mouse. The DF molecules are associated with the cell surface and are normally lost or inactivated slowly as cells capacitate, but they can be removed rapidly from uncapacitated sperm by gentle centrifugation and resuspension in fresh medium. This treatment causes an immediate and significant increase in the fertilizing ability of suspensions, these functional changes being reflected by a rapid transition from the F (uncapacitated) to the B (capacitated) pattern of CTC fluorescence in similarly treated suspensions. The reverse treatment, addition of crude or partially purified DF to capacitated, highly fertile suspensions, causes an immediate drop in fertility; CTC analysis indicates an inhibition of the acrosome reaction and a significant reversion from the B to the F pattern of fluorescence (14). Thus there are strong correlations between CTC patterns, presence or absence of DF and fertilizing ability. Recently we have demonstrated that the addition of partially purified mouse sperm DF to human sperm incubated overnight in a medium known to support human fertilization in vitro promoted a significant reversion from the B to the F pattern after 1 hour (15). These similarities in the CTC responses of both mouse and human sperm to mouse sperm DF suggest that there may be similarities in the underlying mechanisms that control capacitation in the two species.

IONIC REGULATION OF CAPACITATION

The establishment of culture systems that support in vitro capacitation and fertilization in a number of mammalian species has made it possible to address specific ionic requirements for each of these distinct stages, determining whether an ion is required and if so, how much and when. The majority of studies have focussed on cations, especially Ca^{2+}, Na^+, K^+ and H^+, but there is a small amount of information available on anions, especially Cl^-.

While many ions are able to affect sperm function, Ca^{2+} appears to play the pivotal role. Extracellular Ca^{2+} is required for completion of capacitation and for the acrosome reaction, but the concentrations required are species- and stage-dependent. Specifically, relatively little (micromolar concentrations) extracellular Ca^{2+} will support capacitation in at least some species (e.g. guinea pig, mouse), but millimolar concentrations are required for maximal acrosome loss and fertilization in all. At least some of this Ca^{2+} needs to be internalized, indicating that the important factor is probably changes in the intracellular Ca^{2+} concentration ($[Ca^{2+}]i$). Indeed, treatment of sperm in a Ca^{2+}-containing medium with a Ca^{2+} ionophore will promote rapid capacitation and acrosome loss; if used carefully to minimize negative effects on motility, ionophore-treated cells are immediately highly fertile (16).

Temporally, capacitation and the acrosome reaction are quite distinct, the former taking hours but the latter occurring within minutes. Therefore, mechanisms involved in modulating $[Ca^{2+}]i$ may well differ during these two stages. Current evidence indicates that modest changes in $[Ca^{2+}]i$ occur during capacitation. For example, an increase in $[Ca^{2+}]i$ was detected in hamster sperm during incubation in vitro for several hours under capacitating conditions (17). In mouse sperm, a rise in $^{45}Ca^{2+}$ accumulation was observed during the first hour of incubation under conditions known to support capacitation and fertilization in vitro (18). While the latter approach only provides an indirect indication of Ca^{2+} movements, it suggests that there is an increase in intracellular Ca^{2+} over the time period evaluated. In marked contrast, the acrosome reaction is associated with a rapid and relatively large influx of Ca^{2+}. Consistent with these apparent differences in magnitude of $[Ca^{2+}]i$ associated with capacitation and the acrosome reaction, Ca^{2+} ionophore treatment of mouse sperm in medium containing micromolar Ca^{2+} will promote the F to B transition only, but in millimolar Ca^{2+} will promote both F to B and B to AR transitions (19). At present, three mechanisms have been identified in mammalian sperm cells that might modulate $[Ca^{2+}]i$: (1) a Ca^{2+}-ATPase that could act as a Ca^{2+} extrusion pump; (2) a Na^+/Ca^{2+} exchanger that has been proposed to effect a Na^+ out/Ca^{2+} in exchange; (3) Ca^{2+} channels capable of permitting a large influx of Ca^{2+} (20).

Of these three mechanisms we feel that the case is strongest for a Ca^{2+}-ATPase playing the major role during capacitation. Indeed, we have hypothesized that mouse sperm DF controls capacitation by modulating Ca^{2+}-ATPase activity in the sperm head (18): when present DF would stimulate enzyme activity, thereby maintaining a low $[Ca^{2+}]i$, but as DF is lost, Ca^{2+}-ATPase activity would decline and $[Ca^{2+}]i$ would rise. This hypothesis is based on several pieces of evidence, both indirect and direct.

Drugs such as quercetin, known to inhibit somatic cell Ca^{2+}-ATPase, have been shown to accelerate capacitation, as evidenced by changes in CTC patterns, in mouse, human and bull sperm during relatively short incubations in vitro (8, 15, 19). Most somatic cell Ca^{2+}-ATPases are calmodulin-sensitive and incubation of sperm suspensions in the presence of calmodulin inhibitors such as trifluoperazine and W-7 have been shown to accelerate the F to B transition in bull, human and mouse sperm suspensions (8, 15, 19) and to stimulate $^{45}Ca^{2+}$ accumulation in mouse sperm during the early stages of capacitation (18). Such responses are consistent with sperm having a calmodulin-regulated Ca^{2+}-ATPase. These various results suggest that inhibition of Ca^{2+}-ATPase activity, either directly or indirectly via inhibition of calmodulin, accelerates capacitation. As confirmation, mouse sperm suspensions incubated in the presence of trifluoperazine for a short interval are significantly more fertile than untreated counterparts (21). Thus, there is considerable indirect evidence that Ca^{2+}-ATPase plays a major role during capacitation.

Very recently we have obtained direct evidence to support our hypothesis. Using a $[(\gamma-^{32}P]ATP$ hydrolysis assay and membranes prepared from isolated mouse sperm heads and tails, we have demonstrated the presence of Ca^{2+}-dependent ATPase activity that is further stimulated by the addition of calmodulin and partially purified DF, both individually and in combination. Interestingly, these effects were only obtained with head membranes, with no obvious responses being detected in tail membranes. In addition, the introduction of DF to DF-depleted suspensions resulted in reduced accumulation of $^{45}Ca^{2+}$ by intact cells over the same time interval when a reversion from the B pattern (capacitated) to F (uncapacitated) was observed (22). These results are consistent with the proposed role for DF acting via stimulation of Ca^{2+}-ATPase activity in the sperm head, with consequent maintenance of a low $[Ca^{2+}]i$. They also suggest that different mechanisms may operate in the head and tail to regulate intracellular ionic composition. Indeed, although addition of DF to capacitated cells inhibits the acrosome reaction and fertilizing ability, there is no obvious inhibition of hyperactivated motility.

In contrast, a recent study on epididymal bull sperm was unable to find evidence for an ATP-dependent Ca^{2+} extrusion mechanism (23). Although the mouse sperm DF is present on epididymal cells it is possible that the molecular equivalent of such a DF in bull sperm is present in seminal plasma and hence only associates with sperm at ejaculation. Certainly, it has been known for some time that epididymal bull sperm accumulate Ca^{2+}, while ejaculated cells do not. CTC analysis of ejaculated bull sperm incubated for a short time in the Ca^{2+}-ATPase inhibitor quercetin indicated an acceleration of capacitation (8), consistent with a role for Ca^{2+}-ATPase in regulating capacitation in this species.

Despite evidence that a Na^+/Ca^{2+} exchanger is present in mammalian sperm, there is relatively little evidence to suggest it plays a major role in controlling $[Ca^{2+}]i$ in most species. In cattle, a low molecular weight protein called caltrin that associates with bull sperm at ejaculation has been isolated and purified. It has been proposed that caltrin initially inhibits the Na^+/Ca^{2+} exchanger, helping to maintain a low $[Ca^{2+}]i$; during transit through the female tract, loss of associated anions may allow conformational changes so that caltrin then stimulates the exchanger and promotes a Ca^{2+} in/Na^+ out movement (24). The fact that the responses of bull sperm to quercetin indicated a role for Ca^{2+}-ATPase during capacitation might suggest that both mechanisms function in this species.

Ca^{2+} channels have been identified in mammalian sperm and they appear to play a very important role in sperm function, but probably during the acrosome reaction rather than during capacitation. This is consistent with the clear differences in $[Ca^{2+}]i$ changes occurring during capacitation (slow and modest) and the acrosome reaction (rapid and large): Ca^{2+} channels provide an effective means for promoting a rapid and large influx of Ca^{2+}. Therefore, Ca^{2+} channels are discussed in greater in detail below.

Of the other cations of particular interest, Na^+ is the most abundant in the sperm's normal extracellular environment during capacitation, whether in vivo or in vitro. Current evidence indicates that Na^+ is necessary for fertilization to occur, reflecting requirements during both capacitation and the acrosome reaction (20). For mouse sperm, a relatively low concentration of Na^+ (~ 25 mM, plus ~ 125 mM choline chloride to maintain osmolality) will support capacitation, but the acrosome reaction and fertilization require > 135 mM Na^+. The fact that the Na^+ ionophore monensin can promote rapid capacitation and acrosome loss in uncapacitated suspensions in high Na^+ medium indicates that internalization of Na^+ occurs during the acquisition of fertilizing ability. In contrast, monensin treatment of cells in medium containing only 25 mM Na^+ stimulates capacitation (F to B transition of CTC fluorescence) but not the acrosome reaction, suggestive of a relatively small rise in $[Na^+]i$ during capacitation, but a large rise during acrosome loss.

Two mechanisms might act as possible regulators of $[Na^+]i$, i.e. a Na^+, K^+-ATPase and a Na^+/Ca^{2+} exchanger; of these more information is available on the former. Mammalian sperm have been shown to have a Na^+, K^+-ATPase that is inhibitable by ouabain (20). Studies on hamster sperm reported an increase in ouabain-inhibitable ATPase activity, assumed to be a Na^+, K^+-ATPase, during capacitation (25). Since this enzyme usually pumps K^+ into and Na^+ out of cells, such a rise in activity should lead to a decrease in $[Na^+]i$. At least with mouse sperm, this would be expected to inhibit, not stimulate, capacitation. When mouse sperm were incubated in the presence of the inhibitor ouabain for a short time, there was a significant shift toward the capacitated B pattern of CTC fluorescence and a longer incubation stimulated the acrosome reaction (20). We have therefore concluded that this enzyme either decreases in activity during mouse sperm capacitation or is relatively inactive throughout. As an attempt to resolve these discrepancies observed with hamster and mouse sperm, it has been pointed out (20) that earlier studies have noted more enzyme activity and ouabain binding in the tail than in the head. Therefore any role played by the enzyme might be more involved with motility than changes in the head. As for a Na^+/Ca^{2+} exchanger, this has not really been investigated as a regulator of $[Na^+]i$. Since mammalian sperm appear to require internalization of both Na^+ and Ca^{2+} to complete capacitation, a major role for this exchanger seems unlikely.

Studies addressing K^+ requirements of hamster and mouse sperm for capacitation and acrosome loss have indicated that extracellular K^+ is not needed for capacitation, but is for the acrosome reaction and fertilization. The apparent lack of a requirement for extracellular K^+ would suggest that Na^+, K^+-ATPase activity to maintain $[K^+]i$ is not particularly important and would be consistent with conclusions drawn regarding this enzyme in relation to changes in $[Na^+]i$. Indeed, it has been reported that the $[K^+]i$ of mouse sperm incubated under capacitating conditions decreased from 122 mM to 30 mM (26), a change that could reflect a decrease in Na^+, K^+-ATPase activity. This is consistent with the ability of the inhibitor ouabain to accelerate capacitation.

In considering $[H^+]$, both extracellular and intracellular, it has been known for some time that extracellular pH can affect sperm function in general. Experiments using media with a pH < 7.0 have revealed markedly reduced acrosome loss, motility and fertilizing ability (16). However, none of those studies specifically addressed the question of whether capacitation can occur in conditions with an acidic pH. Recently, time-dependent changes in CTC patterns in mouse sperm incubated in media buffered with 25 mM HEPES and 10 mM bicarbonate and adjusted to pH 6.8 or 7.8 were assessed. At pH 7.8, cells were able to undergo both capacitation and the acrosome reaction (F to B and AR transition) during a standard incubation period of 2 h, whereas at pH 6.8 the majority of cells (> 80%) were still in the F pattern of CTC fluorescence after 2 h (27). Therefore, an acidic pH will not support capacitation. Perhaps these conditions prevent the rise in intracellular pH (pHi) that is reported to occur during capacitation (28). Interestingly, experimental treatment of sperm to cause a precocious rise in pHi does not accelerate capacitation and the acrosome reaction (20, 27, 29). Therefore, a rise in pHi may be a component of capacitation, but without additional intracellular alterations it is not sufficient to trigger acrosome loss.

In vivo, of course, mammalian sperm undergo functional changes in an alkaline environment where it is likely that bicarbonate ions play an important role in controlling pH of the fluids in the female reproductive tract. Interestingly, HCO_3^- concentrations are considerably higher in these fluids than in serum (30). HCO_3^- is probably functioning as more than just a buffering agent, however, since at a constant alkaline external pH, the concentration of HCO_3^- can significantly alter sperm parameters (9, 31, 32). One possible function for HCO_3^- ions within sperm is stimulation of adenylate cyclase activity, leading to a rise in cAMP (33); introduction of exogenous cAMP or inclusion of a cyclic nucleotide phosphodiesterase inhibitor to inhibit cAMP breakdown has been shown to promote sperm function in many species (34).

To date, few experimental studies have addressed anion requirements during capacitation. We have investigated a possible role for Cl^- transport mechanisms by using 4,4 - diisothiocyanatostilbene - 2,2 disulfonic acid (DIDS - an inhibitor of Cl^-/HCO_3^- exchange), anthracene - 9 - carboxylic acid (A9C - a Cl^- channel blocker) and furosemide (an inhibitor of Na^+/Cl^- and $Na^+/K^+/Cl^-$ co-transport). CTC analysis revealed that, when present continuously, both A9C and furosemide markedly inhibited capacitation, while DIDS had relatively little effect. When added acutely, to capacitated cells, A9C had no detectable inhibitory effect on the acrosome reaction, while furosemide caused a partial inhibition and DIDS a total inhibition of acrosome loss (35). Thus, Cl^- transport may well be important for the acquisition of fertilizing ability, but different mechanisms appear to function during capacitation and the acrosome reaction.

Thus, there is considerable evidence that changes in the concentrations of key ions are important during capacitation of mammalian sperm. Some of the mechanisms involved in regulating these events are summarised in Table I.

MECHANISM	CAPACITATION	ACROSOME REACTION
Ca^{2+}-ATPase		
Ca^{2+} channels	?	Yes
Cl^- channels (different types)	Yes	Yes
Cl^-/HCO_3^- exchanger	?	Yes
Na^+/Ca^{2+} exchanger	Yes (limited species)	?
Na^+/Cl^- and $Na^+/K^+/Cl^-$ Cotransport	Yes	?
Na^+/H^+ exchanger	?	Yes
Na^+, K^+ - ATPase	Yes / No	?

Table I: **Mechanisms possibly involved in capacitation and/or acrosome reaction**

IONIC REGULATION OF THE ACROSOME REACTION

Just as capacitation can be modulated by the availability of extracellular ions, so too can the acrosome reaction. In particular, availability of extracellular Ca^{2+} is an absolute requirement for the acrosome reaction during normal fertilization, with maximal responses requiring millimolar concentrations (20). Indeed, one of the early responses in capacitated cells interacting with oocytes is a rise in $[Ca^{2+}]_i$ (36, 37). As will be discussed at greater length in other chapters, this response can be elicited by sperm interaction with zona glycoproteins (e.g. ZP3 in mouse) and/or progesterone, both components of the oocyte-cumulus complex. The possibility that the acrosome reaction may be initiated by sequential interaction with progesterone and ZP3 has recently been suggested (16).

The majority of evidence currently available indicates that Ca^{2+} channels, particularly those with properties similar to voltage-sensitive L-type channels identified in cardiac and skeletal muscle, play an important role in this agonist-induced Ca^{2+} influx. Binding sites for Ca^{2+} channel antagonists have been identified in bull and ram sperm (38). Furthermore, the zona-induced acrosome reaction in bull sperm (38) and the progesterone-induced response in human sperm (39) can be significantly inhibited by Ca^{2+} channel antagonists. Furthermore, the inclusion of a Ca^{2+} channel blocker just prior to progesterone stimulation of human sperm significantly inhibits the production of diacylglycerol (DAG) (39), one of the early events detected in cells following interaction with progesterone. As discussed in detail in other chapters, DAG is formed following a rise in $[Ca^{2+}]_i$ that stimulates various phospholipases, thereby initiating a complicated series of reactions that produce fusogenic molecules responsible for the membrane fusion events of the acrosome reaction. In mouse sperm, inclusion of a similar antagonist inhibited both influx of $^{45}Ca^{2+}$ and the acrosome reaction, but did not inhibit capacitation per se (cells changed from the F to B pattern of CTC fluorescence, but not from B to AR) (40). Using mouse sperm, other experiments have provided evidence that while Ca^{2+} channel blockers can inhibit fertilization in vitro, this is not due to an inhibition of capacitation (16). Thus all results suggest that Ca^{2+} channels function primarily in relation to the acrosome reaction. The activation of Ca^{2+} channels would lead to a rapid and large influx of Ca^{2+}, kinetics consistent with the measured changes in $[Ca^{2+}]_i$ in stimulated cells. That a large influx is required is demonstrated by the inability of a Ca^{2+} ionophore to elicit the acrosome reaction when the $[Ca^{2+}]_e$ is low (19).

Although evidence indicates that the response in capacitated sperm to agonists capable of triggering the acrosome reaction involves activation of Ca^{2+} channels, the link is not a direct one, i.e. sperm interaction with the agonist initiates a sequence of events culminating in Ca^{2+} channel opening. It is in this sequence that other ions such as Na^+ may play important roles. The acrosome reaction normally only occurs in the presence of high $[Na+]_e$, at least some of which is internalized as evidenced by the ability of monensin to promote both capacitation and the acrosome reaction. Monensin also stimulates a rapid influx of $^{45}Ca^{2+}$ that can be inhibited by the inclusion of a Ca^{2+} channel blocker, indicating that a Na^+ influx precedes Ca^{2+} channel opening (20). It has been proposed (20) that this Na^+ influx is associated with activation of a Na^+-H^+ exchanger which would result in a rise in pHi. Numerous studies have indicated that such changes in pHi do occur and precede the acrosome reaction (36). If high $[Na^+]_e$ is required to promote changes in pHi, then it should be possible to circumvent this need by employing other agents to cause a rise in pHi. Indeed, mouse sperm capacitated in medium containing 25 mM Na^+, insufficient to support the acrosome reaction even in the presence of monensin, can be stimulated to undergo acrosomal loss by treatments such as NH_4Cl, and gramicidin, with these responses being inhibited by Ca^{2+} channel blockers (27). Similar responses under low Na^+ conditions have been obtained with carbonyl cyanide p-trifluoromethoxyphenylhydrazone (FCCP) which can act as a H^+ ionophore and would promote H^+ efflux under the experimental conditions used (i.e., basic pHe). Furthermore, FCCP-treated cells in low Na^+ medium have been shown to be significantly more fertile than controls (41).

Thus experimental treatments that would cause a rise in pHi can trigger exocytosis by stimulating cells at a step upstream of Ca^{2+} channel opening. None of these treatments has been found to produce this response in uncapacitated cells, suggesting that capacitation in some as yet unidentified ways promote changes in responsiveness in the path leading to Ca^{2+} channel activation. In contrast, treatments that would act at points downstream of Ca^{2+} influx have been reported to trigger the acrosome reaction in human sperm, even in uncapacitated cells (42). These differences suggest that 'maturation' of the mechanisms involved in triggering Ca^{2+} channel activation must occur during capacitation.

Recent studies have begun to examine possible roles for anion transport mechanisms in the acrosome reaction. The progesterone-initiated acrosome reaction in human sperm has been reported to involve progesterone interaction with a steroid receptor/Cl^- channel complex, with characteristics similar to a neuronal γ-aminobutyric acid receptor/Cl^- channel complex, leading to activation of Cl^- channels and a large influx of Cl^-. This rise in $[Cl^-]_i$ could activate a Cl^-/HCO_3^- exchanger and produce a Cl^- efflux/HCO_3^- influx (43). Consistent with this, the introduction of DIDS (an inhibitor of Cl^-/HCO_3^- exchange) at low micromolar concentrations to capacitated mouse sperm was able to totally inhibit the acrosome reaction (35). A rise in $[HCO_3^-]_i$ might stimulate the acrosome reaction either by stimulating adenylate cyclase activity and consequent production of cAMP or by contributing to a rise in pHi. Both are known to occur prior to the acrosome reaction (36). At present, it is not possible to discriminate between these two possibilities, or even to know whether they are mutually exclusive, given that the DIDS-induced inhibition of the acrosome reaction could be overcome by inclusion of either dibutyryl cAMP or FCCP (35).

As with capacitation, the evidence indicates that the acrosome reaction occurs as a result of a complicated series of changes involving intracellular ionic composition, the major one being a large rise in $[Ca^{2+}]_i$, primarily by activation of Ca^{2+} channels. Possible mechanisms involved in regulating the intracellular composition, relative to the acrosome reaction, are summarized in Table I

CONCLUSIONS

The transformation of an uncapacitated mammalian sperm into a capacitated cell which can then undergo the acrosome reaction is clearly very complex and involves a wide array of interacting systems that control fluxes of ions and hence their intracellular concentrations. At present, these are only beginning to be understood and we currently have more information about mechanisms that may help to regulate events occurring primarily in the sperm head. Since the head and tail are almost totally separate anatomical regions, it is quite possible that different mechanisms might regulate a given ion in each compartment. Although in this chapter the focus has been on the sperm head, some consideration has been given to changes in motility as well. While capacitation is unique to mammalian sperm, the acrosome reaction is common to many invertebrate and vertebrate species. A somewhat more detailed picture of ionic events has been obtained from studies of invertebrate, particularly sea urchin, sperm and there appear to be a number of similarities with events in mammalian sperm (16, 37). In all sperm, there is an obligatory requirement for extracellular Ca^{2+} and there appears to be an intricate interplay of ion fluxes that contribute to the acrosome reaction and successful fertilization.

Acknowledgements:
Recent original research in the author's laboratory has been supported by the Biotechnology and Biological Sciences Research Council, the Bourn-Hallam Group, the Japan Society for the Promotion of Science and the Wellcome Trust.

REFERENCES

1. Loeb J. On the nature of conditions which determine or prevent the entrance of the spermatozoa into the egg. Amer Nat 1915; 49: 257-85.
   Austin CR. The `capacitation' of the mammalian sperm. Nature, Lond 1952; 170: 326.
2. Yanagimachi R. Mammalian fertilization. In: Knobil E, Neill JD eds. The Physiology of Reproduction, 2nd edition. New York: Raven Press, 1994: 189-317.
3. Bedford JM. Significance of the need for sperm capacitation before fertilization in eutherian mammals. Biol Reprod 1983; 28: 108-20.
4. Caswell AH, Hutchison JD. Visualization of membrane bound cations by a fluorescent technique. Biochem Biophy Res Commun 1971; 42: 43-49.

5. Ward CR, Storey BT. Determination of the time course of capacitation in mouse spermatozoa using a chlortetracycline fluorescence assay. Dev Biol 1984; 104: 287-96.
6. DasGupta S, Mills C L, Fraser, L R. Ca^{2+}-related changes in the capacitation state of human spermatozoa assessed by a chlortetracycline fluorescence assay. J Reprod Fertil 1993; 99: 135-43.
7. Fraser LR, Abeydeera LR, Niwa K. Ca^{2+}-regulating mechanisms that modulate bull sperm capacitation and acrosomal exocytosis as determined by chlortetracycline analysis. Mol Reprod Dev 1995; 40: 233-241.
8. Wang WH, Abeydeera LR, Fraser LR, Niwa K. Functional analysis using chlortetracycline fluorescence and in vitro fertilization of frozen-thawed ejaculated boar spermatozoa incubated in a protein-free chemically defined medium. J Reprod Fertil 1995; in press.
9. Green CM, Cockle SM, Watson PF, Fraser LR. Stimulating effect of pyroglutamylglutamylprolineamide, a prostatic, TRH-related tripeptide, on mouse sperm capacitation and fertilizing ability in vitro. Mol Reprod Dev 1994; 38: 215-21.
10. Green CM, Cockle SM, Watson PF, Fraser LR. FPP, a TRH-like peptide, stimulates capacitation of human spermatozoa in vitro. Human Reprod 1995; in press.
11. Cockle SM, Aitken A, Beg F, Morrell JM, Smyth DG. The TRH-related peptide pyroglutamylglutamylprolineamide is present in human semen. FEBS Letts 1989; 253: 113-117.
12. Oliphant G, Reynolds AB, Thomas T S. Sperm surface components involved in the control of the acrosome reaction. Am Anat 1985; 174: 269-83.
13. Fraser LR, Harrison RAP, Herod JE. Characterization of a decapacitation factor associated with epididymal mouse spermatozoa. J Reprod Fertil 1990; 89: 135-48.
14. DasGupta S, Mills C L, Fraser LR. A possible role for Ca^{2+}-ATPase in human sperm capacitation. J Reprod Fertil 1994; 102: 107-16.
15. Fraser LR. Ionic control of sperm function. Reprod Fertil Dev 1995; in press.
16. White DR, Aitken RJ. Relationship between calcium, cyclic AMP, ATP and intracellular pH and the capacity of hamster spermatozoa to express hyperactivated motility. Gamete Res 1989; 22: 163-77.
17. Adeoya-Osiguwa SA, Fraser LR. A biphasic pattern of $^{45}Ca^{2+}$ uptake by mouse spermatozoa in vitro correlates with changing functional potential. J Reprod Fertil 1993; 99: 187-94.
18. Fraser LR, McDermott CA. Ca^{2+}-related changes in the mouse sperm capacitation state: a possible role for Ca^{2+}-ATPase. J Reprod Fertil 1992; 96: 363-77.

19. Fraser LR. Na^+ requirements for capacitation and acrosomal exocytosis in mammalian sperm. Int Rev Cytol 1994; 149: 1-46.
20. Adeoya SA, Fraser LR. Unpublished observation.
21. Adeoya-Osiguwa S, Fraser LR. Evidence for Ca^{2+}-dependent ATPase activity, modulated by decapacitation factor and calmodulin, in mouse spermatozoa. Reprod Fertil Abstr Ser 1994; 14: 9-10.
22. Vijayaraghavan S, Trautman K, Mishra SK, Hermsmeyer K. Evidence against a functional ATP-dependent calcium extrusion mechanism in bovine epididymal sperm. Mol Reprod Dev 1994; 38: 326-33.
23. Lardy H, San Agustin J. Caltrin and calcium regulation of sperm activity. In: Schatten H, Schatten G, eds. The Cell Biology of Fertilization. New York: Academic Press, 1989: 29-39.
24. Mrsny, RJ, Siiteri J E, Meizel S. Hamster sperm Na^+, K^+-adenosine triphosphatase: increased activity during capacitation in vitro and its relationship to cyclic nucleotides. Biol Reprod 1984; 30: 573-84.
25. Chou K, Chen J, Yuan S, Haug A. The membrane potential changes polarity during capacitation of murine epididymal sperm. Biochem Biophys Res Commun 1989; 165: 58-64.
26. Fraser LR, Gallostra-Barri I. pH and K^+ modifications can modulate mouse sperm capacitation and acrosomal exocytosis. J Reprod Fertil Abstr Ser 1994; 14: 9.
27. Vredenburgh-Wilberg WL, Parrish JJ. Intracellular pH of bovine sperm increases during capacitation. Mol Reprod Dev 1995; 40: 490-502.
28. Working PK, Meizel S. Evidence that an ATPase functions in the maintenance of the acidic pH of the hamster sperm acrosome. J Biol Chem 1981; 256: 4708-11.
29. Brackett BG, Mastroianni L. Composition of oviductal fluid. In: Hafiz ESE, Blandau RJ, ed. The Mammalian Oviduct. Chicago: University of Chicago Press, 1974: 231-50.
30. Suzuki K, Ebihara M, Nagai T, Clarke NGE, Harrison RAP. Importance of bicarbonate/CO_2 for fertilization of pig oocytes in vitro and synergism with caffeine. Reprod Fertil Dev 1994; 6: 221-7
31. Ashworth PJC, Harrison RAP, Miller NGA, Plummer JM, Watson PF. Flow cytometric detection of bicarbonate-induced changes in lectin binding in boar and ram sperm populations. Mol Reprod Dev 1995; 40: 164-176.
32. Okamura N, Tajima Y, Soejima A, Masuda H, Sugita Y. Sodium bicarbonate in seminal plasma stimulates the motility of mammalian spermatozoa through direct activation of adenylate cyclase. J Biol Chem 1985; 260: 9699-705.
33. Fraser LR, Monks NJ. Cyclic nucleotides and mammalian sperm capacitation. In: Whitaker M, Fraser LR, Weir BJ, eds. Cell Messengers at Fertilization. J Reprod Fertil Suppl 1990; 42: 9-21.

34. Fraser LR, Chiu C, Ghaharian K. A role for Cl⁻ transport in mammalian sperm capacitation and acrosomal exocytosis. J Reprod Fertil Abstr Ser 1995; 15: in press.
35. Kopf GS, Gerton GL. The mammalian sperm acrosome and the acrosome reaction. In: Wassarman PM, ed. Elements of Mammalian Fertilization. I. Basic Concepts. Boca Raton, Fl: CRC Press, 1990: 153-203.
36. Ward C R, Kopf GS. Molecular events mediating sperm activation. Dev Biol 1993; 158: 9-34.
37. Florman HM, Corron ME, Kim TD-H, Babcock DF. Activation of voltage-dependent calcium channels of mammalian sperm is required for zona pellucida-induced acrosomal exocytosis. Dev Biol 1992; 152: 304-14.
38. O'Toole CMB, Roldan ERS, Fraser LR. A role for Ca^{2+} channels in progesterone-stimulated human sperm acrosomal exocytosis. J Reprod Fertil Abstr Ser 1995; 15: in press.
39. Fraser LR. Calcium channels play a pivotal role in the sequence of ionic changes involved in initiating mouse sperm acrosomal exocytosis. Mol Reprod Dev 1993; 36: 368-76.
40. Fraser L. Unpublished observation.
41. Bielfeld P, Anderson RA, Mack SR, De Jonge CJ, Zaneveld LJD. Are capacitation or calcium ion influx required for the human sperm acrosome reaction? Fertil Steril 1994; 62: 1255-1261.
42. Wistrom CA, Meizel S. Evidence suggesting involvement of a unique human sperm steroid receptor/Cl⁻ channel complex in the progesterone-initiated acrosome reaction. Dev Biol 1993; 159: 679-690.

Modification of sperm membrane antigens during capacitation

Harry D.M. Moore

Departments of Obstetrics and Gynaecology and Molecular Biology and Biotechnology, University of Sheffield, S10 2UH, United Kingdom

Abstract

Although capacitation involves a continuum of changes within the cell, it is reviewed here as a number of discrete events. These are (1) plasma membrane destabilization; (2) surface antigen expression or modification and (3) protein kinase phosphorylation. It is postulated that much of what is termed capacitation is an intrinsic process which is initiated by membrane destabilization. Priming of a protein tyrosine kinase signal transduction pathway leads to induction of the acrosome reaction and possible hyperactivation.

Bien que la capacitation implique une continuité de changement à l'intérieur de la cellule, elle sera abordée ici comme une série d'événements discontinus. Ceux-ci sont (1) la déstabilisation de la membrane plasmique, (2) l'expression ou la modification d'antigènes de surface, (3) la phosphorylation des protéine kinases. Nous pensons que la capacitation est essentiellement un processus intrinsèque initié par la déstabilisation des membranes. L'initialisation de la voie de transduction de la tyrosine kinase conduit à l'induction de la réaction acrosomique et probablement à l'hyperactivation.

Over 40 years after the discovery of sperm capacitation in mammals the phenomenon remains somewhat of an enigma. In the intervening years, we have learnt a lot about how to induce capacitation *in vitro* in spermatozoa from many species (1,2), but we remain essentially ignorant of this process in spermatozoa within the female tract, and indeed can only speculate why spermatozoa need to undergo capacitation in the first place (3). The original definition referred to the period that spermatozoa must reside in the female tract before they are capable of fertilizing (1,4). This was widened to include the incubation period *in vitro* before fertilization but lack of information regarding sperm status in the female tract means that we still cannot be sure whether the processes *in vitro* and *in situ* are truly equivalent. Exactly when the capacitation process begins and ends is also open to interpretation but it is generally accepted that until spermatozoa are fully capacitated they are incapable of undergoing the acrosome reaction and hyperactivated motility required for fertilization.

Our conceptual uncertainties stem, in part, from the fact that capacitation is an 'umbrella' term for a general transformation of the spermatozoon leading to fertilization and therefore can (and does) encompass many membrane and cytoplasmic events. Furthermore, until comparatively recently, we have had no detailed information about how the acrosome reaction might be triggered and therefore what, at the molecular level, capacitation was in part leading towards. Over the last few years, a much more detailed understanding of the acrosome reaction has begun to emerge and this in turn has led to a greater appreciation of capacitation processes. In particular, the discovery that sperm-egg interactions and the acrosome reaction resemble the extracellular matrix - cell interations and protein kinase signal transduction pathways present in somatic cells (5,6,7) has allowed hypotheses to be tested at the molecular level. Here capacitation is examined as a number of separate cellular events.

CAPACITATION AS A PLASMA MEMBRANE DESTABILIZATION EVENT

Numerous *in vitro* experiments indicate that capacitation involves a destabilization of the sperm plasma membrane leading to reorganization of membrane surface antigens. The increase in the general fluidity of the plasma membrane is reflected at the ultrastructural level by the aggregation of intramembrane particles and the presence of particle-free patches (8). Several studies have shown that the lipid composition of sperm membranes alters during capacitation, particularly, cholesterol/phospholipid ratios. This may be due to a loss of cholesterol to an appropriate extracellular ligand such as albumin (9,10). The presence of bicarbonate ions seems to be essential in this respect perhaps by increasing the turnover of lipids in the membrane and making them available to extracellular acceptor molecules (11). At present it is unclear whether destabilization is mediated solely by changes in membrane lipid ratios or by modification to the underlying cytoskeleton, or both. Certainly, a major consequence of an increase in membrane fluidity is that transmembrane proteins might be capable of oligomerization. As discussed later, this may be important for priming receptor molecules for signal transduction processes.

CAPACITATION AS A SURFACE ANTIGEN EXPRESSION OR MODIFICATION EVENT

Changes to the surface of spermatozoa during capacitation can be clearly detected using a variety of probes. Many reports (1) suggest that membrane determinants may be acquired (unmasked), lost or hidden (masked), are redistributed over a membrane domain (capping), or can migrate from, for example, the tail region to the acrosomal region (12). An early and recurring theme, has been the idea that the removal of sperm coating material constitutes an important event of capacitation and various proteins have been implicated as having decapacitation or membrane stabilization activity (13). While this is an attractive hypothesis, and there seems no doubt that sperm surface changes do occur, it has proved difficult to tell whether such surface modifications play a specific role in the capacitation process, are in response to other capacitation process, or are only important for subsequent sperm-egg interactions. A recent example is the expression of mannose lectin-like receptors on human spermatozoa during capacitation which appears to be regulated by cholesterol depletion of the membrane (10). These molecules are intrinsic to the membrane but become exposed as destabilization occurs. What role they may have in late capacitation events or in subsequent sperm-egg recognition processes remains to be established.

CAPACITATION AS A PROTEIN KINASE PHOSPHORYLATION EVENT

One of the most important findings in recent years was the observation that a 95 kD surface membrane protein (P95) displayed increased phosphotyrosine expression when mouse spermatozoa were incubated under capacitating conditions or when capacitated spermatozoa were exposed to zona protein (5). Subsequent studies have demonstrated the importance of protein phosphorylation during mouse and human sperm capacitation and the acrosome reaction and now besides the P95 several other tyrosine phosphorylated proteins have been identified (14-19). The inhibition of human sperm-egg binding with a monoclonal antibody recognising a similar P95 molecule on human spermatozoa (20) led to the characterisation in human spermatozoa of a novel protein tyrosine kinase as a receptor for the zona component, ZP3 (6). The amino-acid sequence of this trans-membrane receptor (designated zona receptor kinase, ZRK) indicates that it is similar to other phosphotyrosine kinases but has a unique extracellular domain. Under capacitating conditions, ZRK in human spermatozoa becomes increasingly phosphorylated with time to a maximum after about 4-5 hours incubation (6,18). This pattern of phosphorylation is at a relatively low level compared to that induced by recombinant human ZP3 although by 24 hr incubation the level of phosphorylation is similar in the presence or absence of ZP3 (figure 1a).

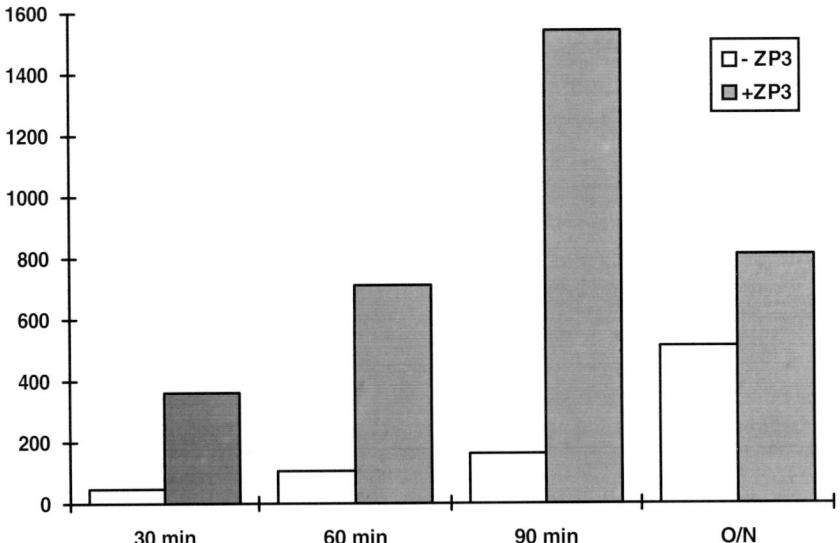

Figure 1a. **Typical relative intensities of chemiluminescent signal of 95 kDa phosphotyrosine expression (Western blot) of capacitated (3h) human spermatozoa incubated for various times in the presence or absence of recombinant human ZP3** *(18). In the absence of ZP3, there is a low but significant increase in phosphotyrosine expression. Addition of ZP3 increases expression markedly. Before capacitation, phosphotyrosine at 95kDa is not detected under similar conditions.*

The increase in phosphorylation induced by ZP3 (but not capacitation), and the subsequent acrosome reaction can be inhibited with monoclonal antibody that recognises ZRK (figure 1b). Other groups have also demonstrated increased expression in a 94-97 kD human sperm protein (presumably ZRK) during capacitation and in response to zona pellucida proteins or other substances (progesterone, PAF). In the mouse, the increase in tyrosine phosphorylation of a 95 kD protein could also be induced by cyclic AMP (21) and recent evidence suggests a whole subset of proteins are phosphorylated during capacitation and regulated by a cAMP-dependent pathway (16). Exactly how such pathways eventually regulate the induction of the acrosome reaction and hyperactivated motility remains to be determined.

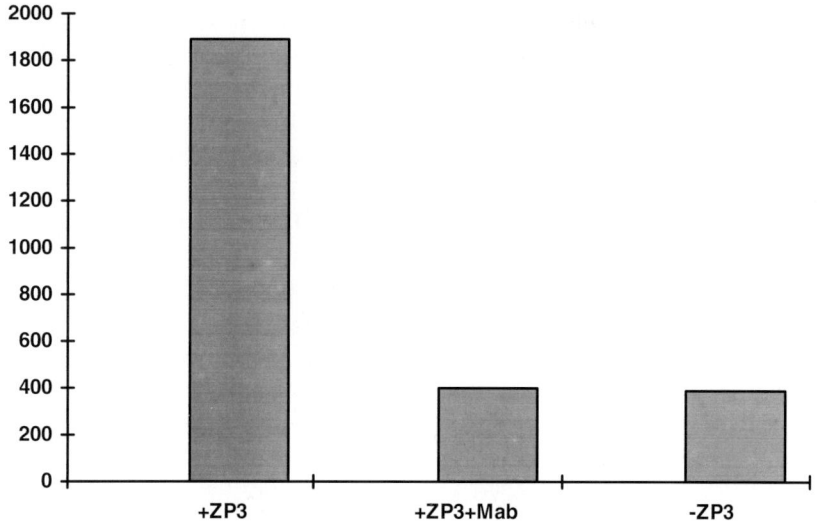

Figure 1b. **Typical relative intensities of chemiluminescent signal of 95 kDa phosphotyrosine expression (Western blot) of capacitated (3h) human spermatozoa incubated for various times in the presence or absence of recombinant human ZP3 and monoclonal antibody 97.25 (18)..** *Addition of ZP3 increases expression markedly and promotes the acrosome reaction. Addition of monoclonal antibody 97.25 that recognises ZRK to spermatozoa inhibits phosphorylation and the acrosome reaction. In the absence of ZP3, there is a low but significant increase in phosphotyrosine expression.*

CAPACITATION AS AN INTRINSIC PRIMING EVENT FACILITATED BY MEMBRANE DESTABILIZATION.

It has been suggested that in response to storage of spermatozoa in the cauda epididymidis in a viable and stable state, capacitation has evolved as a process of destabilisation of sperm membranes so that sperm-egg interactions at fertilization can occur (3). In keeping with this concept is the notion that much of capacitation may be an intrinsic sperm process ultimately leading to fully functional trans-membrane signal transduction pathways that permit the acrosome reaction and hyperactivated motility to occur at the appropriate point for fertilization. Recent evidence now implicates the phosphorylation of ZRK and other protein kinases as a key pathway of late capacitation. Hence, agents such as genistein that inhibit tyrosine phosphorylation also prevent the induction of the acrosome reaction (22). In this model, capacitation may involve an increasing aggregation of receptors due to increased lateral mobility of proteins in a fluid membrane. This process in the presence of appropriate factors leads to increasing autophorylation of protein kinases. When a threshold level is reached, stimulation of ZRK by its natural ligand, ZP3, promotes a massive increase in phosphorylation and the immediate induction of the acrosome reaction. In the absence of an interaction with the zona, the sperm continues capacitation as a slow autophosphorylation process of the signal pathway until a spontaneous acrosome reaction may be elicited by a variety of other factors (figure 2).

Artificially destabilising sperm membranes such as heating or cooling spermatozoa or using chemical perturbation (23-25) may accelerate capacitation by rapidly aggregating receptor molecules.

Although there is an overall increase in phosphoproteins during capacitation it is likely that, as in other cells, this process is in dynamic balance with protein tyrosine phosphatases that dephosphorylate proteins. Therefore conditions that bring about full capacitation may act to enhance the activity of protein tyrosine kinases or suppress tyrosine phosphatase activity (7). Other factors could act in the opposite manner (figure 2). Such a dynamic process may account for the apparent reversibility of capacitation when spermatozoa are for example returned to seminal plasma.. Recent experiments indicate that reactive oxygen species might also act on this equilibrium (26).

There is now persuasive evidence that ZRK is involved in the signal transduction pathway of the acrosome reaction but the molecular mechanisms involved at sperm-egg binding remain unclear. There is considerable evidence that the oligosaccharide side chain of ZP3 (or at least a glycosylated form of ZP3) is required for induction of the acrosome reaction (27). Since receptor kinases such as ZRK act through protein ligands it suggests that additional factors acting through sugar interactions may also play a role. This could be similar to transmembrane signalling by antigen receptors of lymphocytes where complement components bind via oligosaccharides to membrane cofactors to initiate rapid phosphorylation of the receptor (28).

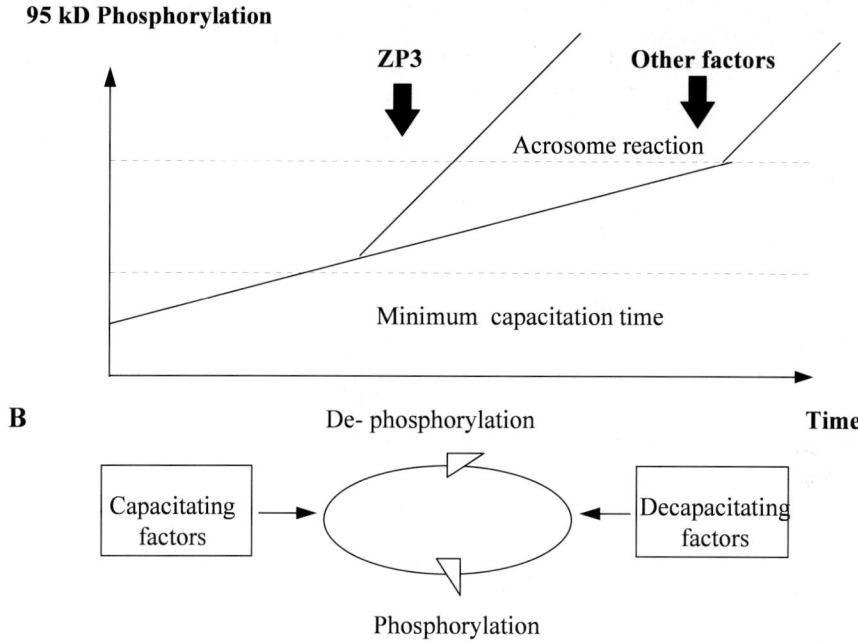

Figure 2. (A) Schematic diagram of a model for protein tyrosine kinase (PTK) phosphorylation during capacitation and the acrosome reaction. *Autophosphorylation of PTKs above a threshold level during capacitation permits ZP3 induction of the acrosome reaction and a rapid phosphorylation. If contact with ZP3 does not occur, then PTK phosphorylation continues until a further threshold level is reached where other factors may trigger the acrosome reaction.*
(B) The rate phosphorylation will vary with various factors acting of the balance between kinase and phosphatase activity.

REFERENCES

1. Yanagimachi R. Mammalian Fertilization. In: Knobil E and Neill JD. Physiology of Reproduction, 2nd edition. New York: Raven Press, 1994: 189-317
2. Dunbar BS, O'Rand MG. A comparative overview of mammalian reproduction. New York:Plenum Press, 1991.
3. Bedford JM. The contraceptive potential of fertilization: a physiological perspective. Human Reprod 1994; 9:842-858.
4. Moore HDM, Bedford JM. The interaction of mammalian gametes in the female. In: Hartmann JF,ed. Mechanism and control of animal fertilization. New York : Academic Press, 1983 : 453-497.

5. Leyton L, Saling PM. 95 kDa sperm proteins binds ZP3 and serve as tyrosine kinase substrates in response to zona binding. Cell 1989; 57: 1123-1130.
6. Burks DJ, Carballada R, Moore HDM, Saling PM. Interaction of a tyrosine kinase from human sperm with the zona pellucida at fertilization. Science 1995; 269: 83-86
7. Van der Greer P, Hunter T, Linberg RA. Receptor protein-tyrosine kinases and their signal transduction pathways. Ann. Rev.Cell Biol.1994; 10: 251-337
8. Koehler JK, Gaddum-Rose P. Media induced alterations of the membrane associated particles of the guinea-pig sperm tail. J.Ultrastruct.Res 1975; 51: 106-118
9. Davis BK. Timing of fertilization in mammals: sperm cholesterol/phospholipid ratio as a determinant of the capacitation interval. Proc.Natl.Acad.Sci. USA 1981; 78: 7560-7564.
10. Benoff S, Hurley I, Cooper GW, Mandel FS, Rosenfeld DL and Hershlag A. Head specific mannose-ligand receptor expression in human spermatozoa is depedent on capacitation-associated membrane cholesterol loss. Human Reprod. 1993; 8: 2141-2154.
11. Harrison RAP, Mairet B, Miller NGA. Flow cytometric studies of bicarbonate-mediated Ca^{2+} influx in boar sperm populations. Mol. Reprod. Dev. 1993; 35: 197-208.
12. Shalgi R; Matityahn A, Gaunt SJ, Jones R. Antigens on rat spermatozoa with a potential role in fertilization. Mol.Reprod.Dev. 1990;25: 286-296.
13. Koehler JK Surface alterations during capacitation of mammalian spermatozoa. Am.J.Primatol. 1981; 1: 131-141.
14. Naz RK, Ahmad K, Kumar R. Role of membrane phosphotyrosine proteins in human spermatozoa function. J.Cell Sci.1991; 99:157-165.
15. Luconi M, Bonnaccorsi L, Krauz C, Gervasi G, Forti G, Baldi E. Stimulation of protein phosphorylation by platelet-activating factor and progesterone in human spermatozoa. Mol.Cell Endo. 1995; 108: 35-42
16. Visconti PE, Moore GE, Bailey JL, Leclerc P, Connors SA, Pan D, Olds-Clarke P, Kopf GS. Capacitation of mouse spermatozoa. II. Protein tyrosine phosphorylation and capacitation are regulated by a cAMP-dependent pathway. Development 1995; 121: 1139-1150
17. Brewis IA, Barratt CLR, Hornby DP, Moore HDM. The signal transduction pathway of the acrosome reaction in response to recombinant human ZP3 involves phosphorylation of a receptor kinase and a rapid influx of Ca^{2+} into human spermatozoa. J.Reprod.Fert. Abs.Ser. 1995; 15: 6
18. Moore HDM, Clayton R, Barratt CLR, Hornby DP. Induction of the acrosome reaction in capacitated human spermatozoa with recombinant

human ZP3 is associated with a 95 kDa phosphotyrosine epitope and is inhibited with a specific monoclonal antibody. J.Reprod.Fert.Abs ser.1995; 15:7

19. Murase T, Roldan ERS. Epidermal growth factor stimulates hydrolysis of phosphatidyl- inositol 4,5- bisphosphate, generation of diacylglyerol and exocytosis in mouse spermatozoa. FEBS Letters 1995; 360: 242-246.

20. Moore HDM, Hartman TD, Bye AP, Lutjen P, De Witt M, Trounson AO. Monoclonal antibody against a sperm M_r 95000 inhibits attachment of human spermatozoa to the zona pellucida J.Immunol. 1987; 11: 157-166.

21. Duncan AE, Fraser LR. Cyclic AMP-dependent phosphorylation of epididymal mouse sperm proteins during capacitation in vitro: identification of an M_r 95 000 phosphotyrosine containing protein. J.Reprod.Fert. 1993; 97: 287-299.

22. Tasarik J, Moos J, Mendoza C. Stimulation of protein tyrosine phosphorylation by a progesterone receptor on the surface of human sperm. Endocrinology 1993; 133: 328-335.

23. Bedford JM, Yanagimachi R. Epididymal storage at abdominal temparatures reduces the time required for capacitation of hamster spermatozoa. J.Reprod.Fert. 1991; 91:403-410.

24. Fuller SJ, Whittingham DG. Capacitation-like changes induced in mouse spermatozoa at low temperatures above freezing. J.Reprod.Fert. Abs. ser. 1995; 15: 95.

25. Graham Jk, Nolan JP, Hammerstedt RH. Effect of dilauroylphosphotidylcholine liposomes on motility, induction of the acrosome reaction and subsequeent egg penetration of ram epididymal sperm. Biol.Reprod. 1991; 44: 1092-1099.

26. Aitken RJ, Paterson M, Fisher H, Buckingham DW, Van Duin M. Redox regulation of tyrosine phosphorylation in human spermatozoa and its role in the control of human sperm function. J.Cell Sci. 1995; 108: 2017-2025.

27. Wassarman P, Profile of a mammalian sperm receptor. Development 1990; 108: 1-17.

28. DeFranco AL. Transmembrane signaling by antigen receptors of B and T lymphocytes. Curr.Opinion Cell Biol. 1995; 7: 163-175.

Human sperm acrosome reaction. Eds P. Fénichel, J. Parinaud.
Colloque INSERM/John Libbey Eurotext Ltd © 1995. Vol. 236, pp. 45-65.

Membrane changes during capacitation with special reference to lipid architecture

R.A.P. Harrison and B.M. Gadella

Department of Development and Signalling, The Babraham Institute, Cambridge CB2 4AT, United Kingdom

ABSTRACT

The physiological « priming » process of capacitation enables the spermatozoon to undergo the acrosome reaction in response to zona pellucida components. It is believed that, during capacitation, modulation of membrane lipid architecture must occur to render the plasma membrane and outer acrosomal membrane potentially mutually fusible and hence allow the acrosome reaction. Using bicarbonate/CO_2 to induce capacitation in boar sperm populations, we have identified, by means of flow cytometry, an important early change in the plasma membrane lipid architecture that manifests itself in increased binding of the lipophilic probe merocyanine 540. This alteration takes place in most cells within 5 minutes of exposure to bicarbonate at 38°C, and appears to result from modulations of an enzymatic process. We have also used nitrobenzoxadiazolyl-aminohexanoyl-(C6NBD-) labeled phospholipid analogues to investigate phospholipid transverse distribution across the plasma membrane bilayer in boar spermatozoa. We have been able to determine that in these cells (as in other cell types) the aminophospholipid phosphatidylserine and phosphatidylethanolamine are essentially incorporated by an energy -dependent process into the inner leaflet whereas phosphatidylcholine and sphingomyelin remain in the outer leaflet. Bicarbonate greatly reduces the rate of incorporation of the aminophospholipids into the inner leaflet though it does not alter their eventual distribution. On the other hand, bicarbonate increases the proportion of phosphatidylcholine found in the inner leaflet. All of these *changes seem independent of any lipid exchange processes that might occur between the sperm cell and its environment, and precede the bicarbonate-induced changes in surface coating described in a previous report from this laboratory (Asworth et al., Mol Reprod Dev 1995; 40: 164-76)*

Le mécanisme de sensibilisation physiologique que représente la capacitation permet au spermatozoïde d'accomplir sa réaction acrosomique en réponse aux composants de la zone pellucide. Il est admis à l'heure actuelle que la modulation de l'architecture lipidique membranaire pendant la capacitation permet aux membranes plasmique et acrosomique externe de fusionner et donc au spermatozoïde de faire la réaction acrosomique. En utilisant le bicarbonate/CO2 comme inducteur de la capacitation chez le verrat, nous avons identifié, grâce à la cytométrie de flux, un changement précoce de l'architecture lipidique membranaire. Elle se manifeste par une augmentation de liaison de la merocyanine 540, une sonde lipophile. Cette modification se produit dans la plupart des cellules au bout de 5 minutes d'exposition au bicarbonate à 38°C, et semble résulter d'un mécanisme de régulation enzymatique. Nous avons également utilisé un analogue phospholipidique marqué, le nitrobenzoxadiazolyl-aminohexanoyl-(C6NBD-), afin d'étudier la distribution transversale des phospholipides constituant la bicouche de la membrane plasmique des spermatozoïdes de verrat. Nous avons pu ainsi déterminer que dans ces cellules (comme dans d'autres types cellulaires) les aminophospholipides, phosphatidylserine et phosphatidylethanolamine, sont incorporés dans le feuillet interne essentiellement par un processus énergie - dépendant alors que la phosphatidylcholine et la sphingomyéline restent dans le feuillet externe. Le bicarbonate réduit de façon importante le taux d'incorporation des aminophospholipides dans le feuillet interne bien qu'il n'altère pas leur distribution définitive. Par ailleurs, le bicarbonate augmente la proportion de phosphatidylcholine trouvée dans le feuillet interne. Ces modifications semblent être indépendantes d'un quelconque processus d'échange lipidique pouvant se produire entre la cellule et son environnement, et précèdent les changements du revêtement de surface induits par le bicarbonate, préalablement décrits par notre laboratoire. (Ashworth et al., Mol Reprod Dev 1995; 40: 164-176)

The essential feature of the sperm acrosome reaction is the extensive Ca^{2+}-dependent fusion between the outer acrosomal membrane and the overlying plasma membrane (1, 2). Such fusion, which involves a merging of the phospholipid bilayers of the two membranes (at least in the fusing regions), rarely occurs spontaneously, regardless of whether the spermatozoa are in the male reproductive tract or freshly deposited within the female tract. It is clear that fusion requires considerable prior modification of the normal membrane architecture.

As will be described by later speakers, the acrosome reaction plays a vital role in fertilization by exposing lytic enzymes for facilitation of the sperm's penetration of the zona pellucida. It is believed that the fertilizing spermatozoon is specifically triggered to undergo its acrosome reaction at the zona surface through binding of specific zona pellucida components (ZP3 in the mouse (3)). By some means, this binding induces an sudden influx of Ca^{2+} (4-6) to trigger a series of subsequent events, several of which are Ca^{2+}-dependent (7). Other physiological factors such as progesterone (8) or serum albumin (9) are also capable of inducing the acrosome reaction; more particularly, they enhance the ability of the zona to induce it (10, 11). On the other hand, such induction is not achievable in spermatozoa freshly removed from the male reproductive tract. The sperm must first complete a relatively lengthy period of incubation either in the female reproductive tract or in a specialized in-vitro environment. This priming process of "capacitation", which has already been alluded to by earlier speakers, is still poorly understood, both in functional and in molecular terms (2).

Capacitation is not an absolutely essential prerequisite for induction of the acrosome reaction. Treatment with Ca^{2+} and a bivalent-metal-cation ionophore will readily and rapidly provoke an acrosome reaction in uncapacitated cells (12 and refs therein). The question is therefore not only what molecular changes occur in the sperm cell during capacitation but also what functional responses these changes serve to modify. Both zona triggering and ionophore triggering appear to set in train similar series of lipolytic processes (11). However, the high concentrations of ionophore and Ca^{2+} that are needed to induce significant numbers of acrosome reactions in uncapacitated cells are severely detrimental to the spermatozoa, whereas it is possible to provoke acrosome reactions with low levels of ionophore in "capacitated" sperm samples without obvious degeneration (e.g. 13, 14). Moreover, the Ca^{2+} increases that accompany progesterone's induction of acrosome reactions in capacitated cells are also relatively modest (e.g. 15). Capacitation can therefore be considered as a sensitising process which specifically renders the acrosomal and overlying plasma membranes potentially fusible.

Studies of capacitation are complicated. There are three particular difficulties. Firstly, several different characteristics are currently being used as parameters for capacitation, though these may not be measuring the same functional state: e.g. surface changes (16) inducibility of the acrosome reaction in response to zona material (17), expression of hyperactivated motility (18), ability to bind to or to penetrate zonae (19). Secondly, relatively lengthy incubation is generally required to achieve a significant level of "capacitation" as measured by such parameters; it is likely that these changes are the culmination of a series of processes taking place sequentially, and sequential events are very hard to characterize via quantitation of the terminal results. Thirdly, there is increasing evidence that sperm populations do not capacitate synchronously (6, 20-22); such heterogeneity adds greatly to the complexities of interpreting data and the kinetics of change.

Our own approach to investigating capacitation has assumed that capacitational changes occur in many cells when they are incubated in media that support in-vitro fertilization whereas few cells undergo capacitation in media that do not support in-vitro fertilization. As Ca^{2+} (23 and refs therein), bicarbonate/CO_2 (24 and refs therein) and serum albumin (25 and refs therein) are all key ingredients of successful in-vitro fertilization media, we have focussed on the effect of these components on sperm membrane and surface characteristics. We have used fluorescent probes in combination with flow cytometry to observe changes in individual cells within the sperm population.

Previous studies in our laboratory (26) have demonstrated that of the three components mentioned it is bicarbonate/CO_2 that induces major detectable changes in the sperm population. Serum albumin enhances the effects of bicarbonate but has little or no effect alone. Ca^{2+} has not yet been found to play any specific role. Several studies, involving a number of animal species (see refs in 24), have indicated the importance of bicarbonate/CO_2 in in-vitro fertilization, and Boatman and Robbins (27) have concluded that in the hamster this component is primarily responsible for provoking in-vitro capacitation.

Many investigations have used lectins to detect changes in the sperm glycocalyx during capacitation. Using fluorescein-conjugated lectins, our group has been able to confirm that bicarbonate provokes surface changes in boar and ram spermatozoa. These changes appear to be due to a loss of coating material with concomitant exposure of underlying components (21). The changes occur essentially over the acrosomal region of the sperm head, and are observed within the sperm population as the development of a sub-group of live cells with enhanced or diminished lectin-binding abilities. Initially, few if any such cells are seen, but, during exposure to bicarbonate, numbers of altered cells increase slowly, reaching a maximum after some 120 min in boar sperm populations (90 min in ram sperm populations). The changes can be inhibited or reversed by addition of seminal plasma. Our flow cytometric analyses have indicated that, even after shorter incubation periods, almost all the individual cells in the new sub-group of spermatozoa show the full extent of surface change (in terms of increase or decrease in lectin binding ability): few cells show intermediate binding properties. It therefore appears that the transition between coating states takes place rather rapidly, but that this response to bicarbonate occurs after widely different delays in individual cells. The heterogeneous functionality of sperm populations is thus clearly illustrated.

The time course of the surface changes corresponds well with estimates of minimum "capacitation times" (earliest times at which fertilization is observable after initiation of gamete co-incubation, probably representing attainment of a threshold concentration of capacitated sperm). However, the slowness, with which the surface changes develop, implies that they depend upon earlier processes. As the major and essential components of the cell plasma membrane are phospholipids, we have sought early effects of our "capacitating" system on plasma membrane lipid architecture in spermatozoa.

The lipophilic fluorescent probe merocyanine 540 has been used in several cell types to indicate changes in membrane fluidity, lipid in a higher state of disorder apparently being capable of binding increased levels of merocyanine (e.g. 28). We have found that boar sperm populations exposed to bicarbonate/CO_2 rapidly develop an enhanced ability to bind merocyanine (29-31). This change is induced in most but not all of the cells. The high-merocyanine-binding sub-group is first seen after about 100 seconds of exposure and maximizes by about 300 seconds. As with the surface changes described above, the new sub-group is rapidly distinguishable within the live population and few cells display intermediate merocyanine-binding characteristics; thus the spermatozoa appear to switch from a "low binding" state to a "high binding" state. The effect is not dependent on external Ca^{2+}, and, although serum albumin enhances the proportion of the population that responds rapidly in this way, the change will take place in its absence.

Merocyanine 540 is a highly lipophilic molecule but it carries a permanent negative charge in the form of a sulphonate group. Previous workers (e.g. 32) have presented evidence to suggest that this probe is impermeant and it has therefore been used to detect changes in the outer leaflet of the plasma membrane (e.g. 33). Our own data (see Fig. 1) shows that the enhanced merocyanine binding is at sites that are inaccessible to the impermeable reducing agent dithionite (34) until the cells are dead or permeabilized (the water-soluble dithionite destroys the merocyanine fluorescence through reduction). At the same time, direct microscopic observation indicates that the enhanced binding takes place all over the sperm cell (data not shown). Whether the merocyanine becomes embedded more deeply within the outer leaflet or whether it actually passes through the bilayer to the inner leaflet, the increased fluorescent staining clearly reflects a major overall change in the sperm plasma membrane lipid.

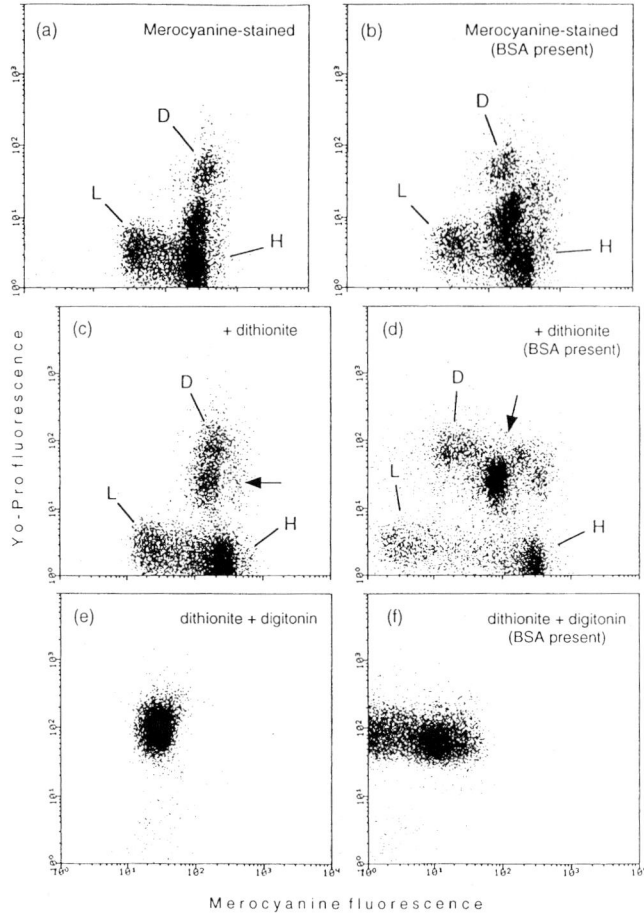

Figure 1. **Dithionite quenching of merocyanine fluorescence in boar sperm populations stimulated by isobutylmethylxanthine.**
Two suspensions of washed spermatozoa were incubated for 20 min at 38°C in a bicarbonate-free Hepes-buffered Tyrode's-based medium (21) containing 1 mg polyvinyl alcohol and 1 mg polyvinylpyrrolidone/ml and 0.5 mM isobutylmethylxanthine; 25 nM Yo-Pro-1 (impermeable nuclear stain: Molecular Probes, Eugene, Oregon, USA) was included as a fluorescent viability probe. After 16 min, bovine serum albumin (3 mg/ml final concentration) was added to one of the suspensions. Merocyanine 540 (2 µM final concentration) was then added and incubation continued for 6 min after which suspensions were analysed on a Becton-Dickinson Facstar flow cytometer ((a) and (b)). Excitation was at 488 nm, and emission was collected using a 530/30 nm bandpass filter for Yo-Pro fluorescence and a 620 nm longpass filter for merocyanine fluorescence.

Sodium dithionite (10 mM final concentration, from a freshly prepared solution) was then added, and the suspensions re-analysed after 2 min ((c) and (d)). Digitonin (20 µg/ml final concentration) was then added, and the suspensions re-analysed after a further 2 min ((e) and (f)).
L represents the low-merocyanine-binding live cells, H the high-merocyanine-binding live cells, D the dead cells. Note the large difference between (c) and (d) in response to dithionite addition: most cell groups in (d) show greatly diminished merocyanine fluorescence. Note also the cells arrowed in (c) and (d) whose Yo-Pro fluorescence has increased after dithionite addition; these represents an especially unstable sub-group.
Addition of the permeabilizing agent digitonin allows dithionite access, in particular, to the merocyanine in the previously stable H subgroup of cells.

Two aspects of this bicarbonate-induced effect are particularly noteworthy. Firstly, it is reversible. The increase in merocyanine binding is manifested at 38°C, disappears as the spermatozoa are replaced at 25°C, and reappears once more as they are re-incubated at 38°C. If the cells are removed from the bicarbonate-containing medium, binding ability declines rapidly and does not re-appear on rewarming; however, replacement of the cells in fresh bicarbonate-containing medium at 38°C induces the response once more. Secondly, the effect (as judged by numbers of high-binding cells after 10 minutes) shows saturation kinetics in relation to bicarbonate concentration, with a half-maximal response at about 4 mM; moreover, similar increases in merocyanine-binding ability can be provoked by general cyclic nucleotide phosphodiesterase inhibitors such as caffeine and isobutylmethylxanthine (IBMX), with an efficacy that approximately matches their published abilities to inhibit the phosphodiesterases. The change in the membrane lipid architecture thus seems to be under metabolic control.

In all cell types that have been studied so far (including spermatozoa), phospholipid classes have been shown to display asymmetric distribution across membrane bilayers (see 35). At the present time, it is believed that aminophospholipids are translocated to the cytoplasmic leaflet by a specific ATP-dependent translocase; other transporters, termed "flippases", may effect more general exchange of phospholipids between the two leaflets (36). Such mechanisms, working in concert, are now considered largely responsible for maintaining the steady-state equilibria observed, and it has been proposed that modulation of these mechanisms may significantly alter membrane function through specific redistribution of phospholipid classes differing not only in head group polarity but also in lipid composition. We have therefore investigated the effect of bicarbonate on phospholipid distribution in the boar sperm plasma membrane, using (6-(7-nitrobenz-2-oxa-1,3-diazol-4-yl)amino)hexanoyl- (C6NBD-) labelled phospholipid analogues as tracers (37). Loading such lipids into the spermatozoa via monomolecular transfer from carrier vesicles, we have assessed the proportion of each class located in the inner membrane leaflet by destroying NBD fluorescence in the outer leaflet with dithionite; by counterstaining dead cells with propidium iodide, we have focussed specifically on the live sperm population. We have been able to show that in boar spermatozoa, as in spermatozoa of ram (38), bull (39) and trout spermatozoa (40), phosphatidylserine is essentially confined to the inner leaflet, while sphingomyelin is confined to the outer leaflet; phosphatidylethanolamine is found mostly in the inner leaflet and phosphatidylcholine is found mostly in the outer leaflet (Table I).

Transfer of added aminophospholipids to the inner leaflet is a very rapid process that is greatly inhibited by depleting sperm ATP levels or by blocking sperm thiol groups with N-ethylmaleimide (Fig. 2a); such sensitivity implies that an enzymatic process is involved in the phospholipid translocation. Although exposure to bicarbonate or to phosphodiesterase inhibitors does not alter the distribution of the aminophospholipids (Table I), there is a strongly inhibitory effect on aminophospholipid transfer (see Fig. 2a). Moreover, during a 60-minutes exposure to these agents, steady-state levels of NBD-phosphatidylcholine in the inner leaflet slowly increase from about 14% to over 30% (Fig. 2b; see also Table I).

Our studies therefore show firstly that the lipid architecture of the sperm plasma membrane is controlled dynamically by complex enzymatic processes, secondly that bicarbonate/CO2, considered the primary agent of capacitation in vitro, induces rapid and important changes in these processes that precede any detectable changes in the surface glycocalyx. The molecular mechanisms involved in the lipid changes remain to be determined. However, certain points can be made.

Treatment	C6-NBD-PHOSPHOLIPID INTERNALIZED (% OF TOTAL INCORPORATED)			
	PtdEth	PtdSer	PtdCho	Sphingomyelin
Control	80.4	96.1	13.6	1.3
Bicarbonate addition	82.9	97.3	32.0	2.1
IBMX addition	81.7	95.3	33.5	3.4
ATP-depletion*	10.5†	21.5†	24.3	trace
Blocking of thiols	9.1†	15.3†	28.0	trace

Table I. **Steady-state distribution of incorporated phospholipid analogues in living boar spermatozoa.**
*ATP content was less than 5% of normal, as detected by a luciferin-luciferase assay.
† These treatments also reduced overall aminophospholipid uptake to less that 25% of control values, whereas uptake of PtdCho and sphingomyelin was unaltered.
Parallel samples of washed boar spermatozoa were pre-incubated for 30 min at 38°C in a protein-free Hepes-buffered Tyrode's-based medium before being mixed with suspensions of vesicles loaded with a given (6-(7-nitrobenz-2-oxa-1, 3-diazol-4-yl) amino-hexanoyl-labelled (C_6-NBD-) phospholipid (PtdEth, phosphatidylethanolamine; PtdSer, phosphatidylserine; PtdCho, phosphatidylcholine) (37). After a further 1 h incubation at 38°C, samples were analysed by flow cytometry before and after brief treatment with 10 mM dithionite to destroy NBD fluorescence located in the sperm plasma membrane outer leaflet (34). Living cells were distinguished by their ability to exclude propidium iodide (26). NBD and propidium iodide fluorescence was collected using respectively a 530/30 bandpass filter and a 620 longpass filter. The relative amount of fluorescence that resisted dithionite destruction in the live cells (i.e. internalized phospholipid) was calculated for each phospholipid type.

The effects of the following additional treatments were tested: (a) inclusion of 15 mM bicarbonate/5% CO_2 in the medium, during both pre-incubation and lipid labelling; (b) similar inclusion of 0.5 mM isobutylmethylxanthine; (c) depletion of sperm ATP content by including 5 mM azide in the medium and replacing glucose with 2-deoxyglucose, during both preincubation and lipid labelling; (d) blocking of cellular thiol groups by inclusion of 2 mM N-ethylmaleimide (NEM) during preincubation (NEM was removed by washing prior to lipid labelling in the standard medium). 5 mM phenylmethylsulfonylfluoride was included in all treatments to minimize *catabolism of the phospholipid analogues (c.f. 41). The results are mean values from 4 experiments.*

Hitherto, ideas regarding capacitation have largely focussed on the characteristics of membrane protein components (e.g. 42-47). The perceived role of the membrane lipid has been principally as a support matrix for the protein components; studies and discussion of lipid behaviour has focussed on lipid fluidity in relation both to membrane fusibility (48, 49) and to mobility of proteins within the membrane plane (50); this latter aspect has been highlighted following the discovery that clustering of zona protein receptors is apparently crucial to the triggering of the acrosome reaction (51; see also 52-54). In turn, consideration of membrane lipid fluidity changes during capacitation has focussed on the modulating effects of sterols on sperm lipid fluidity (55, 56) and on the roles of serum albumin and lipid transfer proteins as carriers in facilitating cholesterol and other lipid transport to and from the sperm plasma membrane (57-59). However, while our studies do not exclude that such transfers may be involved in later stages of the capacitation process, several pieces of evidence argue against lipid exchange between media components and spermatozoa being primarily responsible for the changes we have detected. Firstly, although serum albumin usually enhances the proportion of spermatozoa showing increased merocyanine binding, the increases can be induced in the complete absence of extracellular protein. Secondly, while one might conceive of a lipid exchange mechanism whose equilibrium was reversed by a change in temperature between 38°C and 25°C, it is very difficult to see how such exchange could be reversed by replacement of the cells in fresh medium. Thirdly, it is very difficult to envisage how bicarbonate or phosphodiesterase inhibitors can specifically induce lipid exchange on their own, nor how such exchange can then proceed to completion so rapidly in some cells yet not take place in others. Finally, the presence of sterols smooths out temperature-induced gel-to-liquid lipid phase transitions, making them more continuous (c.f. 60 and refs therein). Although temperature affects the ability of bicarbonate to induce increases in merocyanine binding (see above), the merocyanine binding itself (as judged by fluorescence intensity of either live or dead cell groups in bicarbonate-free media) is unaffected by temperature (Table II). This implies that sperm outer-leaflet lipid disorder is unaltered between 25°C and 38°C and suggests that conventional physicochemical lipid phase changes are not responsible for the change in merocyanine binding.

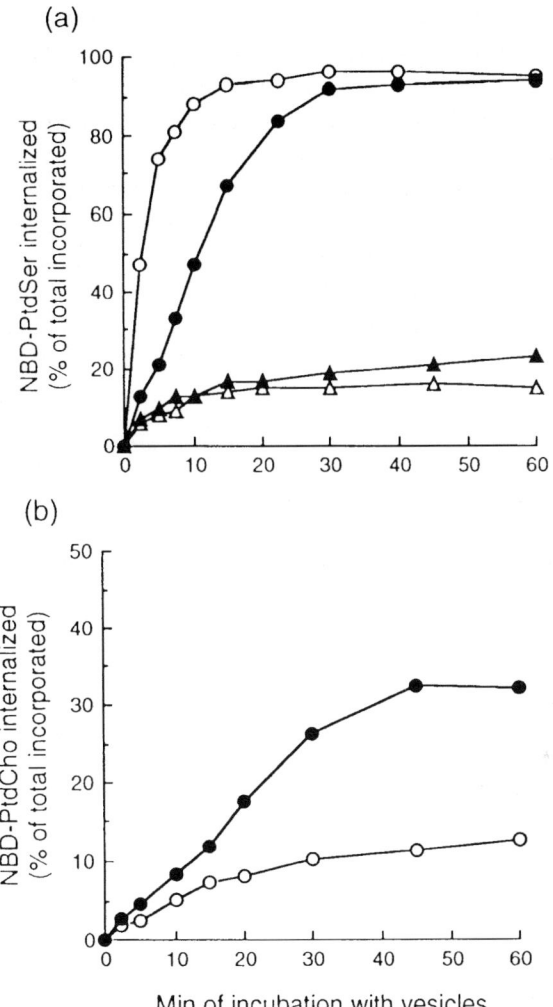

Figure 2. **Time-dependent transfer of C6NBD-labelled phospholipids across the lipid bilayer of the boar sperm plasma membrane.**
Supensions of washed boar spermatozoa were pre-incubated in variations of a Hepes-buffered Tyrode's-based medium before being mixed with vesicles loaded with (a) C6NBD-labelled phosphatidylserine (NBD-PtdSer), (b) C6NBD-labelled phosphatidylcholine (NBD-PtdCho). At intervals during further incubation at 38°C, samples were subjected to flow cytometric analysis before and after brief treatment with dithionite, in order to detect the total amount of C6NBD phospholipid incorporated and the relative amount internalized in the live cells. For further experimental details, see legend to Table I.

○, preincubation and lipid labelling in simple medium; ●, 15 mM bicarbonate/5% CO_2 included during pre-incubation and labelling; Æ, ATP-depleted (azide included in medium and glucose replaced with 2-deoxyglucose); Æ, thiol-blocked (N-ethylmaleimide included during preincubation).

CONDITIONS	% LIVE	MEAN FLUORESCENCE	
		LIVE CELLS	DEAD CELLS
15 min at 38 °C	93.4	26.5	136.1
Then 15 min at 25°C	92.8	25.9	127.7
Then washed (25°C)	88.6	29.0	135.2
Reincubated 15min at 38°C	85.0	23.9	107.9

Table II. **Merocyanine fluorescence in boar sperm populations: response to temperature change.**
Washed spermatozoa were incubated at 38°C in a bicarbonate-free Hepes-buffered Tyrode's-based medium containing 3 mg serum albumin/ml and 25 nM Yo-Pro. After 15 min, samples were taken, stained with merocyanine, and analysed by flow cytometry as described in the legend to Fig. 1. The sperm suspensions were then incubated at 25°C for 15 min before further samples were taken for staining and analysis. Next the spermatozoa were washed through a cushion of sucrose medium (26) at 25°C, replaced in fresh Tyrode's medium and reanalysed. Finally, they were reincubated at 38°C for 15 min before final analysis.
In the absence of bicarbonate or IBMX stimulation, there were essentially only two groups within the sperm population, live low-merocyanine-binding cells and dead cells (Yo-Pro-positive, showing high merocyanine-binding ability). The mean fluorescence (arbitrary units) of the cells in each group was obtained using the Becton-Dickinson Lysys II programme to analyse the data, which was originally collected in logarithmic mode. The results are mean values from 2 experiments.

The role of serum albumin in capacitation and the acrosome reaction has received much attention over the years, since it was discovered to be the major fertilization-promoting component in follicular fluid (9). Serum albumin's ability to bind fatty acids and other lipophilic molecules has been assumed to be a crucial characteristic, enabling it to act as a carrier for such components, thereby transporting them into, or more particularly out of, the sperm cell plasma membrane (see refs in 2). Some recent experiments we have performed, however, indicate that albumin's action may be more subtle, involving close interaction with the sperm surface. When boar spermatozoa were stimulated by the phosphodiesterase inhibitor IBMX and then stained with merocyanine, the cell populations showed an essentially similar pattern whether or not serum albumin was present in the medium (compare Figs 1a and 1b). However, when dithionite was added to quench accessible merocyanine, the two systems showed considerable differences (compare Figs 1c and 1d): relatively little quenching took place in the absence of albumin, whereas extensive quenching took place in its presence. Although albumin binds merocyanine (61), the protein did not appear to be acting as a carrier in this situation, because addition of high levels of albumin alone (10 mg/ml) did not remove merocyanine at all from the low-binding cells and removed it only slowly from the dead cells (deduced from flow cytometric fluorescence data, not shown). Albumin has been shown to bind in a "non-specific" way to spermatozoa (62), thus one explanation of our findings would be that serum albumin binds to and perturbs (either directly or indirectly) the outer leaflet of the lipid bilayer so as to enhance access of the dithionite to the merocyanine. Recent studies of the way in which carrier proteins facilitate transfer of lipophilic molecules across cell membranes have shown that the process is still far from understood, but appears to involve a close association of these proteins with the plasma membrane surface that is not receptor-mediated in the usual sense of the term (63, 64). Despite uncertainties as to mechanism, however, the key point of our experiments is that albumin plays a secondary, facilitating role in the lipid changes we have observed. It does not act as the primary effector. Perhaps albumin's other reported effects on sperm function should be re-evaluated in this light.

The concept of bicarbonate as the essential modulator of capacitation in vitro begs the question as to how such a ubiquitous physiological component could play a similar role in vivo. In fact, there is increasing evidence that bicarbonate's levels can be locally modulated within the animal. In particular, levels of bicarbonate within the epididymal lumen are maintained very much below circulating blood levels (65, 66). It would therefore appear that spermatozoa acquire their fertilizing ability and are then stored in an environment that minimizes potential capacitating changes (the secretion of sperm coating factors may also play an important stabilizing role - see 67). Spermatozoa would encounter increased levels of bicarbonate on ejaculation/deposition in the female tract (c.f. 66, 68), at which point the mechanisms yielding the changes we have described would be initiated. Capacitation should therefore be considered a process which is actively "switched on" in the correct environment.

It has long been axiomatic that capacitation involves a degree of membrane destabilization (e.g. 42, 48, 69). Our group has obtained considerable evidence that the changes induced by bicarbonate/CO2 can indeed destabilize the spermatozoa. An early study demonstrated that bicarbonate induced the appearance of a sub-group of spermatozoa with greatly enhanced intracellular Ca^{2+} levels; the influx of Ca^{2+} was shown to be non-specific and concomitant with increasing leakiness of the plasma membrane (26). We always observe enhanced and increasing levels of cell death (detected by uptake of impermeable nuclear dyes) as spermatozoa are incubated in the presence of bicarbonate and/or phosphodiesterase inhibitors

(26, 31). Part of the sperm population in which high merocyanine binding has been induced is rendered very fragile, easily damaged by (e.g.) dithionite or mechanical manipulation (see Figs 1c and 1d). These observations, coupled with the sequential nature of the bicarbonate-induced changes we have detected in the live cells, have led us to propose that capacitation is an on-going process of membrane destabilization rather than a specifically limited cellular change (31). The functionally capacitated spermatozoon (i.e. one that will undergo the acrosome reaction in response to the zona pellucida) is a cell that is passing through a "window" in the destabilization continuum. While early stages of destabilization may be reversible, later stages are probably irreversible; eventually, cell death will ensue.

In the light of what is currently known of sperm biology at fertilization, how might our findings be integrated into an overall molecular scheme? One possibility might be that the initial changes in merocyanine permeability are brought about via altered interactions between the sperm cytoskeleton and the cytoplasmic face of the plasma membrane phospholipid bilayer (28, 70). The activity of the translocases is modified either directly or indirectly, and transverse phospholipid composition begins to alter. The consequent changes in the lipid characteristics of the bilayer coupled with changed interactions with the underlying cytoskeleton alter surface glycoprotein orientation, diminish mutual affinities and binding constants of coating proteins to membrane proteins and lipids, with the result that coating material is gradually lost (c.f. 21). Lateral mobilities of protein components within the bilayer also increase (c.f. 46). Ion permeabilities across the bilayer also increase, with consequent increases in levels of intracellular Na^+ and Ca^{2+} as outward membrane pump capabilities are overloaded by the influx (c.f. 71, 72). The higher levels of intracellular ions activate enzymes such as phospholipases (73-75), with further destabilizing consequences for membrane structure and function.

If this general scheme is imposed on the highly domained nature of the sperm plasmalemma, it can easily be imagined that at some stage in the process, key domains such as those in the acrosomal region would be sufficiently destabilized/sensitized that a sudden (additional?) influx of Ca^{2+}, brought about through zona binding and clustering of unmasked and/or mobilized membrane receptors, would set in train the key sequence of lipid catabolism to induce the membrane fusion needed for exocytosis. It is noteworthy that recent studies by Roldan and his colleagues have revealed the need for important catabolism of phosphatidylcholine during the acrosome reaction (75, 76). Assuming the Ca^{2+}-dependent phospholipases responsible are intracellular, only after bicarbonate-dependent redistribution of phosphatidylcholine to the inner leaflet (see above) might sufficient substrate be made available to them.

A corollary to this scenario is the implication that, as the changes we are suggesting proceed, a point will come when the acrosome reaction may take place spontaneously, due to increasing intracellular Ca2+ in combination with increasing lipid catabolism. In recent years, emphasis has been placed on distinguishing those acrosome-reacted cells that are still "live" (e.g. 77, 78). If capacitation is viewed as an on-going destabilization process, delineating "live" acrosome-reacted cells as physiologically important and "dead" reacted cells as degenerative may well be an oversimplification.

Much relating to capacitation remains to be elucidated. Indeed, our findings regarding lipid architecture suggest that we are only just beginning to understand the outline of the process. Nevertheless, recognition of capacitation as an on-going cascade of changes that may proceed at widely different rates in individual cells in the sperm population should enable us to design more revealing experiments and lead us to more subtle interpretations of our findings.

REFERENCES

1. Bedford JM, Cooper GW. Membrane fusion events in the fertilization of vertebrate eggs. In: Poste G, Nicolson GL, eds. Membrane Fusion. Amsterdam: Elsevier North-Holland Biomedical Press, 1978: 65-125.
2. Yanagimachi R. Mammalian fertilization. In: Knobil E, Neill JD, eds. The Physiology of Reproduction, Second Edition, Vol I. New York: Raven Press Ltd, 1994: 189-317.
3. Wassarman PM. Profile of a mammalian sperm receptor. Development 1990; 108: 1-17.
4. Florman HM, Tombes RM, First NL, Babcock DF. An adhesion-associated agonist from the zona pellucida activates G protein-promoted elevations of internal Ca2+ and pH that mediate mammalian sperm acrosomal exocytosis. Dev Biol 1989; 135: 133-46.
5. Storey BT, Hourani CL, Kim JB. A transient rise in intracellular Ca2+ is a precursor reaction to the zona pellucida-induced acrosome reaction in mouse sperm and is blocked by the induced acrosome reaction inhibitor 3-quinuclidinyl benzilate. Mol Reprod Dev 1992; 32: 41-50.
6. Florman HM. Sequential focal and global elevations of sperm intracellular Ca^{2+} are initiated by the zona pellucida during acrosomal exocytosis. Dev Biol 1994; 165: 152-64.
7. Harrison RAP, Roldan ERS. Phosphoinositides and their products in the mammalian sperm acrosome reaction. J Reprod Fertil, Suppl 1990; 42: 51-67.

8. Osman RA, Andria ML, Jones AD, Meizel S. Steroid induced exocytosis: the human sperm acrosome reaction. Biochem Biophys Res Commun 1989; 160: 828-33.
9. Lui CW, Cornett LE, Meizel S. Identification of the bovine follicular fluid protein involved in the in vitro induction of the hamster sperm acrosome reaction. Biol Reprod 1977; 17: 34-41.
10. Andrews JC, Bavister BD. Hamster zonae pellucidae cannot induce physiological acrosome reactions in chemically capacitated hamster spermatozoa in the absence of albumin. Biol Reprod 1989; 41: 117-22.
11. Roldan ERS, Murase T, Shi Q-X. Exocytosis in spermatozoa in response to progesterone and zona pellucida. Science, NY 1994; 266: 1578-81.
12. Shams-Borhan G, Harrison RAP. Production, characterization, and use of ionophore-induced, calcium-dependent acrosome reaction in ram spermatozoa. Gamete Res 1981; 4: 407-32.
13. DeJonge CJ, Mack SR, Zaneveld LJD. Synchronous assay for human sperm capacitation and the acrosome reaction. J Androl 1989; 10: 232-9.
14. Aitken RJ, Buckingham DW, Fang HG. Analysis of the responses of human spermatozoa to A23187 employing a novel technique for assessing the acrosome reaction. J Androl 1993; 14: 132-41.
15. Pillai MC, Meizel S. Trypsin inhibitors prevent the progesterone-initiated increase in intracellular calcium required for the human sperm acrosome reaction. J Exp Zool 1991; 258: 384-93.
16. Fraser LR, Harrison RAP, Herod JE. Characterization of a decapacitation factor associated with epididymal mouse spermatozoa. J Reprod Fertil 1990; 89: 135-48.
17. McNutt TL, Killian GJ. Influence of bovine follicular and oviduct fluids on sperm capacitation in vitro. J Androl 1991; 12: 244-52.
18. Kervancioglu ME, Djahanbakhch O, Aitken RJ. Epithelial cell coculture and the induction of sperm capacitation. Fertil Steril 1994; 61: 1103-8.
19. Andrews JC, Nolan JP, Hammerstedt RH, Bavister BD. Role of zinc during hamster sperm capacitation. Biol Reprod 1994; 51: 1238-47.
20. Stewart-Savage J. Effect of bovine serum albumin concentration and source on sperm capacitation in the golden hamster. Biol Reprod 1993; 49: 74-81.
21. Ashworth PJC, Harrison RAP, Miller NGA, Plummer JM, Watson PF. Flow cytometric detection of bicarbonate-induced changes in lectin binding in boar and ram sperm populations. Mol Reprod Dev 1995; 40: 164-76.
22. Vredenburgh-Wilberg WL, Parrish JJ. Intracellular pH of bovine sperm increases during capacitation. Mol Reprod Dev 1995; 40: 490-502.
23. Fraser LR. Minimum and maximum extracellular Ca2+ requirements during mouse sperm capacitation and fertilization in vitro. J Reprod Fertil 1987; 81: 77-89.

24. Suzuki K, Ebihara M, Nagai T, Clarke NGE, Harrison RAP. Importance of bicarbonate/CO2 for fertilization of pig oocytes in vitro, and synergism with caffeine. Reprod Fertil Dev 1994; 6: 221-7.
25. Saeki K, Nagao Y, Hoshi M, Nagai M. Effects of heparin, sperm concentration and bull variation on in vitro fertilization of bovine oocytes in a protein-free medium. Theriogenology 1995; 43: 751-9.
26. Harrison RAP, Mairet B, Miller NGA. Flow cytometric studies of bicarbonate-mediated Ca2+ influx in boar sperm populations. Mol Reprod Dev 1993; 35: 197-208.
27. Boatman DE, Robbins RS. Bicarbonate: carbon-dioxide regulation of sperm capacitation, hyperactivated motility, and acrosome reactions. Biol Reprod 1991; 44: 806-13.
28. Del Buono BJ, Williamson PL, Schlegel RA. Relation between the organization of spectrin and of membrane lipids in lymphocytes. J Cell Biol 1988; 106: 697-703.
29. Harrison RAP, Ashworth PJC, Miller NGA. Rapid effects of bicarbonate/CO2 on boar spermatozoa detected by merocyanine, a probe of lipid packing. J Reprod Fertil, Abstr Ser 1993; 12: 14.
30. Harrison RAP, Ashworth PJC, Miller NGA. The bicarbonate-inducible change in boar sperm plasma membrane lipid architecture. J Reprod Fertil, Abstr Ser 1995; 15: 33.
31. Harrison RAP. Capacitation mechanisms, and the role of capacitation as seen in eutherian mammals. Reprod Fertil Dev 1995; (in press).
32. Schlegel RA, Phelps BM, Waggoner A, Terada L, Williamson P. Binding of merocyanine 540 to normal and leukemic erythroid cells. Cell 1980; 20:321-8.
33. Verhoven B, Schlegel RA, Williamson P. Rapid loss and restoration of lipid asymmetry by different pathways in resealed erythrocyte ghosts. Biochim Biophys Acta 1992; 1104: 15-23.
34. McIntyre JC, Sleight RG. Fluorescence assay for phopholipid membrane asymmetry. Biochemistry 1991; 30: 11819-27.
35. Zachowski A. Phospholipids in animal eukaryotic membranes: transverse asymmetry and movement. Biochem J 1993; 294: 1-14.
36. Zwaal RFA, Comfurius P, Bevers EM. Mechanism and function of changes in membrane-phospholipid asymmetry in platelets and erythrocytes. Biochem Soc Trans 1993; 21: 248-53.
37. Kok JW, Hoekstra D. Fluorescent lipid analogs: applications in cell and membrane biology. In: Mason WT, ed. Fluorescent and Luminescent Probes for Biological Activity, A Practical Guide to Technology for Quantitative Real-Time Analysis. London, UK: Academic Press Ltd, 1993: 100-19.

38. Müller K, Pomorski T, Müller P, Zachowski A, Herrmann A. Protein-dependent translocation of aminophospholipids and asymmetric transbilayer distribution of phospholipids in the plasma membrane of ram sperm cells. Biochemistry 1994; 33: 9968-74.
39. Nolan JP, Magargee SF, Posner RG, Hammerstedt RH. Flow cytometric analysis of transmembrane phospholipid movement in bull sperm. Biochemistry 1995; 34: 3907-15.
40. Müller K, Labbé C, Zachowski A. Phospholipid transverse asymmetry in trout spermatozoa plasma membrane. Biochim Biophys Acta 1994; 1192: 21-6.
41. Wykle RL, Malone B, Blank ML, Snyder F. Biosynthesis of pulmonary surfactant: comparison of 1-palmitoyl-sn-glycero-3-phosphocholine and palmitate as precursors of dipalmitoyl-sn-glycero-3-phosphocholine in adenoma alveolar type II cells. Arch Biochem Biophys 1980; 199: 526-37.
42. O'Rand MG. Changes in sperm surface properties correlated with capacitation. In: Fawcett DW, Bedford JM, eds. The Spermatozoon. Maturation, Motility, Surface Properties and Comparative Aspects. Baltimore: Urban and Schwarzenberg, 1979: 195-204.
43. Voglmayr JK, Sawyer RF. Surface transformation of ram spermatozoa in uterine, oviduct and cauda epididymal fluids in vitro. J Reprod Fertil 1986; 78: 315-25.
44. Villarroya S, Scholler R. Lateral diffusion of a human sperm-head antigen during incubation in a capacitation medium and induction of the acrosome reaction in vitro. J Reprod Fertil 1987; 80: 545-62.
45. Berger T. Changes in exposed membrane proteins during in vitro capacitation of boar sperm. Mol Reprod Dev 1990; 27: 249-53.
46. Jones R, Shalgi R, Hoyland J, Phillips DM. Topographical rearrangement of a plasma membrane antigen during capacitation of rat spermatozoa in vitro. Dev Biol 1990; 139: 349-62.
47. Benoff S, Cooper GW, Hurley I, Napolitano B, Rosenfeld DL, Scholl GM, Hershlag A. Human sperm fertilizing potential in vitro is correlated with differential expression of a head-specific mannose-ligand receptor. Fertil Steril 1993; 59: 854-62.
48. Bearer EL, Friend DS. Modifications of anionic-lipid domains preceding membrane fusion in guinea pig sperm. J Cell Biol 1982; 92: 604-15.
49. Gadella BM, Lopes-Cardozo M, Van Golde LMG, Colenbrander B, Gadella TWJ. Glycolipid migration from the apical to the equatorial subdomains of the sperm head plasma membrane precedes the acrosome reaction. Evidence for a primary capacitation event in boar spermatozoa. J Cell Sci 1995; 108: 935-46.
50. Wolf DE. Lipid domains in sperm plasma membranes. Mol Membrane Biol 1995; 12: 101-4.

51. Leyton L, Saling P. Evidence that aggregation of mouse sperm receptors by ZP3 triggers the acrosome reaction. J Cell Biol 1989; 108: 2163-8.
52. Aarons D, Boettger-Tong H, Holt G, Poirier, GR. Acrosome reaction induced by immunoaggregation of a proteinase inhibitor bound to the murine sperm head. Mol Reprod Dev 1991; 30: 258-64.
53. Macek MB, Lopez LC, Shur BD. Aggregation of beta 1,4-galactosyltransferase on mouse sperm induces the acrosome reaction. Dev Biol 1991; 147: 440-4.
54. McKinnon CA, Weaver FE, Yoder JA, Fairbanks G, Wolf DE. Cross-linking a maturation-dependent ram sperm plasma membrane antigen induces the acrosome reaction. Mol Reprod Dev 1991; 29: 200-7.
55. Go KJ, Wolf DP. The role of sterols in sperm capacitation. Adv Lipid Res 1983; 20: 317-30.
56. Parks JE, Ehrenwald E. Cholesterol efflux from mammalian sperm and its potential role in capacitation. In: Bavister BD, Cummins J, Roldan ERS, eds. Fertilization in Mammals. Norwell, Mass: Serono Symposia, 1990: 155-67.
57. Langlais J, Kan FWK, Granger L, Raymond L, Bleau G, Roberts KD. Identification of sterol acceptors that stimulate cholesterol efflux from human spermatozoa during in vitro capacitation. Gamete Res 1988; 20: 185-201.
58. Ravnik SE, Albers JJ, Muller CH. A novel view of albumin-supported sperm capacitation: role of lipid transfer protein-1. Fertil Steril 1993; 59: 629-38.
59. Ravnik SE, Albers JJ, Muller CH. Stimulation of human sperm capacitation by purified lipid transfer protein. J Exp Zool 1995; 272: 78-83.
60. Hernandez-Borrell J, Keough KMW. Heteroacid phosphatidylcholines with different amounts of unsaturation respond differently to cholesterol. Biochim Biophys Acta 1993; 1153: 277-82.
61. Allan D, Hagelberg C, Kallen K-J, Haest CWM. Echinocytosis and microvesiculation of human erythrocytes induced by insertion of merocyanine 540 into the outer membrane leaflet. Biochim Biophys Acta 1989; 986: 115-22.
62. Blank M, Soo L, Britten JS. Adsorption of albumin on rabbit sperm membranes. J Membrane Biol 1976; 29: 401-9.
63. Uriel J, Torres J-M, Anel A. Carrier-protein-mediated enhancement of fatty-acid binding and internalization in human T-lymphocytes. Biochim Biophys Acta 1994; 1220: 231-40.
64. Trigatti BL, Gerber GE. A direct role for serum albumin in the cellular uptake of long-chain fatty acids. Biochem J 1995; 308: 155-9.

65. Caflisch CR, DuBose TD. Direct evaluation of acidification by rat testis and epididymis: role of carbonic anhydrase. Am J Physiol 1990; 258: E143-50.
66. Rodriguez-Martinez H, Ekstedt E, Einarsson S. Acidification of epididymal fluid in the boar. Int J Androl 1990; 13: 238-43.
67. Bedford, JM. The contraceptive potential of fertilization: a physiological perspective. Human Reprod 1994; 9: 842-58.
68. Okamura N, Tajima Y, Soejima A, Masuda H, Sugita Y. Sodium bicarbonate in seminal plasma stimulates the motility of mammalian spermatozoa through direct activation of adenylate cyclase. J Biol Chem 1985; 260:9699-705.
69. Chang MC, Hunter RHF. (1975) Capacitation of mammalian sperm: biological and experimental aspects. In: Hamilton DW, Greep RO, eds. Handbook of Physiology, Section 7: Endocrinology, Vol. V. Washington, DC: American Physiological Society, 1975: 339-51.
70. Devaux PF. Static and dynamic lipid asymmetry in cell membranes. Biochemistry 1991; 30: 1163-73.
71. Fraser LR, McDermott CA. Ca2+-related changes in the mouse sperm capacitation state: a possible role for Ca2+-ATPase. J Reprod Fertil 1992; 96: 363-77.
72. Fraser LR, Umar G, Sayed S. Na+-requiring mechanisms modulate capacitation and acrosomal exocytosis in mouse spermatozoa. J Reprod Fertil 1993; 97: 539-49.
73. Bennet PJ, Moatti J-P, Mansat A, Ribbes H, Cayrac J-C, Pontonnier F, Chap H, Douste-Blazy L. Evidence for the activation of phospholipases during acrosome reaction of human sperm elicited by calcium ionophore A23187. Biochim Biophys Acta 1987; 919: 255-65.
74. Roldan ERS, Fragio C. Phospholipase A2 activity and exocytosis of the ram sperm acrosome: regulation by bivalent cations. Biochim Biophys Acta 1993; 1168: 108-14.
75. Roldan ERS, Fragio C. Phospholipase A2 activation and subsequent exocytosis in the Ca2+/ionophore-induced acrosome reaction of ram spermatozoa. J Biol Chem 1993; 268: 13962-70.
76. Roldan ERS, Murase T. Polyphosphoinositide-derived diacylglycerol stimulates the hydrolysis of phosphatidylcholine by phospholipase C during exocytosis of the ram sperm acrosome. Effect is not mediated by protein kinase C. J Biol Chem 1994; 269: 23583-9.
77. Cross NL, Morales P, Overstreet JW, Hanson FW. Two simple methods for detecting acrosome-reacted human sperm. Gamete Res 1986; 15: 213-26.

78. Holden CA, Hyne RV, Sathananthan AH, Trounson AO. Assessment of the human sperm acrosome reaction using concanavalin A lectin. Mol Reprod Dev 1990; 25: 247-57.

Lipid transfer protein: a natural stimulator of the sperm capacitation process [1]

Charles H. Muller[1] and Stuart E. Ravnik[2]

[1] *Department of Urology, University of Washington School of Medicine Seattle, Washington 98195, USA and* [2] *Department of Cell Biology and Biochemistry, Texas Tech University, Lubbock, Texas 79430, USA*

Abstract

An important step in the capacitation of sperm prior to the acrosome reaction is the loss of membrane cholesterol. A highly lipophilic plasma protein, Lipid Transfer Protein-I (LTP-I) plays a role in cholesterol exchange among plasma lipoprotein particles. Human and animal reproductive fluids are examined for the presence of this protein, and for its activity. LTP-I and lipid (cholesterol) transfer activity (LTA) are found in many of the fluids, including human follicular fluid (HFF). Both LTA and LTP-I are found as contaminants in commercial albumin preparations which support sperm function tests. Removal of LTP-I from active albumin or HFF destroys this support, which can be recovered by the re-addition of purified LTP-1. Experiments were designed to determine the role of purified LTP-I, in absence of other exogenous protein, on human sperm capacitation. The time-course of acrosome reaction suggests that LTP-I stimulates capacitation, but does not induce an immediate acrosome reaction. LTP-I and other lipid exchange proteins and their inhibitors may have important roles in regulation of sperm function, but whether these proteins are irreplaceable is unknown.

La perte de cholestérol membranaire est une étape importante dans la capacitation des spermatozoïdes. Une protéine plasmatique très lipophile, la Lipid Transfer Protein-I (LTP-I), joue un rôle dans les échanges de cholestérol dans les lipoprotéines plasmatiques. La présence de cette protéine et son activité ont été recherchées dans les sécrétions génitales chez l'homme et chez l'animal. LTP-I et l'activité de transfert lipidique (cholestérol) (LTA) ont été retrouvées dans beaucoup de ces sécrétions, y compris le liquide folliculaire humain. La LTP-I et la LTA contaminent toutes deux les préparations commerciales d'albumine qui sont utilisées pour les tests fonctionnels du sperme. Lorsque l'on enlève la LTP-I de l'albumine ou du liquide folliculaire, on supprime leur effet sur les spermatozoïdes, effet qui peut être retrouvé par l'adjonction de LTP-I purifiée. Le rôle de la LTP-I purifiée, en l'absence d'autre protéine exogène, a été évalué sur la capacitation du sperme humain. La cinétique de la réaction acrosomique montre que la LTP-I stimule la capacitation mais n'induit pas immédiatement la réaction acrosomique. La LTP-I et les autres protéines échangeuses de lipides ainsi que leurs inhibiteurs pourraient avoir un rôle important dans la régulation de la fonction spermatique, mais on ne sait pas si elles sont irremplaçables.

INTRODUCTION

Capacitation is a time-dependent and reversible process required for mammalian sperm to eventually fertilize eggs. This much was confirmed in the early days of fertilization research. But unlike the acrosome reaction there was no obvious morphological change in sperm during capacitation. The process could not be quantified directly, since no one knew what it was at the cellular or biochemical levels. Indeed even the concept itself at times seemed to have gone out of favor. but it is clear that sperm in seminal fluid cannot fertilize or even acrosome react, so it follows that something must happen to sperm to allow these events. The dramatic membrane fusions occurring during acrosome reaction must be preceded by permissive changes in membrane structure. At its simplest, capacitation must include these changes leading to fluid and therefore fusible plasma and outer-acrosomal membranes. It undoubtedly includes other equally important changes such as expression, exteriorization or modification of surface ligands essential for sperm-zona pellucida recognition and binding. One or several of these surface ligands must transduce the zona's signal to induce the acrosome reaction. And capacitation includes or at least is contemporaneous with profound changes in sperm motility patterns. The process is an intriguing mystery; functional changes occurring in isolated cells over a matter of minutes to hours, in the absence of nuclear or macomolecular synthetic activity, under the control of unknown external or internal signals.

Each of the major aspects of capacitation (surface ligands, motility, and membrane fluidity) is receiving at least modest attention. However the basic concepts of temporal relationships to fertilization and reversibility have not been sufficiently addressed. Also all of the molecular players in the capacitation game are not known, but new possibilities seem to appear monthly. Thus, the possibility of profound redundancy of molecular pathways leading to each of the events in fertilization must be seriously considered. And after all, what even in life is more important to safeguard with redundant mechanisms?

Here we address one small part of the mystery: It is possible to demonstrate the presence and activity of a naturally occurring signal or effector involved in the membrane fluidity changes that must precede the acrosome reaction ?

Membrane lipids change during sperm development

Membrane fluidity is predominately a function of the membrane's specific lipid content. In particular, the amount of cholesterol (and its esters), the cholesterol/phospholipid ratio and the structure of the fatty acid chains of the phospholipids are the most relevant. All of these can be altered by enzymatic activity, exchange phenomena, or physical conditions such as temperature changes. At body temperature, cholesterol, the predominant sterol in many cells, imparts a stiffening of low fluidity effect on biological membranes. Lipid composition of the germ cell plasma membrane is altered during spermatogenesis and sperm maturation, and these changes are particularly notable in the sperm head overlying the acrosome. Evidence exists that there is an increase in the cholesterol/phospholipid ratio in this region, which may be a result of decreases in membrane phospholipids or exchange of cholesterol during epididymal sperm maturation (1). The result of these lipid changes appears to be a maintenance or accentuation of the regionalized differences in lipid diffusibility found in testicular sperm. The plasma membrane of the acrosomal region of the sperm head is believed to be relatively highly loaded with cholesterol, and therefore has a low fluidity.

Seminal fluid has well-known inhibitory effects on sperm fertilizing ability. Some of this action is due to " decapacitation factors ", which include cholesterol/phospholipid vesicles and cholesterol itself, present in high concentrations (69mg/dl) in human seminal fluid (2,3). The result of sperm maturation and exposure to seminal fluid is a cholesterol-rich sperm membrane that is rigid and unable to allow acrosome reaction.

Changes in sperm membrane lipid composition during capacitation

Obvious morphological changes are not seen during capacitation, but some modifications of the membrane are identified with ultrastructural methods. Freeze fracture images of sperm during capacitation show a clustering of proteins, seen as redistribution of intramembranous particles, and patchy clearing of membrane cholesterol is demonstrated for sperm labeled with filipin, an electron dense molecule that binds beta-hydroxy-sterols (4,5,6). Using fluorescence recovery after photobleaching (FRAP), a membrane lipid analogue is found to diffuse faster in the sperm head plasma membrane of capacitated sperm than in non-capacitated sperm (7).

Evidence has also accumulated demonstrating compositional changes in sperm membrane lipids. Davis (9) found an increase in the amount of phospholipids in rat sperm during capacitation and reported that albumin present in the medium was able to transfer radiolabeled phospholipids to the sperm. These changes could lead to a decrease in the cholesterol/phospholipid ratio, increasing the fluidity of the membrane during capacitation.

More evidence has implicated a loss of sperm membrane cholesterol. During in vitro capacitation, in several species including human, cholesterol is reportedly removed from the sperm membranes (9-12). Such an alteration should lead to increased membrane fluidity. A concern regarding studies such as these is that it is not possible to determine from which membrane, nor from which part of the sperm, the lipids have been extracted for analysis. Nevertheless, there is now ample evidence for a net loss of cholesterol from the sperm cell during capacitating incubations.

Evidence also exists for the reversibility of this cholesterol loss. Studies of rat, rabbit, bull and human sperm have demonstrated that cholesterol, presented as a dispersion, in liposomes, or albumin-bound, can inhibit capacitated sperm functions associated with fertilization (9, 10, 11, 13, 14).

Finally, data suggest that the cholesterol/phospholipid ratio in sperm is related to the time required for capacitation in different species (8). Variation in cholesterol levels has been linked to normal vs abnormal sperm function or infertility (2, 15, 16). One study of eight normospermic men concludes that cholesterol/phospholipid ratio of sperm is related to capacitation time as determined by the sperm penetration assay (17). Whether or not cholesterol levels or ratios in sperm (or semen) from different men can be closely tied to the sperm capacitation times in those men awaits further study. Sperm membrane cholesterol may be a major factor determining both the time-dependence and reversibility phenomena of capacitation. Understanding the control of cholesterol loss and gain by sperm membranes is therefore of critical interest, since this may lead to an unraveling of the mystery, and a mean of predicting and modifying capacitation itself.

Effectors of cholesterol loss from the sperm membrane

The mechanisms of the sperm lipid compositional changes during in vivo capacitation are not known. Changes in phospholipid structure may increase membrane fluidity, which in turn could result in increased cholesterol loss from the membrane by mechanisms which may or may not require actual transfer of cholesterol. For example, increased amounts of 22:6 fatty acid chains, or the formation of lysophospholipids by phospholipase both are known to increase membrane fluidity. Clearly, an understanding of the entire suite of lipid changes occurring during capacitation will be needed.

Albumin, among its many putative roles in sperm function, is reported to donate phospholipids to sperm (18, 19). To date no further evidence for the addition of phospholipids to sperm has been presented.

The removal of sperm membrane cholesterol has been explored in more detail. Cholesterol removal from sperm is attributed to albumin (11, 18), albumin from uterine fluid (20), or lipoproteins from either serum (15) or reproductive fluids such as follicular fluid (15) and oviductal fluid (21). An elegant model of sperm cholesterol removal has been proposed by Langlais and Roberts (12). This model hypothesizes the cleavage of sperm cholesteryl sulfate by a sterol sulfatase, present in the female reproductive tract, and subsequent removal and transfer of cholesterol to endogenous lipid acceptors, such as albumin or high density lipoproteins (HDL). The modification of cholesteryl sulfate in the sperm membrane has, however been shown for only a few species and it is probably the free sterol that is generally acted upon. However, cholesteryl ester is reported to be transferred from the sperm membrane to albumin fractions isolated from the capacitation media (18). It was not clear, at the time of these studies, how the cholesterol was transported from the sperm membrane to albumin or HDL.

Many of the components suggested to be involved in phospholipid and cholesterol transfers to and from sperm, namely HDL, lecithin-cholesterol acyltransferase (LCAT), albumin and certain apolipoproteins, have been recognized for many years to be involved in plasma lipid transport and in the events leading to atherosclerosis (22). However, a specific lipid transfer protein, LTP-I, is also present in plasma to transfer lipids (primarily cholesteryl esters and, to a lesser extent, phospholipids) between the plasma lipoproteins (23, 24). It is conceivable that a lipid transfer protein such as LTP-I is present in reproductive fluids to facilitate the lipid transfer associated with sperm capacitation.

Lipid transfer proteins
Lipid transfer protein, isolated from the plasma of many species, transiently bind and transfer lipids between liposomes, cells and lipoproteins. One of the better studied lipid transfer proteins, LTP-I (or cholesteryl ester transfer protein, CETP), facilitates the exchange and net mass transfer of cholesteryl ester, triglycerides, and phospholipids, between plasma lipoproteins. Lipid transfer proteins in plasma have a role in remodeling of lipoproteins, by

transfer and exchange of various lipids among the lipoprotein particles (24, 25).

The LTP-I is a fairly ubiquitous protein, present in the plasma of several species and synthesized and secreted from several different cell types. The gene for LTP-I has been cloned, and LTP-I mRNA has been found in abundance in small intestine, adrenal and spleen, with lower amounts in liver (26). Sequence analysis reveals that LTP-I is a unique protein, one of the most hydrophobic known.

The major role of LTP-I may be in "reverse cholesterol transport", the transfer of extra-hepatic cholesterol from HDL to VLDL (very low density lipoproteins) en route back to the liver. Biochemical studies reveal an inverse relationship between plasma HDL cholesterol and plasma LTP-I activity. The regulation of this interaction is cofounded and probably intricately controlled by the presence of a lipid transfer inhibitor protein (27).

The LTP-I and its inhibitor are part of unique subclasses of HDL (27). High density lipoproteins are typically small lipid/protein multi lamellar vesicles with molecular weights averaging around 150,000 daltons. Particular subclasses of HDL that contain apolipoprotein A-I but not A-II, have the majority of lipid transfer activity. Thus, although LTP-I is active in its free state, it is probably usually a component of an HDL subclass.

We considered LTP-I to be a likely candidate for the missing link in sperm cholesterol efflux during capacitation for the following reasons. It is fairly common in its tissue distribution, so it may be synthesized in the male or female reproductive tract. Even if not, it is present in plasma and therefore would possibly be present in partly plasma-derived fluids such as follicular fluid. It is associated with HDL, which is known (while LDL and VLDL are not) in follicular fluid. And finally, having an assay for cholesterol exchange (developed for LTP-I) in hand, we could screen fluids and chromatographic fractions of them for lipid exchange activities, and subsequently attempt protein identification. We believe our results show the merits of this approach.

MATERIALS AND METHODS

All methods are previously published (28-33), except as noted.

Human spermatozoa
Healthy, normospermic donors collected semen which was allowed to liquefy for 20 minutes at 37°C. Spermatozoa were prepared for assays either by direct swim-out from semen, or, in some earlier experiments, by 3-times washing as follows. Semen was diluted 1:2 with Biggers, Whitten and Whittingham medium (BWW) containing either 0.4 % bovine serum

albulmine (BSA, Sigma #4503) or 0.4 % polyvynil alcohol (PVA) and centrifuged at 225xg for 8 minutes. Half of the supernatant was removed and the sample resuspended with 5ml of BWW-BSA or-PVA, centrifuged for 5 minutes, then washed once more with 5ml of fresh medium. Highly motile (>96%) preparations of sperm were obtained by allowing sperm to directly swim out of 0.5ml semen layered under 3ml medium for one hour at 37°C, 1% CO2. Following incubation, the supernatant containing motile sperm was centrifuged as above for 5 minutes. In both methods, sperm were resuspended to a concentration of 10×10^6 sperm/ml.

Sperm were incubated in medium for 45 minutes to 1 hour at 37°C, 1%CO2. After incubation, 200μl of sperm suspension were added to 50 μl of the sample to be tested (eg., follicular fluid, fractions of purified LTP) and incubated for 12 minutes at 37°C, 1%CO2. Controls had 50μl of HEPES saline or medium in place of sample as appropriate. Sperm were then washed once with 400μl of medium, resuspended in 200μl of medium, and 95μl of the suspension (approx. 10^6 sperm) were added to a 5μl drop of medium under oil and incubated for 1 hour.

Assays

1. Lipid transfer activity

Lipoproteins were isolated from human plasma by differential ultracentrifugation, and the HDL_3 (here referred to as HDL) and plasma proteins, was dialyzed overnight and used to make ^{14}C-labeled cholesteryl ester (CE) lipoprotein donor as described by Albers et al (23). A final centrifugation separated HDL from the majority of the plasma proteins with 99% of the label remaining in the HDL fraction.

Each assay was performed in triplicate at the donor/acceptor ratio which yielded maximum activity after a 3 hour incubation at 37°C. Unlabeled LDL were incubated with ^{14}C-CE-HDL without (control) or with added lipid transfer activity (FF, serum, albumin). A typical assay had 50μl of labeled HDL, 200μl of unlabeled LDL (approximately 100μg CE), and 25-200μl of transfer factor to be assayed, made to final volume of 0.6ml with HEPES saline. Following incubation, LDL were removed by dextran sulfate: $MgCl_2$ precipitation of apoB-containing lipoproteins, and the supernatants were counted greater than 90% of the total counts could be recovered. Lipid transfer activity (LTA) is defined in this assay as the percentage of labeled lipid transferred (% Transfer), and was measured as a decrease in counts in the HDL supernatant compared to the control. Values are obtained using the following equation, which sets control values to zero:

$$100 - ((\text{Test cpm/control cpm}) \times 100)$$

2. Sperm penetration assay

The human sperm, hamster zona pellucida-free oocyte penetration assays (SPA) were performed with one important modification: sperm were preincubated only 1-2h prior to their addition to the eggs. Results were scored for the percentage of eggs penetrated (% Penetration) and the number of decondensed sperm heads divided by the total number of eggs (Penetration Index: PI). We named this type of sperm penetration assay an "ultra short" SPA because of the very short capacitation times involved, before sperm-egg coincubation.

3. Acrosome reaction assessment (ARA)

In some experiments, acrosomal status of spermatozoa was analyzed using the PSA lectin staining method modified from Cross et al (34). At the indicated times, 1×10^6 sperm from each treatment were incubated 10 minutes with 1µg Hoechst 33258 dye/ml and centrifuged through 2% polyvinylpyrollidone (PVP) in Ham's F-10 medium without protein. Sperm were resuspended in 100µl cold 100% ethanol, and kept at 4°C for at least 30min. Aliquots of 20µl were dried on slides, hydrated with 20µl FITC-PSA (25µg/ml) in HEPES saline containing 0.1mM $CaCl_2$ and 0.01mM $MnCl_2$. After 20-30 min, the slides were washed in distilled water, mounted in 90% glycerol, and 1200-200 sperm which had excluded the Hoechst dye were scored for acrosomal loss.

Purification methods

1. Purification of LTP-I

Lipid transfer activity was purified from human follicular fluid (hFF) based on the method of Albers et al (23) for LTP-I. This involved removal of follicular fluid lipoproteins by ultracentrifugation, sequential column chromatography on Phenyl Sepharose, DEAE Sepharose, Heparin Sepharose, Carboxymethyl cellulose and Hydoxyl apatite. This purification scheme was based on the rationale that hFF-LTA eluted from an S-300 gel filtration column in similar size fractions as LTP-I.

Aliquots of the Heparin Sepharose LTA-active pool were applied to an S-300 gel filtration column for size determination and to a chromatofocusing column for determination of the isoelectric point. At least every second fraction was assayed for LTA and every third fraction was assayed for protein. Fractions with LTA, and some without LTA, were tested for stimulation of sperm penetration as described previously. The final Hydroxyl apatite fractions were dialyzed against 150mM NaCl, 20mM HEPES, pH 7.4 and assayed for lipid transfer activity. Prior to assaying aliquots of active pools in the sperm penetration assay, aliquots were dialyzed against a buffer containing BWW salts. Washed human sperm were treated for 15 minutes with 50µl of each dialyzed fraction.

2. Preparation of LTP-free HSA or hFF.

Human serum albumin depleted of LTP-I was derived from crystallized-HSA (C-HSA; Sigma #8763) since this preparation had a high level of LTA. Human follicular fluid depleted of LTP was derived from pooled samples of individual patient's follicular fluid. Removal of LTP-I was performed by passage of C-HSA or hFF over an anti-LTP-I sepharose antibody column (3.5ml of gel), prepared with affinity purified goat anti-human LTP-I antibody and CnBr activated Sepharose. A control antibody was prepared in the same manner except affinity purified goat anti-human IgG was coupled to the gel.

Following equilibration in 0.15M NaCl, 0.01M Tris, pH 7.4 (Tris saline), 4 mls of a 40mg/ml C-HSA solution or 4 mls of 1:4 diluted hFF was recirculated through each column (anti-LTP-I or anti-IgG) for 1 hour at a flow rate of 30mls/hr. The columns were washed with 30mls of TRIS saline and eluted with 30mls of 3M NaSCN. Fractions of 3mls were collected. Wash fractions were assayed for LTA and slot immunoblotted for detection of LRP-I. Elution fractions were immediately dialyzed against HEPES saline and then assayed for LTA and slot immunoblotted.

Fractions containing LTA from the anti-IgG column and the corresponding fractions from the anti-LTP-I column were dialyzed against BWW salts and concentrated back to 40 mg/ml, or the original hFF protein concentration. The concentrated material was assayed in the ultra-short SPA and for ARA.

RESULTS

Identification of lipid transfer activity and SPA activity in human follicular fluid

We assayed hFF for LTA and for the ability to stimulate human sperm penetration of zona pellucida-free hamster oocytes, in short incubation SPA. The rationale for this "ultra short" Spa was to assay for the response of sperm to molecules capable of enhancing sperm capacitation as opposed to immediate acrosome reaction (35). We performed a minimum of three replicates for each experiment and sperm penetration assays were performed with at least 3 different semen donors. From our analysis of human follicular fluid, we observed an average 4-fold increase in sperm penetration with hFF-treated sperm versus control sperm (this finding has been confirmed in hundreds of hFF-stimulated SPAs for our clinical patients). The same hFF samples were also assayed for LTA. The samples had an average of 18% transfer of labeled lipid. In addition, there was a time- and dose- dependent response of lipid transfer activity in hFF.

Preliminary purification of the LTA in hFF was carried out using gel filtration chromatography. Fractions from the gel filtration column which had LTA were assayed in the SPA, and these significantly stimulated sperm penetration above control, non treated sperm. The fraction with the highest LTA and Spa inducing activity had an apparent molecular weight of 64 kD.

Based on these results we reached the following conclusion: 1) hFF does have lipid transfer activity and stimulates human sperm penetration of zona-free hamster oocytes; and 2) Gel filtration fractions of hFF that have LTA stimulate an increase in sperm penetration above control, particularly fractions eluting with a molecular weight of approximately 64kD. These results were the first evidence of lipid transfer activity in reproductive fluids and provided the foundation for this research (29).

Identification of LTP and LTA in reproductive fluids

While follicular fluid is able to stimulate sperm capacitation and acrosome reaction, it remains to be determined if this plays a significant role in vivo. Follicular fluid may be present only in very small amounts between the cells of the cumulus mass, rather than present in bulk in the reproductive tract.

Species	Fluid Sources	LTA	Anti-LTP-I Immunoblot +	Stimulated SPA Activity
Human	Follicular	++	++	++
	Uterine flushes	+	+	±
	serum	++	++	+*
Hamster	Uterine flushes	+	++	±
	Oviduct	±	+	ND
Mouse	Uterine flushes	±	ND	ND
	Cauda epididymis	+*	ND	±*
Rabbit[1]	Uterine	+	ND	ND
	Oviduct	±	+	ND
Bovine[2]	Follicular	+*	++	+*
	Serum	-	++	-
	Fertile phase oviduct	++	++	++
	Luteal phase oviduct	+	+	+

Table I. **LTP-I and stimulation of human sperm penetration in different species' reproductive fluids.**
* The fluid was active only after partial purification by S-300 gel filtration;
[1] Rabbit fluids courtesy of Dr T. Thomas.
[2] Bovine fluids courtesy of Dr G. Killian.

To begin addressing this problem, we assayed LTA, immunoreactive LTP-I, or stimulation of human sperm penetration in oviduct and uterine fluid, the probable in situ sites of capacitation. We assayed reproductive fluids from five different species (Table I). Strikingly, in those fluids tested, if LTP was present and active the fluid generally stimulated human sperm in the SPA.

Interestingly, some of the fluids (e.g. bovine FF) had immunoreactive LTP, but had no LTA., nor did they significantly stimulate human sperm. In some of these cases, LTA can be found in gel filtration fractions of the fluid, and these active fractions are able to stimulate human sperm. Experiments were performed with bovine FF to determine the cause of this phenomenon. We discovered that bovine FF contained a lipid transfer inhibitor protein in fractions corresponding to 160,000 daltons, which also was able to inhibit LTP-induced sperm penetration This is similar to the molecular weight of an inhibitor protein/HDL complex present in human serum. After fractionation of the bovine FF and isolation of the LTA-rich material, we found substantial SPA-stimulating activity. Similar SPA results were found for human serum, although it has strong LTA even in the presence of the inhibitor. (We have not yet studied human oviductal fluid). These results raise the interesting possibility of regulation of LTP action by a specific inhibitor during capacitation and the acrosome reaction.

Oviduct fluid from rabbits and cows (collected by indwelling catheter) and uterine fluid flushes from humans and hamsters have active LTP. In addition, bovine oviduct fluid has more LTA in fluid from cows in fertile (non-luteal) period than oviduct from cows during the luteal phase. This raises the possibility of hormonal regulation of LTP action at the site of capacitation.

Isolation of LTP-I from human follicular fluid

Knowing that HFF contained LTA of approximately the molecular weight of LTP-I, and that it cross-reacted with anti- LTP-I on immunoblots, we proceeded with the isolation and characterization of the activity. The LTA eluted from Sephacryl S-300 just ahead of the calibrated albumin peak, with an approximated molecular weight of 64,000 daltons. Chromatofocusing of the Heparin sepharose non-binding pool demonstrated an LTA peak at a pH of 5.0. An aliquot of the Heparin Sepharose active pool was used for further purification.

The final two chromatographic steps produced an LTA fraction that was greater than 20,000-fold purified for % lipid transfer/µg protein. Sperm penetration inducing activity was purified greater than 28,000-fold. The resulting purified protein from HFF which had LTA and stimulated sperm penetration, showed a single band by SDS-PAGE. This purified protein was recognized by an antibody raised in goat against plasma LTP-I. The elution profiles and physico-chemical characteristics of HFF LTA using this purification protocol were very similar to those reported for plasma LTP-I.

We conclude that 1) the activity isolated from HFF is indeed LTP-I; and 2) the lipid transfer activity co-purifies with capacitation-inducing activity (21).

Identification of LTP-I as a contaminant in serum albumin

It is well known that different commercial albumin preparation differ greatly in their support of human sperm capacitation. In addition, albumin has previously been implicated in cholesterol and phospholipid exchange to or from sperm, as well as in other activities affecting sperm capacitation and acrosome reaction. We verified the presence or absence of sperm capacitation support by many different albumins in the ultra-short SPA, the tested whether these differences were related to LTA or even to presence of LTP-I in albumin preparations. Our results were clear-cut and surprising (32).

In five experiments, we measured LTA in eight albumin preparations obtained from Sigma Chemical Co; 4 of BSA and 4 of HSA. Of the BSA preparations, only Fraction V (frV) #4503 had detectable LTA at all the concentrations tested (4, 8, 16, or 32 mg/ml final protein concentration). In contrast, each of the HSA preparation had LTA. FrV-HSA#2386 and C-HSA#8673 had the highest LTA amounts, and were the only ones if these eight to exhibit a dose response. In different experiments, albumin preparations from other companies also exhibited LTA (assayed at 16mg/ml), although in widely variable amounts.

Each Sigma albumin preparation (BSA or HSA) was also tested for the ability to support or enhance in vitro sperm capacitation and acrosome reaction, measured using ultra-short SPA. Similar to LTA results, BSA preparations supported only a low to moderate level of SPA activity. The HSA preparations overall did better than BSA in supporting the ultra-short SPA, and there were significant differences in the responses to different preparations.

These data appeared to show a relationship between the ability of an albumin preparation to support capacitation and the amount of LTA present in that preparation. When LTA was plotted against PI for each of the albumin preparations there was a significant correlation between the two ($r = 0.76$, $P < 0.001$).

The differences in LTA and capacitation support between albumin preparations may be explained in part by compositional differences or by contamination with other proteins such as LTP-I. In silver stained SDS-PAGE gels, a high degree of contamination by other proteins in the albumin preparations is demonstrated. To test if LTP-I was a contaminant in the albumin preparations, FrV-HSA#2386 (high LTA, high PI) was western blotted after SDS-PAGE, and probed with anti- LTP-I antibodies. This analysis revealed a reactive bad at approximately 64 kD, the reported size of LTP-I on SDS-PAGE. We also carried out quantitative immunoblot analysis of each HSA to determine the relative LTP-I immunoreactivities of each. Albumins with highest anti-LTP-I immunoreactivity also had the highest LTA and the highest SPA PI.

Removal of LTP-I from albumin and HFF preparation
In these experiments, we studied the requirement of LTP-I contamination in an albumin preparation for support of capacitation, and the role of LTP-I in HFF. We employed anti- LTP-I affinity chromatography to remove LTP from C-HSA#8763 and from three different HFF, and assayed the resulting preparations for support of sperm SPA and ARA activities. Passage of a 4% albumin solution (LTA = 6.8% Transfer) aver an anti- LTP-I Sepharose column removed all of the LTA, while 85ù of LTA (5.8% transfer) was recovered from a control column (anti-human IgG Sepharose). Lipid transfer protein eluted from the anti- LTP-I column with 3 M NaSCN had 3.19% Transfer, a 47% recovery, while this elution from the control column had no activity. HFF recovered from the anti- LTP-I column did not have detectable LTA. These results were confirmed by western blotting of the unbound fractions.

Penetration activity in LTP-free albumin and HFF preparations
We next assayed the affinity column treated HFF and HSAs (unbound fractions) for their abilities to support human sperm capacitation and acrosome reaction. Sperm were washed in BWW containing FrV-BSA#4503 (baseline control), control HSA (anti-IgG column recovered), or LTP-free HSA (anti- LTP-I column recovered) each at a final concentration of 0.4% and incubated for 2 hours before adding sperm to eggs to assess their penetration ability. In 4 experiments, significantly ($P < 0.01$) more sperm penetrated eggs when incubated with control HSA than with LTP-free HSA or with BSA. In addition, at 0, 1, 2, and 18 hours an aliquot from each treatment was prepared for AR assessment. Significantly more sperm were acrosome reacted at 1, 2, or 18 hours when incubated with control HSA, than when the sperm were incubated with LTP-free HSA ($P < 0.05$, n = 3). Support of sperm functions was restored to the LTP-free HSA when purified LTP-I was added to it.

Control HFF and anti-IgG column recovered HFF treated sperm were not different from each other, but each penetrated significantly more eggs in the SPA than either control sperm or anti- LTP-I column-recovered-HFF-treated sperm.

Therefore, we found that some commercial preparations of serum albumin have LTP-I as a contaminant. Albumins which effectively support sperm capacitation and acrosome reaction (as determined by SPA and ARA) have more lipid transfer activity than those that have lower levels of support. In addition, if LTP-I is removed from albumin or HFF, the degree of support is significantly reduced. It is likely that in LTP-I contaminated albumin, the albumin molecule itself has a role as a lipid acceptor in the absence of other appropriate molecule such as HDL.

Effect of purified LTP-I on human sperm capacitation: time course, dose response and synergistic relation with albumin

The action of highly purified LTP-I, in the absence of any additional macromolecule, during capacitation was explored by determining the dose response and time course of the SPA- and ARA-activity. In addition, the interaction between purified LTP-I and LTP-free albumin was investigated. Most of these results were recently published (33).

In all of these experiments, sperm were directly swim-up in BWW-PVA for 1hr and then treated with purified LTP-I. In the first experiment, sperm were treated for 15 min with 3.5 µg of LTP-I in 50 µl, washed, and incubated for 2 hrs. At 0, 15, 30, 45, 60, and 120 minutes later, the treated sperm were processed for ARA. Control, buffer-treated sperm were also analyzed. Control sperm did not show any significant changes over the entire incubation period, and treated sperm did not undergo AR until approximately 45-60 min, when significantly more sperm were acrosome reacted. Between 45 and 120 min, there was a linear increase in % AR for treated sperm; Only % AR was recorded for this experiment because of the technical impossibility of performing the SPA every 15 min. These results were similar to those seen for raw HFF in that immediate acrosome reactions were not stimulated, rather there was about a one hour lag.

Next, we assayed purified LTP-I in the SPA and for sperm AR over a range of doses, using sperm that were incubated in BWW-PVA for 1 hr, treated 15 min with LTP-I, and further incubated for 1 hr, prior to adding eggs or processing for ARA. The amounts of LTP-I used were 0, 0.35, 0.7, 1.4, 2.0, and 3.5µg protein / 50µl. There was a slight response at 0.7µg, but only 1.4µg LTP-I or more were able to significantly stimulate sperm penetration. Similar results were seen for % AR at the same doses.

The results from these two experiments indicated that there were time and dose thresholds at which LTP-I was able to stimulate sperm capacitation in the absence of other exogenous macromolecules. That purified LTP-I alone was able to stimulate capacitation was somewhat surprising, since it is thought that LTP-I action is dependent upon lipid acceptor molecule. Perhaps higher amounts of LTP-I provide sufficient support for the induction of sperm capacitation, in the absence of lipid acceptor.

To begin to address this point, a constant amount of LTP-I (0.35 µg) was added to sperm with different amounts of LTP-free HSA. HSA can act as a sperm lipid acceptor and LTP-free HSA alone does not stimulate sperm penetration at any dose tested. Swim-up sperm were in BWW containing 0, 0.05, 0.1, 0.2, 0.4, and 2.0% LTP-free HSA. Sperm were resuspended treated for 15 min with resuspended treated for 15 min, washed, and resuspended in BWW-PVA. As above, LTP-I alone at 0.35 µg did not stimulate sperm penetration. However, when increasing amounts of LTP-free HSA, as a possible lipid acceptor, were added, the combination was able to stimulate sperm, except at the lowest amount of albumin. Similar results were seen for sperm AR. Based on these results, the above time course experiment was repeated using 0.35 µg LTP-I alone, 0.4% LTP-free HSA alone, and 0.35 µg LTP-I with 0.4% LTP-free HSA. In contrast to a higher dose if LTP-I (3.5 µg), the low doses did not stimulate capacitation and acrosome reaction even after 2 hours, unless albumin was included.

DISCUSSION

We have begun to characterize a novel, endogenous activity in reproductive fluids that may have an important role in human and mammalian sperm capacitation. These findings may explain the time-dependence and reversibility of the capacitation process. They may eventually assist in the diagnosis and possible treatment of some forms of sperm dysfuncions with male infertility.

It is clear that more than one molecule, and more than one process is likely involved in capacitation. Other stimulators of the process must exist, and other steps in capacitation may be unrelated to cholesterol efflux. It is interesting, however, to speculate that cholesterol loss and the subsequent increase in membrane fluidity may be the necessary key step in setting into motion all the other events leading to hyperactivated motility, opening of calcium channels, expression of zona-binding ligands and eventual ability to acrosome react.

One of the best characterized stimulatory agents purified from follicular fluid is progesterone. Meizel and co-workers showed that HFF could stimulate the acrosome reaction within 15 sec to a few minutes (36). A number of arguments can be made for differences between LTP-I stimulated acrosome reactions and those of progesterone. First, HFF fractions from the phenyl Sepharose columns that have LTA and stimulate sperm penetration, have progesterone concentrations of less than 0.1 ng/ml, at the limit of detection for the assay. The lowest level of progesterone that stimulated the acrosome reaction in human sperm was 250 ng/ml. Second, and most important, are the differences in time-course between LTP-I- and progesterone-stimulated acrosome reactions. Progesterone (and HFF) stimulates the acrosome reaction within minutes after sperm are exposed, providing the sperm have capacitated (typically at least a few hours to overnight). In fact, progesterone does not stimulate acrosome reactions in uncapacitated sperm. These results contrast sharply with the effects of

LTP-I, which we believe accelerates capacitation by assisting cholesterol efflux. This accelerated efflux may then lead to « spontaneous » acrosome reactions about an hour later. The important issue here is not whether the acrosome reactions are spontaneous or stimulated, rather that the capacitation process was accelerated.

It will be intersting, and challenging, to piece together the many prts of a process which, by its nature may have built in a good deal of redundancy.

Acknowledgments
This research was supported in part by NIH Grant HD-16211 and the NIH Population Center Grant HD-12629.

REFERENCES

1. Parks JE, Hammerstedt RH. Development cahnges accurring in the lipids of ram epididymal spermatozoa plasma membrane. Biol Reprod 1985; 32:653-668.
2. Cross NL. Human seminal plasma prevents sperm from becoming acrosomally responsive; cholesterol is the major inhibitor. Biol Reprod 1995; in press.
3. Huacuja L, Delgado NM, Calzada L, Wens A, Reyes R, Pedron N, Rosado A. Exchange of lipids between spermatozoa and seminal plasma in normal and pathological human semen. Arch Androl 1981; 7:343-349.
4. Bearer EL, Friend DS. Modifications of anionic-lipid domains preceding membrane fusion in guinea pig sperm. J Cell Biol 1982; 92:604-615.
5. Suzuki F, Yanagimachi R. Changes in the distribution of intramembranous particles and filipin-reactive membrane sterol during in vitro capacitation of golden hamster spermatozoa. Gamete Res 1989; 23:335-347.
6. Tesarik J, Flechon J-E. Distribution of sterols and anionic lipids in human sperm plasma membrane: effect of in vitro capacitation; J Ultrastruct Mol Struct Res 1986; 97:227-237.
7. Wolf DE, Hagopian SS, Ishijima S. Changes in sperm plasma membrane lipid diffusibility after hyperactivation during in vitro capacitation in the mouse. J Cell Biol 1986; 102:1372-1377.
8. Davis BK. Timing of fertilization in mammals: sperm cholesterol/phospholipid ratio as a determinant of the capacitation interval. Proc Natl Acad Sci USA 1981; 78:7560-7564.
9. Benoff S, Cooper GW, Hurley I, Mandel FS, Rosenfeld DL. Antisperm antibody binding to human sperm inhibits capacitation induced changes

in the levels of plasma membrane sterols. Am J Reprod Immunol 1993; 30:113-130.
10. Ehren wald E, Parks JE, Foote RH. Cholesterol efflux from bovine sperm. I. Induction of the acrosome reaction with lysophosphatidylcholine after reducing sperma cholesterol. Gamete Res 1988; 20: 145-157.
11. Go KJ, Wolf DP. Albumin-mediated changes in sperm sterol content during capacitation. Biol Reprod 1985; 32:145-153.
12. Langlais J, roberts KD. A molecular model of sperm capacitation and the acrosome reaction of mammalian spermatozoa. Gamete Res 1985; 12:183-224.
13. Davis BK. Inhibitory effect of synthetic phospholipid vesicles containing cholesterol on the fertilizing ability of rabbit spermatozoa. Proc Soc Exp Biol Med 1976; 152:257-261.
14. Fayrer H-RA, Brackett BG, Brown J. Reversible inhibition of rabbit sperm-fertilizing ability by cholesterol sulfate. Biol Reprod 1987; 36:878-883.
15. Langlais J, Kan FWK, Raymond L, Bleau G, Roberts KD. Identification of sterol acceptors that stimulate cholesterol efflux from human spermatozoa during in vitro capacitation. Gamete Res 1988; 20:185-201.
16. Benoff S, Hurley I, Cooper GW, Mandel FS, Rosenfeld DL, Hershlag A. Head-specific mannose ligand receptor expression in human spermatozoa is dependent on capacitation-associated membrane cholesterol loss. Hum Reprod 1993; 8:2141-2154.
17. Hoshi K, Aita T, Yanagida K, Yoshimatsu N, Sato A. Variation in the cholesterol/phospholipid ratio in human spermatozoa and its relationship with capacitation. Hum Reprod 1990; 5:71-74.
18. Davis BK, Byrne R, Hungund B. Studies on the mechanism of capacitation. II Evidence for lipid transfer between plasma membrane of rat sperm and serum albumin during capacitation in vitro. Biochem Biophys Acta 1979; 558:257-266.
19. Davis BK, Byrne R, Bedigan K. Albumin-mediated changes in plasma membrane lipids during in vitro capacitation. Proc Natl Acad Sci USA 1980; 77:1546-1550.
20. Davis BK. Uterine fluid proteins bind sperm cholesterol during capacitation in the rabbit. Experientia 1982; 38:1063-1064.
21. Ehrenwald E, Foote RH, Parks JE. Cholesterol efflux from bovine sperm: bovine oviductal fluid components and their potential role in sperm cholesterol efflux. J Androl 1989; 10:P-21.
22. Phillips MC, Johnson WJ, Rothblat GH. Mechanisms and consequences of cellular cholesterol exchange and transfer. Biochem Biophys Acta 1987; 906:223-276

23. Albers JJ, Tollefson JH, Chen C-H, Steinmetz A. Isolation and characterization of human plasma lipid transfer proteins. Arteriosclerosis 1984; 4:49-54.
24. Barter P, Rye K-A. Cholesteryl ester transfer protein: its role in plasma lipid transport. Clin Exper Pharmacol Physiol 1994; 21:663-672.
25. Tall AR. Plasma cholesteryl ester transfer protein. J Lipid Res 1993; 34:1255-1273.
26. Drayna D, Jarnagin As, McLean J, Henzel W, Kohr W, Fielding C, Lawn R. Cloning and sequencing of human cholesteryl ester transfer protein cDNA. Nature 1987; 327:632-634.
27. Nishide T, Tollefson JH, Albers JJ. Unhibition of lipid transfer by a unique high density lipoprotein subclass containing an inhibitor protein. J Lipid Res 1989; 30:149-158.
28. Muller CH. Precision, reliability and biological variability in human sperm function measured by penetration of zona-free hamster oocytes. Int J Androl 1986; Suppl 6:31-41.
29. Ravnik SE, Zarutskie PW, Muller CH. Lipid transfer activity in human follicular fluid: relation to human sperm capacitation. J Androl 1990; 11:216-226.
30. Muller CH. The andrology laboratory in an assisted reproductive technologies program: quality assurance and laboratory methodology. J Androl 1992; 13:349-360.
31. Ravnik SE, Zarutskie PW, Muller CH. Purification and characterization of a human follicular fluid lipid transfer protein that stimulates human sperm capacitation. [published erratum appears in Biol Reprod 1993; 48:214] Biol Reprod 1992;47:1126-1133.
32. Ravnik SE, Albers JJ, Muller CH. A novel view of albumin-supported sperm capacitation: role of lipid transfer protein-I. Fertil Steril 1993; 59:629-638.
33. Ravnik SE, Albers JJ, Muller CH. Stimulation of human sperm capacitation by purified lipid transfer protein. J Exp Zool 1995; 272:78-83.
34. Cross NL, Morales P, Overstreet JW, Hanson FW. Two simple methods for detecting acrosome-reacted human sperm. Gamete Res 1986; 15:213-226.
35. Muller CH, Zaruskie PW, Stenchever MA, Soules MR. The sperm penetration assay: one of the best methods we have. Obstet Gynecol Report 1990; 2:414-420.
36. Yudin AI, Gottlieb W, Meizel S. Ultrastructural studies of the early events of human sperm acrosome reaction as initiated by human follicular fluid. Gamete Res 1988; 20:11-24.

Chapter II
Chapitre II

Physiological induction of acrosome reaction
Induction physiologique de la réaction acrosomique

Sperm interaction with the zona pellucida: the role of ZRK

P.M. Saling, D.J. Burks, M.R. Carballada, C.A. Dowds, L. Leyton, S.B. McLeskey, A. Robinson and C.N. Tomes

Departments of Obstetrics and Gynecology and Cell Biology, Duke University Medical Center Durham, NC 27710, USA

ABSTRACT

To fertilize an egg, mammalian sperm must first bind to the egg's extracellular matrix, the zona pellucida (zp). Once bound, sperm undergo the acrosome reaction (AR), an essential exocytotic event that permits the sperm to penetrate this matrix and gain access to the egg plasma membrane directly. The zp glycoprotein ZP3 serves both as ligand for sperm binding and as trigger for acrosomal exocytosis. We have identified a 95 kd mouse sperm membrane protein with characteristics of a tyrosine kinase as a receptor for ZP3, and have termed this protein ZRK (zona receptor kinase). The evolutionary conservation of receptor tyrosine kinases (RTKs), as well as the demonstrated conservation of the corresponding ligand, ZP3, suggested the existence of a ZP3-binding RTK homolog in human sperm. We have identified a sperm-specific cDNA, hu9, that encodes a novel RTK-like protein. Polyclonal antibodies generated using a synthetic peptide (K16) corresponding to a non-conserved sequence in the predicted intracellular domain of Hu9 identify a 95 kd tyrosine-phosphorylated human sperm protein that is distinct from hexokinase. Functional analyses suggest that hu9 encodes human ZRK (i. peptides corresponding to regions of the Hu9 extracellular domain inhibit human sperm-zp interaction and ii. human ZP3 stimulates the kinase activity of immunoprecipitated Hu9) and that tyrosine kinase activity is essential for acrosomal exocytosis. In addition, a monoclonal antibody (LL95) directed against murine ZRK mimics the effects of the natural ligand ZP3 on sperm-zp binding and acrosome reaction triggering.

Collectively, these results suggest that ZRK is an important component of the signalling complex involved in the stimulating acrosomal exocytosis. A simple model of adhesion followed by signalling is proposed to place ZRK in the context of other findings on sperm-ZP3 interaction.

Pour féconder, le spermatozoïde de mammifère doit d'abord se lier à la matrice extracellulaire de l'oeuf, la zone pellucide (ZP). Une fois lié, il fait la réaction acrosomique (RA), un processus d'exocytose qui lui permet de traverser la matrice et d'accéder directement à la membrane plasmique ovocytaire. La glycoprotéine pellucidaire ZP3 sert à la fois de ligand pour la liaison du spermatozoïde et d'inducteur pour la réaction acrosomique. Nous avons identifié, dans le spermatozoïde de souris, une protéine membranaire de 95kd, possédant les caractéristiques d'une tyrosine kinase, comme étant le récepteurs pour ZP3 et nous l'avons appelée ZRK (zona receptor kinase). La conservation, pendant l'évolution, des récepteurs tyrosine kinase (RTKs), ainsi que celle du ligand correspondant ZP3, suggèrait l'existence d'un RTK spécifique de ZP3 dans le spermatozoïde humain. Nous avons identifié un cDNA, spécifique du spermatozoïde, hu9, qui code une nouvelle protéine de type RTK. Des anticorps polyclonaux, formés en utilisant un peptide synthétique (K16) correspondant à une séquence non conservée dans le domaine intracellulaire supposé de Hu9, identifie une protéine tyrosine phosphorylée de 95 kd dans le spermatozoïde humain, distincte de l'hexokinase. Les études fonctionnelles suggèrent que hu9 code pour la ZRK humain (i. les peptides correspondant aux régions du domaine extracellulaire de Hu9 inhibent l'interaction spermatozoïde humain-ZP et ii. la ZP3 humaine stimule l'activité kinase des immunoprécipités Hu9) et que l'activité tyrosine kinase est indispensable à la réaction acrosomique. De plus, un anticorps monoclonal (LL95) dirigé contre le ZRK murin reproduit les effects de ZP3 sur la liaison spermatozoïde-ZP et sur l'induction de la réaction acrosomique. Au total, ces résultats suggèrent que le ZRK est une composante importante dans les voies de transmission du signal impliquées dans l'exocytose acrosomique. Un modèle simple de liaison-transmission du signal est proposé pour mettre en place le ZRK au sein des connaissances sur l'interaction spermatozoïde-ZP3.

INTRODUCTION

Initial gamete interaction occurs between receptors on the sperm plasma membrane and the egg-specific extracellular matrix, the zona pellucida (zp) (1,2). Determining the molecular basis of productive sperm-zp interaction is fundamental to understanding the process of fertilization, since these events comprise the initial, requisite interactions between mammalian gametes. Mouse zp have been studied extensively, and shown to consist principally of three sulfated glycoproteins, ZP1, ZP2 and ZP3 (3,4). Using mouse gametes, it has been shown that ZP3 serves as ligand for initial sperm binding and as trigger for the regulated exocytotic event (the acrosome reaction, [AR]) that occurs as a consequence of zp binding (1). However, many questions concerning these events and their underlying mechanisms remain unresolved, such as *i)* how does ZP3 bind to the sperm plasma membrane to serve as the primary ligand? *ii)* what is the relationship of the various ZP3-binding proteins that have been identified? *iii)* how does ZP3 binding to sperm initiate the signalling cascade that results in acrosomal exocytosis? and *iv)* what signalling pathway(s) and cellular mechanisms are employed by sperm to achieve regulated exocytosis? Our work is directed toward answering these questions, incorporating the concept that, for fundamental processes like transmembrane signaling and exocytosis, sperm are likely to use mechanisms and proteins that are highly conserved across phyla (5).

Work on molecular dissection of zp glycoproteins and their interaction with sperm was first conducted with mouse gametes, and the conclusions resulting from that work have greatly influenced the general thinking in this area. That basic paradigm specifies that *O*-linked oligosaccharides of ZP3 are responsible for primary binding to sperm plasma membrane receptors, whereas ZP2 is utilized in secondary binding to components of the acrosomal granule once the AR is triggered (1,2). In favor of accepting this paradigm are both cell and molecular biological observations. At the cellular level, interaction between sperm and egg appears to follow a conserved course: 'filtering' of sperm through the cumulus matrix permits transit of only capacitated, plasma membrane-intact cells → primary zp binding [acrosome-intact sperm binding to the zp] → triggering of the AR → secondary zp binding [acrosome-reacting/reacted sperm binding to zp] → limited proteolytic digestion through the zp matrix (2). At a molecular level, mouse, hamster and human ZP3 proteins are well conserved evolutionarily (6-8), and in mice and hamsters, ZP3 has been shown to be responsible for primary zp binding as well as for AR triggering (9,10). At odds with ZP3 being defined as the exclusive ligand for primary binding are findings principally from studies with porcine and rabbit zp proteins. In pigs, both ZP3α and ZP3β have been reported to serve as the ligands for primary sperm binding (11-13), and both *O*-linked and *N*-linked glycans of porcine ZP3α and β demonstrate ligand activity (14, 15), suggesting another scheme for sperm-zp interaction. Additionally, antibodies generated using synthetic peptides that correspond to regions of porcine ZP3α and ZP3β block sperm-zp binding in pigs, suggesting direct interaction of zp peptide(s) with sperm (16, 17); it should be noted that controls to discount steric hindrance or affinity differences were included in this study. Finally, molecular cloning studies reveal that porcine ZP3α exhibits 66% homology with a 55 kd rabbit zp protein (17, 18) that is also expressed in granulosa cells (19). This r55 is related to another rabbit zp protein, r75, which itself is homologous to murine ZP2 (20). However, a 25-mer region of porcine ZP3β that carries sperm-binding O-linked oligosaccharides displays ~80% homology with mouse/hamster/human ZP3 (11, 21). Thus, a variety of unanswered questions remain, such as whether ZP2 and ZP3 bind to non-overlapping sets of sperm proteins and whether O-linked carbohydrate is the exclusive sperm-binding portion of ZP3.

The protein structure of the zp, with only 3-4 components identified to date, is considerably simpler than that of sperm. Nevertheless, considerable progress is being made in characterizing the complementary sperm proteins that function in gamete recognition and binding. Work in our laboratory has defined a 95 kd receptor protein for ZP3 (22), termed ZRK (zona receptor kinase), which has the structure of a receptor tyrosine kinase (RTK). Two other mouse ZP3-binding proteins have been identified by other labs: galactosyltransferase (23) and sp56 (24). The FA-1 antigen of human sperm has been reported to bind ZP3, but in a heterologous system (25). Additionally, many other sperm proteins or enzymatic activities have been implicated in zp binding, but the zp component(s) with which each interacts has not yet been defined (26).

Of the various zp receptors identified so far, only ZRK has intrinsic signalling potential, with the structure and activity of a RTK. During the last decade, an enormous amount of information has been learned about the signalling pathways initiated in response to RTKs binding their ligands (27). Space considerations prohibit more than the briefest review of this rapidly developing area. Upon ligand binding and dimerization, RTKs autophosphorylate (Figure 1). Most have multiple autophosphorylation sites that are recognized by the *src* homology 2 (SH2)-domains of specific signalling components, such as phospholipase Cγ (PLCγ) or phosphatidylinositol 3-kinase (PI 3-K). In many cases, these enzymes also become tyrosine-phosphorylated and thereby activated. However, several SH_2-containing proteins (Grb-2, Shc, Crk) that associate with tyrosine-phosphorylated receptors lack enzymatic activity but act as adaptors, linking other components to the receptors. In several signalling pathways, these adaptors propagate the signalling cascade to the *ras* family of low molecular weight G-proteins via GTPase-activating proteins (*ras*Gap) or guanine nucleotide exchange factors (Sos). In turn, activated *ras* stimulates the raf kinase which activates additional kinase pathways that affect the growth and differentiation characteristics of cells. It has also become

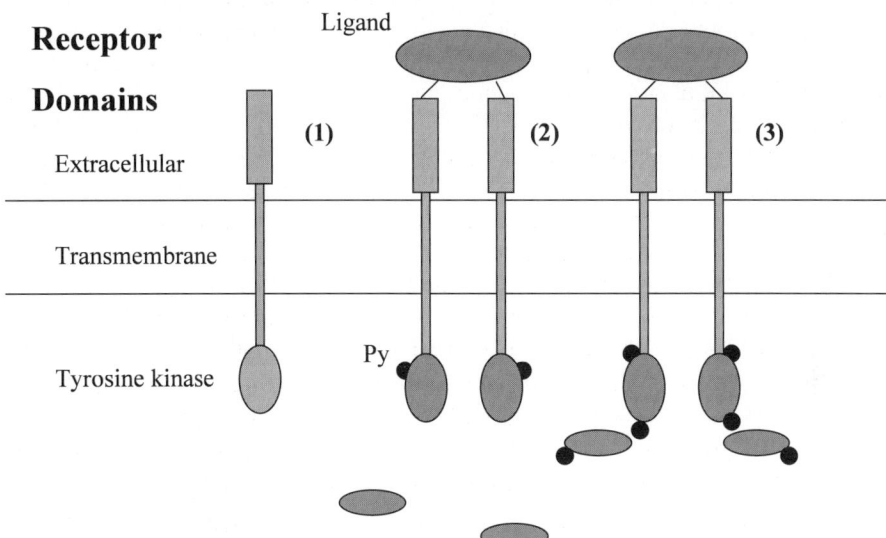

Figure 1: **Generalized scheme for activation of receptor tyrosine kinases (RTKs).** *In non-activated form, RTKs exist as single-pass transmembrane proteins (1). Activated receptors are found as oligomers (2) in which autophosphorylation is responsible for the appearance of phosphotyrosine (PY) residues in the intracellular domain of the activated receptor. If located in the appropriate motifs, these PY residues may become binding sites for cytosolic components that are themselves signalling proteins or adaptor proteins that link the activated RTK to other signalling pathways (3).*

evident that protein tyrosine phosphatases (PTPases) have critical regulatory roles in signalling pathways involving tyrosine phosphorylation. In addition to modulating signalling pathways by removing tyrosine phosphates from the substrates of RTKs, PTPases have also been shown to exhibit complex interactions with RTKs themselves, either activating or inhibiting them. Recently, a PTPase has been found to link a RTK to Grb-2, thus serving an adaptor function (28).

In addition to tyrosine kinase-mediated signalling pathways in sperm, which we and others (29, 30) have studied, there is evidence that G-proteins, particularly G_i-proteins, are also involved in zp-activated signalling (31). At present, it is unclear whether these two pathways are linked, but there is certainly considerable precedent for that possibility (32-38). One example of signalling pathway cross-talk is the regulated release of histamine from basophils (39). In this system, crosslinking of $Fc_\varepsilon RI$ receptors by IgE activates receptor-associated tyrosine kinases, initiating the cascade that leads to histamine release. As is the case in sperm, pertussis toxin blocks secretory granule release, implicating involvement of a G_i- or G_o-protein in these events (40, 41). Current studies of secretion suggest that both heterotrimeric G-proteins as well as monomeric G-proteins are used, that both operate late in the process, and that the cellular machinery employed to accomplish secretion is highly conserved from yeast to mammals (5,42-44). Despite this conservation of the machinery, complete definition of the signalling pathways that are responsible for regulated exocytosis has not yet been achieved for any system.

EVIDENCE FOR A HUMAN ZRK HOMOLOG

Our previous work with mouse gametes suggested a ZP3 receptor with the structure of a RTK (22). Given the evolutionary conservation of this receptor family as well as the demonstrated conservation of the receptor's corresponding ligand, ZP3, we predicted that a related receptor would be present in other mammalian species and therefore began examining human sperm. The presence of phosphotyrosine (PY)-containing proteins in human sperm was addressed by Western analysis using an anti-PY antibody (45). In parallel with findings in mice (22), a 95 kd protein that is tyrosine-phosphorylated is present in human sperm and its level of PY increases with capacitation (46), a final maturational process that primes sperm for zp-triggered ARs (26). Tyrphostin pretreatment of cells eliminates the capacitation-dependent PY increase, suggesting activation of a tyrosine kinase during this process.

Several years ago, Moore and colleagues described the generation and use of mAb 97.25 that *(i)* recognizes a human sperm plasma membrane protein of 95 kd and *(ii)* blocks human sperm interaction with human zp (47). Use of mAb 97.25 allowed us to investigate the possibility that mAb 97.25 recognizes ZRK. Indirect immunofluorescence of live sperm reveals that mAb 97.25 is restricted to the mouse sperm plasma membrane overlying the acrosome (48), co-localizing with anti-PY Ab immunofluorescence. On human sperm, mAb 97.25 also localizes to the sperm surface over the acrosome (46). Using immunoblot analysis, we have found that mAb 97.25 recognizes a 95 kd human sperm protein that is tyrosine-phosphorylated (46).

MOLECULAR CLONING: DETERMINING THE SEQUENCE OF ZRK

We have utilized an anti-PY antibody (PY20) and mAb 97.25, targetted respectively to putative intracellular and extracellular domains of ZRK, as sequential probes in a cloning strategy designed to elucidate the primary structure of ZRK (46). From a human testis cDNA expression library, we have isolated a clone, *hu9*, that is reactive with both antibodies. Sequencing of the 2.2-kb insert revealed an open reading frame of 1,800 nucleotides, predicting a protein of 600 amino acids with a molecular weight of ~68,000 (Figure 2). Comparison of *hu9* with sequences in the Genbank and Swiss Protein data bases revealed that this cDNA encodes a novel RTK. The predicted amino acid sequence of *hu9* contains motifs found in all tyrosine kinases (49), including the highly conserved ATP-binding site (GEGEKG, residues 249-254) and conserved sequences from the major catalytic subdomains of these molecules. Two potential autophosphorylation sites lie within 20 residues upstream of the Ala-Pro-Ile consensus triplet. The deduced amino acid sequence of the Hu9 catalytic domain is most similar (55% identity) to that of c-Eyk, a receptor-like protein tyrosine kinase identified recently as the proto-oncogene of v-*eyk* (v-*ryk*) (50). Hu9 contains other structural features common to RTKs, including a sequence of hydrophobic amino acids (residues 162-182) capable of serving as a transmembrane region (51) and an amino terminal extracellular domain that could possess the ligand binding site(s). However, comparison of the Hu9 extracellular domain with other database-logged sequences yielded no significant homology.

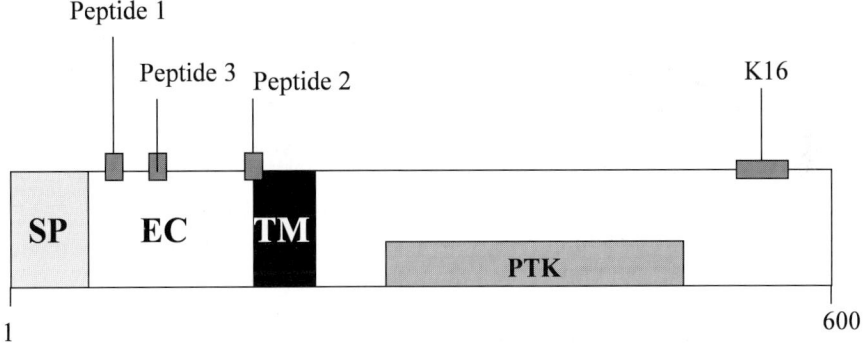

Figure 2: **Predicted structure of ZRK, based upon the sequence of *hu9*.** *The approximate location of the synthetic peptides discussed is indicated. SP, signal peptide; EC, extracellular domain; TM, transmembrane domain; PTK, protein tyrosine kinase domain.*

FUNCTIONAL CHARACTERIZATION OF ZRK

Several lines of evidence (as described below) indicate that *hu9* encodes human ZRK, and for convenience throughout this manuscript, we will refer to the *hu9*-encoded protein as ZRK.

An antibody directed against a region of the Hu9 intracellular domain (K16) recognizes a 95 kd tyrosine-phosphorylated human sperm protein (46).

We have raised an antibody in rabbits against a synthetic peptide (K16; See Figure 2) that corresponds to residues 539-553 of the deduced amino acid sequence of *hu9*. Immunoblots (46) indicate that K16 recognizes a 95 kd human sperm protein that is distinct from hexokinase. Immunoprecipitation with K16 followed by blotting with anti-PY shows that this 95 kd protein is tyrosine-phosphorylated; immunoprecipitation with mAb 97.25 followed by blotting with K16 indicates that the two probes recognize the same protein.

Peptides corresponding to regions of the Hu9 extracellular domain inhibit human sperm-zp binding (46).

We examined the putative receptor function of the *hu9*-encoded polypeptide in a competitive sperm-zp binding assay, using a hemi-zona assay design (52). Based on algorithms to identify regions that might be important in ligand-receptor interaction, 3 peptide sequences found in the Hu9 extracellular domain (Hu9-X) were synthesized (see Figure 2). ZP surrounding non-viable unfertilized human eggs were bisected with a micro-scalpel, and matched zp halves were used subsequently. Half A was preincubated with Ham's F-12 containing 7.5% serum, whereas Half B was preincubated with the same medium (control samples) or with peptides 1, 2, or 3 (10 µM). Capacitated human sperm interaction with the hemi-zonae was terminated after 30 min. Two of the peptides tested (pep1 and pep3) caused significant inhibition of sperm-zp interaction, blocking binding by 69% and 80%, respectively (46). In contrast, a third peptide (pep2) produced no effect on binding levels. These results suggest that portions of Hu9-X are important in sperm-zp interaction, but are only an initial step in attempting to define ZP3-binding epitopes of ZRK. Further work is aimed at refining our analysis of Hu9-X using a complete set of overlapping peptides that describe the full extracellular domain of ZRK.

Human ZP3 stimulates the kinase activity of ZRK in capacitated, but not in uncapacitated, sperm (46).

We have used the K16 pAb, which was generated against residues 539-553 of Hu9, in immune complex kinase assays to examine intrinsic and ligand-dependent kinase activity of ZRK. Solubilized non-capacitated or capacitated human sperm were used as the starting material for immunoprecipitation with K16 pAb. Immune complexes incubated with or without human ZP3 in the presence of ^{32}P-γ-ATP to assess kinase activity. The basal level of kinase activity in K16 immunoprecipitates from non-capacitated sperm is stimulated to a small degree by exposure to human ZP3, however exposure of capacitated sperm proteins precipitated by K16 pAb to human ZP3 significantly increases the amount of ^{32}P incorporated into protein. Results of this assay demonstrate 2 important concepts:

1) human ZP3 is capable of stimulating sperm kinase activity, indicating its expected activity as a ligand, and 2) K16 immunoprecipitates a zona responsive kinase, suggesting that *hu9* encodes ZRK.

Tyrosine kinase activity regulates sperm-zp interaction in mouse and human gametes.

Since activation of RTKs appears essential for their signalling action, specific inhibitors of tyrosine kinase activity constitute important research tools in studying the mechanisms responsible for the resulting pleiotropic responses (53). Given similarities between ZRK and members of the RTK family, we investigated the effect of the tyrosine kinase inhibitor tyrphostin RG-50864 (54) on isolated ZRK, on sperm membranes, and in living cells. We found that mouse zp proteins stimulated the kinase activity of ZRK *in vitro*, and that pre-exposure to tyrphostin prevented the zp-dependent stimulation in kinase activity (55). In capacitated mouse sperm, we found that tyrphostin as well as genistein block zp-triggered ARs (55). In capacitated human sperm, tyrphostin also blocks human ZP3-triggered ARs. Collectively, these results indicate that inhibition of ZP3-induced tyrosine phosphorylation of ZRK parallels inhibition of ZP3-induced ARs, demonstrating a direct role for tyrosine kinase activity in regulating the acrosomal exocytosis.

mAb LL95 serves as a ZP3 mimic (56).

Since receptor oligomerization by ZP3 is essential for acrosome reaction triggering (57), we hypothesized that application of an external cross-linking agent will lead to the acrosome reaction, even in the absence of the natural ligand ZP3. To test this hypothesis, we generated a mouse mAb against murine ZRK. This antibody, named LL95, is unusual in that it is expressed in two forms, LL95-I and LL95-II. The former bears the structure of an immunoglobulin (H_2L_2), whereas the latter corresponds to free κ-light chain. Both LL95-I and LL95-II bind indistinguishably to the acrosomal region of live mouse sperm. Most importantly, they mimic the natural ligand, ZP3, in functional assays. LL95-I (0.05 μg/ml) inhibits primary sperm-zp binding by 90% and, at 1 μg/ml, triggers acrosome reactions in 50% of the population, equivalent to the maximal percentage triggered by solubilized zp. In contrast, monovalent LL95-II inhibits sperm-zp binding, but does not induce acrosome reactions unless crosslinked by an additional bivalent antibody, indicating that LL95 behaves as predicted for an anti-receptor antibody (Figure 3). Immunolocalization reveals that the LL95 antigen is restricted to the sperm head surface in the acrosomal region of live cells (56). Thus, LL95 fulfills several criteria predicted for an antibody that recognizes a sperm receptor for ZP3. However, in standard immunoblot analysis, LL95 mAb shows no specific reactivity with sperm proteins. As an alternative detection method, we tested LL95 with a technique that has been described to study ligand-receptor, rather than antigen-antibody, interactions on a blot. This method, termed ligand blot analysis (58) consists of treating proteins with 3% NP-40 after transfer to a nitrocellulose membrane, thereby facilitating protein renaturation and refolding of conformational epitopes. Using this technique, we found that, under non-reducing conditions, LL95 reacted with a broad band at 95 kd; when samples were separated in the presence of 5% ß-mercaptoethanol, ^{125}I-LL95 recognized two protein bands, principally one at 105 kd, and a minor band at 130 kd (56).

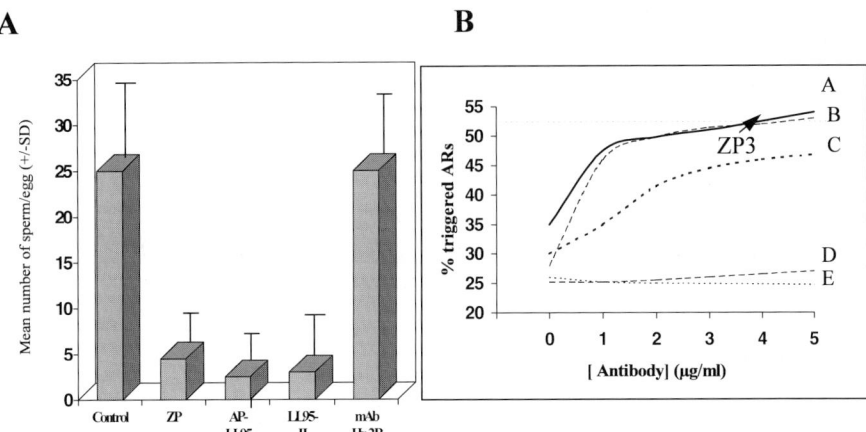

Figure 3: **Comparison of the effects of LL95 and anti-hexokinase antibodies on gamete interaction.** *(A) Capacitated sperm were incubated for 15 min with in vitro fertilization medium alone (control), solubilized zp proteins (2 zp/µl), affinity-purified LL95 (0.05 µg/ml), LL95-II (2 µg/ml), or anti-hexokinase mAb 2B (0.5 µg/ml), and then added to cumulus free, zp-intact mouse eggs. After an additional 15 min, loosely attached sperm were removed and the number of sperm bound were counted after glutaraldehyde fixation. The average number of sperm bound per egg ± SD was calculated from 3 replicate experiments.*
(B) Induction of the acrosome reaction by LL95. Capacitated sperm were incubated with increasing concentrations of: LL95-I (A); affinity-purified LL95 (B); 2 µg/ml LL95-II, followed 30 min later with increasing concentrations of rat mAb ant-mouse κ–chain (C); mAb anti-hexokinase 2B (D); LL95-II alone (E). Acrosomal status was determined 30 min later. These results represent the mean ± SD calculated from 5 different experiments.
(Data redrawn from (56).

ZRK IS NOT HEXOKINASE

A recent report from Kopf and co-workers (59) suggested that the 95 kd ZP3-binding protein that we study is hexokinase. Using 4 different approaches, we have determined that this is not the case.

Localization
Anti-hexokinase antibodies localize exclusively to the sperm tail in both human and mouse sperm (56) whereas a ZP3-binding protein is predicted to demonstrate localization on the sperm head, as does 97.25 mAb (46,48), anti-PY (22), or LL95 mAb ((56)).

Sequence analysis
Sequence comparison of *hu9* with hexokinase (peptide, FASTA) reveals that the two are unrelated. Three unique spermatogenic cell-specific hexokinase type-I cDNAs have been cloned recently (60), and sequence analysis indicates close identity between the sperm and somatic isoforms of hexokinase.

Functional assays
Using mouse gametes, sperm-zp binding and AR triggering are unaffected by anti-hexokinase antibodies, either mAb or pAb (56). In contrast, the LL95 mAb demonstrates significant bioactivity for both of these events (see above).

Biochemistry
To our knowledge, hexokinase from mouse sperm is unusual, though not unique, in bearing residues recognized by anti-PY antibodies; a mouse hepatoma cell line also contains a tyrosine-phosphorylated hexokinase (60). In sperm from 2 other species that have been examined, cat and human, hexokinase is not tyrosine-phosphorylated (Cat: pers. comm., B. Pukazhenthi and J. Howard, National Zoo). In contrast to hexokinase however, ZRK is consistent in its tyrosine phosphorylation among the species that have been examined. Figure 4, showing the results of an immunoprecipitation experiment using capacitated human sperm, addresses this topic. Immunoblots, probed with anti-PY or with anti-hexokinase Abs (lanes 1 and 5, respectively), demonstrate the presence of reactive proteins in a detergent extract. When immunoprecipitates using these same Abs are cross-probed, it is evident that hexokinase is not detected in the PY immunoprecipitate (lane 4), nor is ZRK -- or any tyrosine phosphorylated protein -- present in the hexokinase immune complex (lane 8). Based on the absence of immunoreactivity in the supernatant fractions remaining after the immuno-reactive pellet is sedimented, it appears as though these immunoprecipitations are quantitative. Use of K16, the pAb generated using residues 539-553 of Hu9, compared with anti-hexokinase also reinforces this distinction between ZRK and hexokinase in human sperm (46). In mouse sperm, the distinction between ZRK and hexokinase cannot be made on the basis of anti-PY reactivity; however, the two proteins can be distinguished by the use of specific antibodies. Whereas the two proteins run at 95 kd under non-reducing conditions, under reducing conditions hexokinase

migrates at 116 kd and murine ZRK migrates at 105 kd (56). Analysis of these two proteins with respect to the sperm's physiology also reveals that the tyrosine-phosphorylation of hexokinase is unchanged (61), whereas the tyrosine phosphorylation of ZRK increases approximately 2-fold as a function of capacitation (22,46).

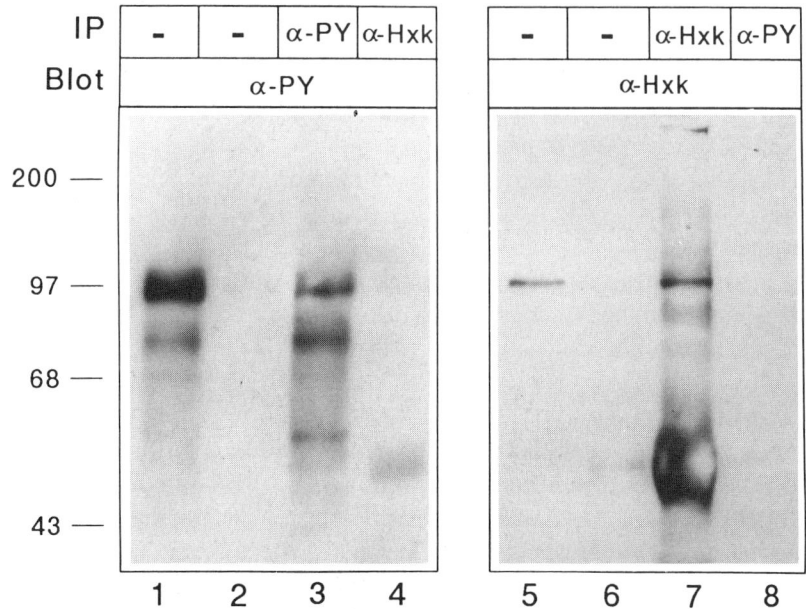

Figure 4: **Immunoprecipitation and immunoblot analysis of human sperm proteins using anti-phosphotyrosine and anti-hexokinase antibodies.** *Capacitated sperm were either solubilized directly in sample buffer (lanes 1, 2, 5, 6), or extracted in RIPA buffer and then incubated with either rabbit antihexokinase antibody (lanes 4, 7) or PY20-agarose (lanes 3, 8; Signal Transduction Laboratories) overnight at 4°C. The anti-hexokinase immune complex was subsequently incubated with Protein-A Sepharose. Following washing with RIPA, proteins in the immune complexes were separated by SDS-PAGE under disulfide-reducing conditions, transferred to nitrocellulose, probed with the antibodies indicated, and developed using ECL (Amersham). Immunoprecipitated proteins were evaluated by immunoblot for phosphotyrosine (lanes 1-4) or hexokinase (lanes 5-8). The human sperm extract before immunoprecipitation contained ZRK, in addition to other tyrosine phosphorylated proteins (lane 1), and also hexokinase (lane 5). Probing of supernatants following immunoprecipitation using PY20 (lane 2) or anti-hexokinase (lane 6) failed to detect proteins of interest, suggesting that both antibodies immunoprecipitate quantitatively. When the PY20 immunoprecipitate was probed with an anti-PY antibody (lane 3), ZRK and other phosphotyrosine proteins are evident. Likewise, anti-hexokinase antibodies recognize hexokinase in the anti-hexokinase immunoprecipitate (lane 7). However, when the anti-hexokinase immunoprecipitate was probed with anti-PY (lane 4) or when the anti-PY immunoprecipitate was probed with anti-hexokinase antibodies (lane 8), no proteins (other than the IgG heavy chain in lane 4) were detected.*

SIGNALLING THROUGH ZRK

Given the role that we propose for ZRK in sperm-zp interaction, the intracellular domain of the receptor is predicted to couple to other signalling components and activate the cascade which results in acrosomal exocytosis (see Figure 1). Examination of the sequence of the intracellular domain encoded by *hu9* reveals that many of its tyrosine residues are in consensus motifs for the binding of SH2-containing proteins to activated RTKs (62) (Figure 5). SH2-containing proteins that are involved directly in signalling, such as PLCγ, as well as adaptor proteins, such as Grb-2, Shc, and 3BP2, that link RTKs with G-protein signalling pathways, are thus predicted to potentially bind to ZRK. We plan to base our investigation of the signalling potential of ZRK in regulated exocytosis on these structural considerations.

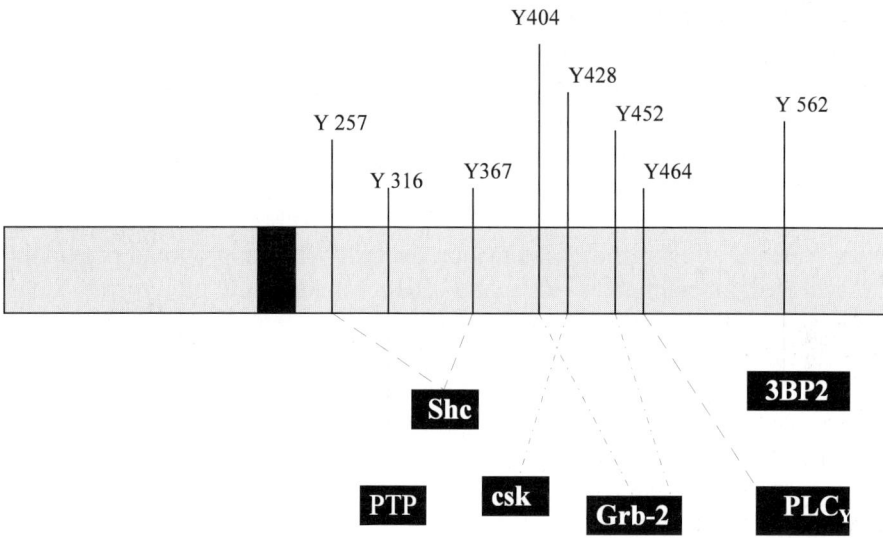

Figure 5: **Identification of consensus motifs in ZRK for potential binding of *src* homology 2 (SH2) domain-containing signalling proteins.**

A WORKING HYPOTHESIS FOR ZP3-STIMULATED ACROSOMAL EXOCYTOSIS

To facilitate our overall investigation, we have developed a working model for ZP3-stimulated acrosomal exocytosis. From our preliminary work as well as by analogy with other ligand-induced cellular responses, we suggest that acrosomal exocytosis is triggered by the activation of aggregated ZP3 receptors in the sperm's plasma membrane. We have identified ZRK as one receptor for ZP3. However, based on numerous results reported in the literature concerning sperm-zp interaction as well as results concerning somatic cell interactions, we suggest that ZRK is but one of several proteins in the sperm plasma membrane that forms a multimeric adhesion/signalling complex resulting in acrosomal exocytosis. At present, ZRK is the only candidate protein with signalling potential.

One consequence of capacitation is the accumulation of PY residues on ZRK. Available PY residues in the appropriate motifs may permit coupling of ZRK to intracellular signalling pathways (e.g., via PLCγ). Capacitation is also reported to increase the fluidity of the membrane and, if not pre-existing, may allow the formation of multimeric complexes consisting of adhesion components (e.g., sp56, galactosyltransferase) and signalling components (e.g., ZRK). Low affinity, high capacity binding of *O*-linked oligosaccharides of ZP3 may mediate initial interaction for positioning and orienting the sperm with ZP3 ligands; the summation of ZP3 binding with multiple sperm proteins may generate a high affinity interaction overall. When appropriate positioning is achieved, interaction of ZP3 and ZRK would result in tyrosine kinase activation, with stimulation of intracellular signalling components that are required for exocytosis.

This two-stage strategy of adhesion-followed-by-signalling may be similar to the pattern exhibited by various somatic cells in which numerous studies indicate that both carbohydrate- and peptide-mediated interactions occur, often in a sequential manner. In capillaries, for instance, endothelial cells and leukocytes initially interact using selectins (carbohydrate-mediated), which is followed by integrin-mediated (protein-mediated) interaction. It is thought that the high capacity, low affinity selectin-mediated binding slows down the fast-moving leukocyte, allowing it to orient properly for more precise, high affinity protein-protein interaction. In this system, cell interaction can be blocked by a large variety of different sugars, as well as the appropriate peptide sequences (63). It may also be pertinent to recall that, in sea urchins, simple sugars effectively block sperm interaction with the vitelline membrane, and it was presumed for decades that a lectin-like interaction was solely responsible. Recently, the bindin receptor of eggs has been cloned and sequenced, and studies at the molecular level reveal that low affinity carbohydrate-mediated interaction precedes high affinity peptide-peptide interaction between ligand and receptor (64-66).

Once stimulated, we propose that the machinery of acrosomal exocytosis (the docking and fusing components; the cytoskeletal elements) is similar to that used in other exocytotic systems, and will be modulated by the cascade set into motion by ZP3 activation of ZRK. Our present work is directed toward determining key initiating features of the sperm-ZP3 interaction that result in exocytosis. What is the nature of the interaction between ZRK and ZP3? Can linear sequences of a ZP3-receptor like ZRK be mapped for ZP3 binding? Do such sequences confer species specific interaction with ZP3? Which intracellular pathways are activated by ZRK? These and many more questions require detailed answers before our understanding of sperm-zp interaction can be considered complete.

Acknowledgements

Dr J. Wilson, Univ of Michigan, kindly provided the rabbit anti-rat hexokinase antibodies used. Work in our laboratory is funded by grants from the NICHD (HD18201 and HD29125) and the Andrew W. Mellon Foundation.

REFERENCES

1. Wassarman PM. Gamete interactions during mammalian fertilization. Theriogenology 1994; 41: 31-44.
2. Saling PM. Gamete interactions leading to fertilization in mammals: Principles, paradigms, and paradoxes. In: Adashi EY, Rock JA, Rosenwaks Z, eds. Reproductive Endcrinology, Surgery, and Technology. New York:Raven Press, 1995 : in press.
3. Bleil JD, Wassarman PM. Structure and function of the zona pellucida:Identification and characterization of the proteins of the mouse oocyte's zona pellucida. Dev Biol 1980; 76: 185-202.
4. Shimizu S, Tsuji M, Dean J. In vitro biosynthesis of three sulfated glycoproteins of murine zonae pellucidae by oocytes grown in follicle culture. J Biol Chem 1983; 258 : 5858-5863.
5. Bennett MK, Scheller RH. The molecular machinery for secretion is conserved from yeast to neurons. Proc Natl Acad Sci, USA 1993; 90 : 2559-2563.
6. Chamberlin ME, Dean J. Human homolog of the mouse sperm receptor. Proc Natl Acad Sci, USA 1990; 87 : 6014-6018.
7. Kinloch RA, Ruiz-Seiler B, Wassarman PM. Genomic organization and polypeptide primary structure of zona pellucida glycoprotein hZP3, the hamster sperm receptor [published erratum appears in Dev Biol 1991 May;145(1):203]. Dev Biol 1990; 142 : 414-421.

8. Ringuette MJ, Sobieski DA, Chamow SM, Dean J. Oocyte-specific gene expression: molecular characterization of a cDNA coding for ZP3, the sperm receptor of the mouse zona pellucida. Proc Natl Acad Sci, USA 1986; 83 : 4341-4345.
9. Moller CC, Bleil JD, Kinloch RA, Wassarman PM. Structural and functional relationships between mouse and hamster zona pellucida glycoproteins. Dev Biol 1990; 137 : 276-286.
10. Bleil JD, Wassarman PM. Sperm-egg interactions in the mouse: Sequence of events and induction of the acrosome reaction by a zona pellucida glycoprotein. Dev Biol 1983; 95 : 317-324.
11. Bagavant H, Yurewicz EC, Sacco AG, Talwar GP, Gupta SK. Block in porcine gamete interaction by polyclonal antibodies to a pig ZP3β fragment having partial sequence homology to human ZP3. J Reprod Immunol 1993; 25: 277283.
12. Yurewicz EC, Pack BA, Armant DR, Sacco AG. Porcine zona pellucida ZP3α glycoprotein mediates binding of the biotin-labeled M_r 55,000 family (ZP3) to boar sperm membrane vesicles. Mol Reprod Dev 1993; 36 : 382-389.
13. Töpfer-Petersen E, Mann K, Calvete JJ. Identification of porcine oocyte 55 kDa α and β proteins within the zona pellucida glycoprotein families indicates that oocyte sperm receptor activity is associated with different zona pellucida proteins in different mammalian species. Biol Chem Hoppe Seyler 1993; 374 : 411-417.
14. Yurewicz EC, Pack BA, Sacco AG. Isolation, composition, and biological activity of sugar chains of porcine oocyte zona pellucida 55K glycoproteins. Mol Reprod Dev 1991; 30 : 126-134.
15. Noguchi S, Hatanaka Y, Tobita T, Nakano M. Structural analysis of the N-linked carbohydrate chains of the 55kDa glycoprotein family (PZP3) from porcine zona pellucida. Eur J Biochem 1992; 204 : 1089-1100.
16. Yurewicz EC, Zhang S, Sacco AG. Generation and characterization of site directed antisera against an amino terminal segment of a 55 kDa sperm adhesive glycoprotein from zona pellucida of pig oocytes. J Reprod Fertil 1993; 98 : 147-152.
17. Bagavant H, Yurewicz EC, Sacco AG, Talwar GP, Gupta SK. Delineation of epitopes on porcine zona pellucida relevant for binding of sperm to oocyte using monoclonal antibodies. J Reprod Immunol 1993; 23 : 265-279.
18. Yurewicz EC, Hibler D, Fontenot GK, Sacco AG, Harris J. Nucleotide sequence of cDNA encoding ZP3α, a sperm binding glycoprotein from zona pellucida of pig oocyte. Biochim Biophys Acta Gene Struct Expression 1993; 1174 : 211-214.

19. Lee VH, Dunbar BS. Developmental expression of the rabbit 55 kDa zona pellucida protein and messenger RNA in ovarian follicles. Dev Biol 1993; 155 : 371-382.
20. Lee VH, Schwoebel E, Prasad S, Cheung P, Timmons TM, Cook R, Dunbar BS. Identification and structural characterization of the 75kDa rabbit zona pellucida protein. J Biol Chem 1993; 268 : 12412-12417.
21. Yurewicz EC, Pack BA, Sacco AG. Porcine oocyte zona pellucida Mr 55,000 glycoproteins: Identification of O-glycosylated domains. Mol Reprod Dev 1992; 33 : 182-188.
22. Leyton L, Saling P. 95 kd Sperm proteins bind ZP3 and serve as tyrosine kinase substrates in response to zona binding. Cell 1989; 57 : 1123-1130.
23. Miller DJ, Macek MB, Shur BD. Complementarity between sperm surface β-1,4-galactosyl-transferase and egg-coat ZP3 mediates spermegg binding. Nature 1992; 357 : 589-593.
24. Cheng A, Le T, Palacios M, Bookbinder LH, Wassarman PM, Suzuki F, Bleil JD. Sperm-egg recognition in the mouse: Characterization of sp56, a sperm protein having specific affinity for ZP3. J Cell Biol 1994; 125 : 867-878.
25. Naz RK, Sacco AG, Yurewicz EC. Human spermatozoal FA-1 binds with ZP3 of porcine zona pellucida. J Reprod Immunol 1991; 20 : 43-58.
26. Yanagimachi R. Mammalian Fertilization. In: Knobil E, Neill JD, eds. The Physiology of Reproduction. New York : Raven Press, Ltd., 1994 : 189-317.
27. Pawson T, Hunter T, Eds. Curr Opin Genet Dev 1994; 4 (February) : see complete volume.
28. Li W, Nishimura R, Kashishian A, Batzer AG, Kim WJH, Cooper JA, Schlessinger J. A new function for a phosphotyrosine phosphatase: Linking GRB2-Sos to a receptor tyrosine kinase. Mol Cell Biol 1994; 14 : 509-517.
29. Tesarik J, Moos J, Mendoza C. Stimulation of protein tyrosine phosphorylation by a progesterone receptor on the cell surface of human sperm. Endocrinology 1993; 133 : 328-335.
30. Naz RK, Ahmad K, Kumar R. Role of membrane phosphotyrosine proteins in human spermatozoal function. J Cell Sci 1991; 99 : 157-165.
31. Ward CR, Kopf GS. Molecular events mediating sperm activation. Dev Biol 1993; 158 : 9-34.
32. Caro JF, Raju MS, Caro M, Lynch CJ, Poulos J, Exton JH, Thakkar JK. Guanine nucleotide binding regulatory proteins in liver from obese humans with and without type II diabetes: Evidence for altered "cross-talk" between the insulin receptor and G_i proteins. J Cell Biochem 1994; 54 : 309-319.
33. Hadcock JR, Port JD, Gelman MS, Malbon CC. Cross-talk between tyrosine kinase and G protein-linked receptors. Phosphorylation of $β_2$ adrenergic receptors in response to insulin. J Biol Chem 1992; 267 : 26017-26022.

34. Gardner AM, Vaillancourt RR, Johnson GL. Activation of mitogen-activated protein kinase/extracellular signal-regulated kinase kinase by G protein and tyrosine kinase oncoproteins. J Biol Chem 1993; 268 : 17896-17901.
35. Imoto M, Sujikai I, Ui H, Umezawa K. Involvement of tyrosine kinase in growth factor-induced phospholipase C activation in NIH3T3 cells. Biochim Biophys Acta Lipids Lipid Metab 1993; 1166 : 188-192.
36. Bourgoin S, Poubelle PE, Liao NW, Umezawa K, Borgeat P, Naccache PH. Granulocyte-macrophage colony-stimulating factor primes phospholipase D activity in human neutrophils in vitro: Role of calcium, G proteins and tyrosine kinases. Cell Signal 1992; 4 : 487-500.
37. Harnett M, Rigley K. The role of G proteins versus protein tyrosine kinases in the regulation of lymphocyte activation. Immunol Today 1992; 13 : 482-486.
38. Iwashita S, Kobayashi M. Signal transduction system for growth factor receptors associated with tyrosine kinase activity: Epidermal growth factor receptor signalling and its regulation. Cell Signal 1992; 4 : 123-132.
39. Gomperts BD, Hide I, Bennett JP, Pizzey A, Tatham PER. Part VII. Secretory cell models: Intracellular signaling, second messengers, and exocytosis. The exocytotic reaction of permeabilized rat mast cells. An all-or-none response. Ann NY Acad Sci 1994; 710 : 217-231.
40. Koffer A. Calcium-induced secretion from permeabilized rat mast cells: Requirements for guanine nucleotides. Biochim Biophys Acta Mol Cell Res 1993; 1176 : 231-239.
41. Aridor M, Traub LM, Sagi-Eisenberg R. Exocytosis in mast cells by basic secretagogues: evidence for direct activation of GTP-binding proteins. J Cell Biol 1990; 111 : 909-917.
42. Burgoyne RD, Morgan A. Regulated exocytosis. Biochem J 1993; 293 : 305-316.
43. Popov SV, Poo M. Synaptotagmin: A calcium sensitive inhibitor of exocytosis. Cell 1993; 73 : 1247-1249.
44. Tsunoda Y. Receptor-operated Ca^{2+} signaling and crosstalk in stimulus secretion coupling. Biochim Biophys Acta Rev Biomembr 1993; 1154 : 105-156.
45. Glenney JR, Zokas L, Kamps MP. Monoclonal antibodies to phosphotyrosine. J Immunol Meth 1988; 109 : 277-285.
46. Burks DJ, Carballada R, Moore HDM, Saling PM. Interaction of a tyrosine kinase from human sperm with the zona pellucida at fertilization. Science 1995; 269 : 83-86.
47. Moore HDM, Hartman TD, Bye AP, Lutjen P, De Witt M, Trounson AO. Monoclonal antibody against a sperm antigen Mr 95,000 inhibits attachment of human spermatozoa to the zona pellucida. J Reprod Immunol 1987; 11 : 157-166.

48. Bunch DO, Saling PM. Generation of a mouse sperm membrane fraction with zona receptor activity. Biol Reprod 1991; 44 : 672-680.
49. Hanks SK, Quinn AM, Hunter T. The protein kinase family: Conserved features and deduced phylogeny of the catalytic domain. Science 1988; 241 : 42-54.
50. Jia R, Hanafusa H. The protooncogene of v-eyk (v-ryk) is a novel receptor-type protein tyrosine kinase with extracellular Ig/FN-III domains. J Biol Chem 1994; 269 : 1839-1844.
51. Kyte J, Doolittle RF. A simple method for displaying the hydropathic character of a protein. J Mol Biol 1982; 157 : 105-132.
52. Burkman LJ, Coddington CC, Franken DR, Krugen TF, Rosenwaks Z, Hodgen GD. The hemizona assay (HZA): development of a diagnostic test for the binding of human spermatozoa to the human hemizona pellucida to predict fertilization potential. Fertil Steril 1988; 49 : 688-697.
53. Yaish P, Gazit A, Gilon C, Levitzki A. Blocking of EGF-dependent cell proliferation by EGF receptor kinase inhibitors. Science 1988; 242 : 933-935.
54. Lyall RM, Zilberstein A, Gazit A, Gilon C, Levitzki A, Schlessinger J. Tyrphostins inhibit epidermal growth factor (EGF)-receptor tyrosine kinase activity in living cells and EGF-stimulated cell proliferation. J Biol Chem 1989; 264 : 14503-14509.
55. Leyton L, LeGuen P, Bunch D, Saling PM. Regulation of mouse gamete interaction by a sperm tyrosine kinase. Proc Natl Acad Sci, USA 1992; 89 : 11692-11695.
56. Leyton L, Tomes CN, Saling PM. LL95 monoclonal antibody mimics functional effects of ZP3 on mouse sperm: Evidence that the antigen recognized is not hexokinase. Mol Reprod Dev 1995; in press.
57. Leyton L, Saling P. Evidence that aggregation of mouse sperm receptors by ZP3 triggers the acrosome reaction. J Cell Biol 1989; 108 : 2163-2168.
58. Grissom F, Rivero-Crespo F, Lindgren B, Hall K. Ligand blot analysis: Validation of quantitative capabilities and utilization for measurement of truncated insulin-like growth factor regulation of Hep-G2 insulin-like growth factor binding protein production. Anal Biochem 1993; 212 : 412-420.
59. Kalab P, Visconti P, Leclerc P, Kopf GS. p95, the major phosphotyrosine containing protein in mouse spermatozoa, is a hexokinase with unique properties. J Biol Chem 1994; 269 : 3810-3817.
60. Mori C, Welch JE, Fulcher KD, O'Brien DA, Eddy EM. Unique hexokinase messenger ribonucleic acids lacking the porin-binding domain are developmentally expressed in mouse spermatogenic cells. Biol Reprod 1993; 49 : 191-203.

61. Visconti PE, Bailey JL, Moore GD, Pan DY, Olds-Clarke P, Kopf GS. Capacitation of mouse spermatozoa. 1. Correlation between the capacitation state and protein tyrosine phosphorylation. Development 1995; 121 : 1129-1137.
62. Songyang Z, Shoelson SE, McGlade J, Olivier P, Pawson T, Bustelo XR, Barbacid M, Sabe H, Hanafusa H, Yi T, Ren R, Baltimore D, Ratnofsky S, Feldman RA, Cantley LC. Specific motifs recognized by the SH2 domains of Csk, 3BP2, fps/fes, GRB-2, HCP, SHC, Syk, and Vav. Mol Cell Biol 1994; 14 : 2777-2785.
63. Cummings RD, Smith DF. The selectin family of carbohydrate-binding proteins: Structure and importance of carbohydrate ligands for cell adhesion. BioEssays 1992; 14 : 849-856.
64. Foltz KR, Lennarz WJ. The molecular basis of sea urchin gamete interactions at the egg plasma membrane. Dev Biol 1993; 158 : 46-61.
65. Lennarz WJ. Fertilisation in sea urchins: how many different molecules are involved in gamete interaction and fusion?. Zygote 1994; 2 : 1-4.
66. Ohlendieck K, Lennarz WJ. Role of the sea urchin egg receptor for sperm in gamete interactions. Trends Biochem Sci 1995; 20 : 29-33.

Human sperm acrosome reaction. Eds P. Fénichel, J. Parinaud.
Colloque INSERM/John Libbey Eurotext Ltd © 1995. Vol. 236, pp.105-122.

Induction of the human acrosome reaction by rhuZP3

Christopher L.R. Barratt[1,] and David P. Hornby[2]

[1] University Department of Obstetrics and Gynaecology, Jessop Hospital for Women, Sheffield S3 7RE, United Kingdom; [2]Krebs Institute, Department of Molecular Biology and Biotechnology, University of Sheffield, P.O. Box 594, Firth Court, Western Bank, Sheffield, S10 2UH, United Kingdom

ABSTRACT

The primary aim of our research is to understand the cellular and molecular basis of human gamete interaction. The nature of human sperm zona interaction remains largely unknown. We report the expression and documentation of biological activity of recombinant ZP3 produced in (1) Escherichia coli as a fusion protein with gluthatione-S transferase (2) Chinese hamster ovary cells (3) in an in vitro transcription/translation system. The purified fusion protein expressed in E.coli did not induce the acrosome reaction in capacitated human spermatozoa. The supernatant from CHO transfected ZP3 was found to be a potent inducer of the acrosome reaction, compared to the well established acrosome reaction inducers, A 23187 and human follicular fluid. Experiments with the in vitro transcription/translation system demonstrated a significant induction of the acrosome reaction only after incubation with ZP3 for 18 hours. These experiments demonstrate the essential role of post translational modifications in the activity of recombinant human ZP3 and lend support to a role for human ZP3 in the early stages of fertilisation. The availability of rhu-ZP3 will lead to greater insight into the structure and function of this glycoprotein.

Le premier objectif de nos travaux de recherche est de comprendre les bases cellulaires et moléculaires de l'interaction gamétique chez l'homme. L'interaction entre le spermatozoïde et la zona reste encore méconnue. Nous rapportons ici l'expression et les caractéristiques biologiques de la ZP3 recombinante produite soit (1) dans Escherichia coli obtenu par fusion avec la gluthatione S transferase (2) dans des cellules ovariennes de hamster, (3) dans un système de transcription/ translation in vitro. La protéine de fusion exprimée dans E. coli n'induit pas la réaction acrosomique de spermatozoïdes préalablement capacités. Le surnageant de CHO transfectées par ZP3 s'avère être un inducteur potentiel de la réaction acrosomique quand on le compare à des inducteurs classiques de la réaction acrosomique tels que l' A23187, ou le liquide folliculaire. Les expériences menées avec le système de transduction/ translation in vitro montrent une induction significative de la réaction acrosomique, uniquement après une incubation avec la ZP3 pendant 18 heures. Ces expériences montrent le rôle essentiel des modifications post-translationnelles dans l'activité de la ZP3 recombinante et penchent pour un rôle de la ZP3 humaine dans les étapes précoces de la fécondation. La disponibilité de la rhuZP3 permettra d'avoir une meilleure approche de la structure et la fonction de cette glycoprotéine.

INTRODUCTION

Complementary gamete recognition between spermatozoa and the zona pellucida has been extensively studied in mice, pigs, rats and rabbits; however, there is a paucity of data on humans (1-4). The major problem in studying human sperm zona interaction is obtaining sufficient quantities of zona pellucida. Interestingly, two recent studies have clearly shown that large quantities of recombinant mouse zona pellucida glycoprotein 3 (ZP3) can be produced *in vitro*.(5; 6). This recombinant product was biologically active i.e. possessed sperm receptor activity and induced the acrosome reaction. The production of biologically active recombinant human ZP3 is a critical first step in detailing the cellular/molecular basis of human gamete recognition.

The molecular composition of the zona pellucida has been well studied in the mouse (1), rabbit (4, 7), pig (2, 8, 9) and rat (3). The zona pellucida from the species studied to date, consists of three or four electrophoretically distinct glycoproteins, each appearing to possess distinct structural and functional roles in the sperm- egg interaction process. The most extensive studies have been carried out in the mouse where ZP3 is the primary sperm receptor, mediating both the initial recognition event and the subsequent triggering of the acrosome reaction via the complementary receptor(s) on the sperm (1, 10). Carbohydrate moieties on ZP3 are of importance for sperm binding although the nature of these carbohydrates (mannose, galactose and/or N-acetylglucosamine) is still open to debate (11, 12, 13). The integrity of the murine ZP3 peptide backbone is necessary for induction of the acrosome reaction - probably by facilitating receptor cross-linking (14). It is clear that the cloning of the cDNAs encoding mouse ZP2 and ZP3 (15-17) will allow a more detailed structural and functional analysis to be carried out in the rodent system.

Less information is available for the human zona pellucida. However, it is known to comprise at least three charge heterogeneous glycoproteins: ZP1, ZP2 and ZP3, with both ZP3 and a ZP2:ZP1 complex displaying affinity for sperm proteins. Intact and solubilised human zonae possess the ability to trigger the acrosome reaction (AR) in capacitated human sperm (18, 19) Interestingly, clinical studies using non-physiological agonists such as the calcium ionophore A23187, demonstrate that defects in the acrosome are likely to be a major cause of infertility in some groups of men (see review 20). At present it remains difficult to interpret experiments that do not use the natural agonist of the human acrosome reaction. Recent attention has been drawn to a putative biological agonist - progesterone. This steroid is in high concentration around the ovulated egg in the cumulus mass and can influence the initiation of the human acrosome reaction in a small proportion of human spermatozoa. Tesarik and colleagues have shown that progesterone acts via a surface receptor which undergoes aggregation when stimulated (21). Progesterone stimulates an increase in intracellular free calcium in the spermatozoa and Fastelli and colleagues have reported a defective increase in intracellular calcium stimulated by progesterone in 18% of men with oligozoospermia (22). Although progesterone may play a role in acrosome induction it is clear that at any one time it stimulates only a small number of sperm and the pathway of induction is separate to that caused by the human zona (23). Interestingly, Liu and colleagues have demonstrated a disordered zona pellucida induced acrosome reaction in a subgroup of patients who have normal semen parameters (24). In such patients ICSI is a suitable form of treatment. Subsequent studies using ZP material as the biological agonist of the AR are necessary to dissect the pathways involved in the AR and identify the nature of these lesions in defective spermatozoa.

One critical process of the AR is capacitation. Surprisingly, despite intensive investigation over the last three decades there is still much confusion about this process (25). It is generally accepted that exocytosis in response to zona agonists is the hallmark of acquisition of the capacitated state (10). Bovine and murine spermatozoa require a time period of incubation under capacitating conditions before they undergo a zona-induced acrosome reaction (10). In bulls for instance, ejaculated sperm required 4 hours incubation for capacitation, but after this time induction of the acrosome reaction is rapid (a half -life of less that 10 min) and is dependent on the concentration of zona pellucida protein (26). Using single cell imaging of capacitated bull spermatozoa an elevation of calcium and pH preceded the zona-induced acrosome reaction. Such changes are not observed in uncapacitated sperm.(27). Equivalent data, which are very basic to our understanding of capacitation and the zona induced human acrosome reaction are simply not available. Experiments using either solubilised zona pellucida or intact zona have all incubated sperm under capacitating conditions for a number of hours (18). Bypassing the membrane-mediated signalling mechanism in human sperm by using ionophore A23187 can induce an acrosome reaction with minimal incubation under capacitation conditions (20). This would suggest that exocytotic second messenger pathways in the sperm cytoplasm are functional at an early stage but that the agonist/receptor interaction (at the level of the plasma membrane) may require a capacitation process. Interestingly, one recent study has obtained significant levels of ZP induced AR in human spermatozoa after a minimal period of capacitation (28).

It is difficult to ascertain the relevance of the above studies on capacitation (and AR) to the in vivo transport circumstances. There is a marked paucity of data on the synchronisation and activation of spermatozoa in the human female reproductive tract. The site of the in vivo AR is yet to be determined, as is the physiological role of FF and ZP3. Recent studies in our laboratory have shown that human oviductal fluid (hOF) provides an optimal environment for sperm survival and can modulate the physiological status of spermatozoa (29, 30). For example, the follicular fluid (FF) induced acrosome reaction appears to be delayed (30) when compared to the responses of spermatozoa incubated in a simple media. This latter point is important. It suggests that either hOF acts to delay the AR in vivo (an observation in contrast to studies in bovines where BOF accelerates capacitation) or, that FF is not a physiological inducer of the AR in vivo. Interestingly a 54 kDa protein (31), has been shown to be a major component of hOF during the peri-ovulatory period (31) and binds to the acrosome of spermatozoa (32). It was suggested, although no data was presented, that this factor may act to delay the AR. The ability to use both rhZP3 and FF in the same experiment would clarify the respective roles for these agonists in inducing the 'natural' acrosome reaction *in vivo*. This is a question which remains controversial since both FF and ZP3 can stimulate high numbers of spermatozoa to acrosome react (at least during *in vitro* experiments), and both are present at the site of fertilisation.

The aims of our experiments were thus two fold (1) to express human ZP3 in several different systems enabling a comprehensive examination of the role of rhuZP3 on the human AR, and,. (2) to use biologically active rhuZP3 as a tool to investigate the role of reproductive tract fluids on sperm function with particular reference to hOF.

MATERIALS AND METHODS

Human ZP3 expression vectors

The cDNA encoding the full length human ZP3 (hu ZP3) was a generous gift from Professor J. Dean (NIDDK, USA). The polymerase chain reaction (PCR) was employed to engineer convenient restriction sites at the 5' and 3' ends of the huZP3 open reading frame (ORF) to allow insertion into the glutathione-S-transferase (GST) fusion vector pGEX-KG (33) and the mammalian expression vector pcDNA1/NEO (Invitrogen Corp., USA). *E. coli* JM109 cells were transformed with the pGEX-KG expression construct (pHZP3GEX1) and E Coli. MC1061/P3 cells (Invitrogen Corp) were transformed with the pcDNA1/NEO expression construct (pHZP3NEO1) by the method of Nishimura (34).

Protein expression in Escherichia coli

JM109 cells harbouring the plasmid pHZP3GEX1 were grown in Luria Broth (LB) at either 30 C or 37 C to mid log phase and protein expression induced by the addition of IPTG. The cells were harvested and lysates analysed by SDS-PAGE. Purification of induced GST and GST-ZP3 fusion protein was carried out by affinity chromatography as described by Guan and Dixon (33). RhuZP3 produced in *Escherichia coli* would not be in a glycosylated form. Using this form of rhuZP3 addresses the importance of glycosylation for the induction of the AR. Conventional wisdom suggests that correct glycosylation is essential, at least in the mouse (1)

Production of Polyclonal Antiserum and Western Blot Analysis

Adult male New Zealand white rabbits were immunised subcutaneously with ~5 µg of GST-ZP3 fusion protein prepared by electroelution from a preparative polyacrylamide gel as described by Harlow & Lane (35). Pre-immune serum was collected prior to immunisation. Serum was prepared from blood (35) aliquoted and stored at -20°C until required. Anti-porcine ZP3 polyclonal antiserum was a kind gift of Prof. A. Sacco, Univ. of Michigan, USA. For Western blot analysis, proteins were separated by SDS PAGE using standard procedures (36).

Cell culture and transfection

Chinese Hamster Ovary cells (CHO) were cultured in Glasgow's MEM (GMEM: GIBCO/BRL BHK21) supplemented with L-Glutamine and penicillin/streptomycin and 10% (v/v) foetal calf serum. Cells were transfected with 10 µg CsCl-pure pHZP3NEO1.1 using the $CaPO_4$ precipitation method (Sambrook et al 1989). Following incubation and selection ZP3 secreting clones were detected using either anti-porcine ZP3 antiserum (the kind gift of Prof. A. Sacco, Univ. of Michigan, USA) or anti-human GST-ZP3 antiserum. Supernatants were removed and concentrated 20-fold then subsequently stored at -20°C in 100 µl aliquots.

In vitro transcription and translation of human ZP3.

Recombinant plasmid huZP3 was used to programme a coupled *in vitro* transcription/translation extract (TNT coupled reticulocyte lysate systems, Promega, Southampton, UK) according to the manufacturers instructions. Products from the reaction were detected either by fluorography following incorporation of ^{35}S- methionine (Amersham) into newly synthesised protein or following SDS PAGE by Western blotting with anti-porcine ZP3 antiserum In order to purify the ZP3 a strep tag was attached to the C terminus. This was a 10 amino acid sequence which had a high affinity for streptavidin ($K^a = 10^{-14}$) and thus enabled the ZP3 protein to be attached to steptavidin coated agarose beads (60-130µm in diameter). Quantification of the rhuZP3 attached to beads was performed using scintillation counting. Our calculations suggest that 0.15ng of ZP3 as attached per bead. Previous experiments have demonstrated that rhuZP3 produced using the in vitro transcription and translation system is folded and has some degree of core glycosylation (37). The production of biologically active rhuZP3 using the in vitro transcription/translation system would allow rapid mutagenesis studies to be performed. It would then be possible to determine the domains of rhuZP3 for sperm binding and the AR.

Sperm preparation and detection of the AR

In order to evaluate the biological activity of recombinant ZP3, samples were tested for their ability to induce the acrosome reaction. Semen was obtained from fertile semen donors. The semen characteristics of the donors were: Sperm concentration $\geq 80 \times 10^6 ml^{-1}$, $\geq 60\%$ ideal forms, $\geq 65\%$ sperm motility (>10 µm.sec^{-1}.). Semen samples were obtained by masturbation after a period of 48-72 h sexual abstinence. Specimens were allowed to liquefy (> 30 min) at 37°C and semen analysis was performed, including analysis of sperm motion characteristics, using the Hamilton Thorn Research Motility Analyser (HTM model 2030; Hamilton Thorn Research, Danvers, MA, U.S.A.). Spermatozoa were separated using a direct swim-up technique: 0.5 ml of semen was gently overlaid with 0.5 ml Earle's balanced salt solution (EBSS; GIBCO/BRL) supplemented with human serum albumin (HSA; Sigma, Poole, Dorset UK) and incubated at 37°C in 5% CO_2 in air for 45 min. The upper half of the supernatant was carefully aspirated and sperm motility analysed (T=0). The motile sperm concentration was adjusted to ~10 x 10^6/ml. The sperm suspension was incubated (in 5% CO_2 in air at 37°C) for a further 3 h (T=3). At T=3 an aliquot was taken and added to the various controls and preparations of recombinant ZP3 as described below.

For GST-huZP3 experiments :

Semen was obtained from 9 fertile donors and spermatozoa prepared as above. Following the 3h incubation, 40 μl aliquots of capacitated spermatozoa were incubated for 15 minutes (5% CO_2 in air at 37°C) with either: GST (final volume 30% GST), GST-huZP3 (final volume 30% GST-huZP3); the ionophore A23187 (10 μM final concentration), follicular fluid (final concentration 20%) or EBSS supplemented with 3.5% HSA.

For the CHO experiments :

Semen was obtained from 9 fertile donors and spermatozoa prepared as above. Following the 3h incubation 40 μl aliquots of capacitated human spermatozoa were incubated for 15 minutes (5% CO_2 in air at 37C) with 120 μl concentrate supernatant from one of three ZP3 secreting positive clones (CHO-ZP3 final concentration 30% CHO secreting clone[1.6, 1.8, 1.12]), supernatant from cells not transfected with ZP3 (control CHO, final concentration 30%); the ionophore A23187 (10 μM final concentration); follicular fluid (final concentration 20% hFF) or EBSS supplemented with 3.5% HSA.

A23178 and hFF are well documented inducers of the acrosome reaction and were used as positive controls. Spermatozoa in EBSS, GST and CHO not expressing rhuZP3 served as negative controls. After 15 min incubation the tubes were mixed well and two 5 μl aliquots were removed and spotted onto Horwell slides for subsequent acrosome status staining. An aliquot of spermatozoa was checked for sperm motility on the HTM Analyser. Only samples with progressive motility >90% after incubation in the tests solutions were analysed for acrosomal status.

The acrosomal status of human spermatozoa was evaluated using the technique described by Zhu et al (1994b) using primary monoclonal antibody 18.6 (Moore et al 1987) and indirect immunofluorescence. Spermatozoa displaying fluorescence over the acrosome region were scored as acrosome intact. Acrosome reacted cells were those displaying fluorescence over the equatorial segment, patchy fluorescence or no fluorescence.

For the vitro transcription/translation experiments :

Spermatozoa were obtained as described above. Two different experiments were performed. Firstly spermatozoa, from 5 donors, were capacitated for 3 hours (see above) and then incubated for 30 minutes with rhuZP3 beads, biotin controls (beads coated with biotin) or uncoated beads. In the second experiment following a three hour capacitation the spermatozoa, from 12 donors, were incubated with rhuZP3 beads, biotin controls or uncoated beads for a further 18 hours. All incubations were at 37C in a 5% CO2 incubator. The AR was evaluated as above except that the HOS test was used to detect viable spermatozoa.

Role of Human Oviductal Fluid on the acrosome reaction
Spermatozoa from 5 healthy donors were isolated as follows : an aliquot of 0.2 ml semen was placed in the Eppendorf tube and gently overlaid with either 0.2 ml 100% hOF or EBSS containing HSA. Swim-ups were incubated at 37°C, in a 5% CO_2 incubator for 20-30 minutes after which approximately 150 µl of the supernatant (exhibiting a sperm motility ≥ 95% and density over 20×10^6/ml) was harvested and transferred to another tube. These supernatants were incubated for up to 3 hours at 37°C in a 5% CO_2 incubator.

Directly after swim up (0 hours) and after 3 (3 hours) of incubation, a 20 µl aliquot of each sample was challenged with either rhZP3 or FF at a final concentration of 50% and 20% respectively. As a control for rhZP3 the supernatant from CHO cells (not transfected with ZP3 - see above) was added to the sperm suspension; this was carried out at after 3 hours capacitation . After 30 minutes incubation at 37°C, 5% CO_2, an aliquot of 10 µl was removed for the measurement of sperm kinematic characteristics and another 10 µl was placed on a multispot slides for acrosomal staining. The measurement of acrosome staining have been described above (Zhu *et al.*, 1994a,b).

Hormone and Total Protein Levels in the Human Oviductal Fluid
Human oviductal fluid (hOF) was provided by Professor Lippes (State University of New York, Buffalo, USA). The hOF used in this experiment was collected from a 38 year old woman on day 17 of her menstrual cycle. This patient had no history of serious medical illness. The detailed collection of hOF has been described previously (32). The hormone levels of oestradiol (E_2) and progesterone in the hOF used in this experiment were 210 pg/ml and 2.9 ng/ml respectively. In addition, the concentration of total protein in this sample of hOF is 66 mg/ml.

RESULTS

Purification, expression and biological activity of human ZP3 expressed in Escherichia coli.
Expression and purification of the human ZP3-GST fusion protein was only possible when the *argU* gene was also expressed at higher than normal levels in the same cells. The data presented in Table 1 clearly demonstrate that bacterially expressed recombinant human ZP3 (i.e. free from post-translational modifications) does not induce the AR in capacitated human sperm.

Treatments	N[A]	% AR[B]
EBSS	9	5 (2-12)
GST	9	4 (1-19)
GST-rhuZP3	9	5 (1-20)
A23187	8	34[c] (31-63)
20% hFF	8	28[c] (22-54)

Table 1: Percentage acrosome reaction (AR) in fertile donor spermatozoa capacitated for 3 hours and then challenged for 15 minutes with GST, GST rhuZP3 fusion protein, EBSS, A 23187 or 20 % human follicular fluid (hFF). a Number of semen samples tested where progresssive motility >90% *after incubation with treatment;* [b] *Median (range);* [c] *Significantly different to EBSS, GST, GST-rhuZP3, P<0.01.*

Treatment	N[A]	% AR[B]
EBSS	9	12 (10-22)
CHO	9	14 (10-22)
CHO-rhuZP3		
1.6	9	50[c] (20-58)
1.8	9	45[c] (28-67)
1.12	9	77[d,e] (28-90)
A 23187	6	27[c] (21-60)
hFF	7	31[c] (24-40)

Table 2: Percentage acrosome reaction (% AR) in fertile donors *capacitated for 3 hours (EBSS) and then challenged for 15 minutes with supernatants from CHO cells (controls), CHO rhu.-ZP3 (CHO cells expressing ZP3), A 23187 or 20% human follicular fluid (hFF).* [a] *Number of semen samples tested where progresssive motility >90% after incubation with treatment;* [b] *Median (range);* [c] *Significantly different to EBSS and CHO P<0.01;* [d] *Significantly different to EBSS and CHO P<0.005;* [e] *Significantly different to A 23187 and hFF P<0.01;* * *Three cells lines tested (1:6, 1:8, 1:12*

Transfection, expression and biological activity of human ZP3 from transfected CHO cells.

Three cell lines were identified as secreting rhuZP3 - 1.6, 1.8 and 1.12. The supernatants from transfectants 1.6, 1.8, 1.12, when analysed by SDS-PAGE did not appear significantly different than control supernatants when stained for protein. Indeed, analysis of the supernatants is significantly hampered by the presence of excessive amounts of serum albumin. However, Western blot analysis of cell supernatants with the anti-porcine ZP3 antibody does reveal the presence of a species of M_R c.55 000.

There was no significant difference between the percentage of AR that had been incubated in control CHO supernatant compared to the EBSS control (Table 2). Both incubation with A23187 and 20% FF resulted in significantly higher percentage of acrosome reaction than controls ($P < 0.01$). However, the highest acrosome reaction levels were recorded in the samples which had been incubated with supernatants containing rhuZP3. Interestingly, there were noticeable differences between the AR in the 3 supernatants (Table2). Spermatozoa incubated in supernatant #1.12 had the highest levels of AR ($P < 0.005$ compared to controls and $P < 0.01$ compared to A23187 and 20% hFF).

In vitro transcription/translation.
Using ^{35}S-methionine for detection, a single species of molecular weight 55,000 Da is produced.

TREATMENT	N^A	% AR^B
ZP3 beads	5	7 (3-12)
Uncoated beads	5	7 (3-16)
Biotin beads	5	8 (2-18)
N° beads	5	4 (1-12)

Table 3. **Percentage live acrosome reaction (AR) in fertile donor spermatozoa** *capacitated for 3 hours and then incubated for 30 minutes with rhuZP3 attached to the beads, biotin controls, uncoated beads and no beads. ZP3 produced using the TnT in vitro transcription/translation system. a number of semen tested; b median (range). All reacted cells are live as judged using the HOS test.*

When the lysate containing in vitro translated ZP3 is analysed by Western blotting, using the anti-porcine ZP3 antibody, a species of this size is detected only when the reaction mixture is programmed with a plasmid encoding human ZP3. This is similar in molecular weight to that expressed in CHO cells. Interestingly, no significant induction in the AR were observed when capacitating the sperm for 3 hours (Table 3), however, significant induction of the AR were observed when the sperm were incubated with the ZP3 beads for 18 hours ($P < 0.01$; Table 4).

Treatment	N [A]	% AR [B]
ZP3 beads	12	53 (35-63)*
Uncoated beads	12	18 (8-44)
Biotin beads	12	19 (19-34)
N° beads	12	14 (8-24)

Table 4. **Percentage live acrosome reaction (AR) in fertile donor spermatozoa** *capacitated for 3 hours and then incubated for a further 18 hours with rhuZP3 attached to the beads, biotin controls, uncoated beads and no beads. ZP3 produced using the TnT in vitro transcription/translation system. *$P<0.01$ significantly different to other treatments (Student's t test applied after normalising the data). a number of semen samples tested;. b Median (range. All reacted cells are live as judged using the HOS test.*

Role of hOF on the AR

Spermatozoa incubated in control (EBSS) alone or hOF alone showed no increase in the AR.. RhuZP3 was a potent inducer of the acrosome reaction at both time points (Table 5), with the level of AR being significantly ($P<0.001$) higher than that observed in both control and FF challenged incubations. Interestingly, spermatozoa showed an ability to undergo the AR immediately after preparation from semen when challenged with rhZP3. In addition, a higher (although not significant) AR was observed in spermatozoa incubated in hOF and challenged with rhuZP3 compared to the EBSS controls (Table 5).

Treatment	Capacitation Time	
	0 Hours	3 Hours
EBSS	3.6 ± 0.6	6.8 ± 1.1
EBSS-ZP3	32.4 ± 4.6*	35.8 ± 7.2*
EBSS-FF	9 ± 1.4	16.6 ± 2.0
CHO		6.6 ± 1.3
HOF	4.2 ± 0.9	6.2 ± 2.0
HOF-ZP3	51.8 ± 7.2*	64.6 ± 4.2*
HOF-FF	11.4 ± 1.4	30.9 ± 9.8

Table 5: **Percentage acrosome reaction (%AR) in fertile donor spermatozoa in each treatment group.**
Capacitation times: 0 Spermatozoa obtained directly after swim up and incubated with treatments groups for 30 minutes.

3 Spermatozoa obtained directly after swim up and incubated at 37°C in a 5% CO2 incubator for 3 hours before incubation with treatment group.

EBSS: Earle's balance salt solution; HOF: human oviductal fluid, CHO: supernatant not transfected with ZP3, ZP3 Recombinant human ZP3 from CHO (1:12) cells, FF: Follicular fluid (final concentration 20%).

All data are mean ± SEM (n=5).* $P< 0.0001$ Compared with the relevant control and FF groups at same time point (Sheffe test).

DISCUSSION

This study clearly demonstrates the successful expression of rhuZP3 in CHO cells. RhuZP3 produced in the CHO system was a potent agonist of the AR (Table 2, 5). Glycosylation appears necessary for the AR as the protein backbone (produced in *Escherichia coli*) did not induce the AR at least under the experimental conditions outlined. Interestingly, a limited amount of core glycosylation of the rhuZP3 (in vitro transcripton/translation) will induce significant AR when the product is in contact with the spermatozoa for long periods (compare Table 3 and 4). These results although preliminary, clearly demonstrate the successful production of biologically active rhuZP3 in more than one form. The use of rhuZP3 will lead to more rigorous studies on human sperm egg interactions in the near future.

It was interesting that the purified bacterial fusion protein did not induce the AR in human spermatozoa. In all these experiment only fertile donors, whose spermatozoa were able to undergo an acrosome reaction *in vitro*, were used. The levels of AR were consistently low in the controls (Table 1) and each donor showed a positive response to induction with A23187 and FF, yet no induction was seen with rhuZP3 GST fusion protein. It would appear therefore that non glycosylated recombinant ZP3 does not induce the human AR. At this stage we cannot exclude other possible reasons for the inert biological properties of GST-huZP3. For example, the recombinant fusion protein may simply be incorrectly folded. Further experimental evidence, for example, deglycosylation of rhuZP3 produced from CHO cells is necessary to confirm our observations. It is of course possible that fusion of rhuZP3 to GST inhibits the activity of rhuZP3. Interestingly, the fusion of a hexahistidine tail to the N- or C terminus of human ZP3, also produced a protein which was also biologically inert i.e., no AR induction (unpublished observations Whitmarsh, Barratt, Moore & Hornby). At present we do not know if the GST fusion protein is capable of binding to the sperm membrane however, preliminary data indicates that overexpression in E Coli does induce an increase in phosphorylation of a 95 kDa membrane protein as assessed by the *in vitro* kinase assay (Brewis et al this symposium). At present we have yet to perform critical experiments to refute or accept the hypothesis that the protein backbone has no role in induction of the human AR.

Using Western blot analysis the molecular weight of the glycoprotein secreted by the transfected CHO cells was established to be approximately 55 kDa. This was a similar molecular weight to the in vitro transcription/translation product, the native zona (Hornby unpublished observations) and to glycosylated recombinant ZP3 produced by other groups (41). Shabanowitz [1990] solubilised human zona and detected ZP3 on Western blots using rabbit anti-porcine ZP and a mouse anti-human-ZP antiserum showing two distinct species, one of which had the same molecular weight as that shown in our studies. Cross reactivity of zona glycoproteins and anti-zona antisera in pigs and humans has been previously documented suggesting that ZP3 is a highly conserved glycoprotein.

It is evident that rhuZP3 is present at low levels in CHO supernatants and therefore the relatively high levels of serum albumin, which dominate the supernatant (and SDS-PAGE profiles), present a very significant hurdle in purification of the rhuZP3. Clearly not all transfected CHO cells produce rhuZP3 and, not all supernatants which appear to contain ZP3, are biologically active (similar variable results have been obtained by Van Duin and colleagues (41). At present there is an urgent need to understand this production system in more detail and obtain a purified product. Nevertheless, despite the apparent low levels of expression of rhuZP3 in the CHO supernatants, rhuZP3 from these cells can be an extremely potent inducer of the acrosome reaction compared with other known inducers (Table 3). Supernatants from CHO cells not transfected with ZP3 showed the same level of acrosome reaction as the negative controls. This data clearly indicate that biologically active rhuZP3 was produced using our system. Interestingly, subsequent studies in our laboratories using rhuZP3 produced by the CHO system have demonstrated that an AR is accompanied by an influx of calcium (42) and that rhuZP3 probably acts via a 95kDa protein at the sperm plasma membrane surface (43; Moore and colleagues - this symposium). RhuZP3 is therefore a very useful tool to investigate the AR in humans.

The high levels of acrosome reaction induced by the rhuZP3 was similar to those in spermatozoa that are bound to the zona pellucida (for example see 24) but higher than those induced by solubilised zona (19, 28, 44). It is not certain why higher percentages of acrosome reaction were recorded using rhuZP3 compared to solubilised material, however, chemical processing of the zona may alter the AR properties of the zona.

One question that our laboratory has been exploring for some time is the mythical nature of human sperm transport from the cervix to the oviduct *in vivo* (see 45; 46). Previous experiments using hOF had suggested that hOF provides an optimal milieu for sperm survival eg maintenance of progressive sperm motility and a low level of hyperactivated motility (see 29, 30). In addition, we observed a delay in the induction of the FF induced AR when sperm had been incubated in hOF. This added to the evidence that hOF (and by inference the oviduct) acts to prolong/maintain sperm function, however, the alternative hypothesis was that FF was not the natural agonist *in vivo*. Data presented in Table 5 supports the latter hypothesis and demonstrates the importance of using an appropriate agonist to study the physiological acrosome reaction It was also interesting that a highly significant induction of the AR was observed in spermatozoa that had been obtained direct from a swim up (see Table 5). This preliminary result requires confirmation yet limited data supporting this observation exist (see 28) when induction of the AR was observed using solubilised ZP in spermatozoa that had only been capacitated for a minimal period. Such results challenge the conventional wisdom that a long period of capacitation is necessary for the biological AR to occur at least in human spermatozoa. Such observations will ignite a serious debate on capacitation of human spermatozoa.

At present we are currently delineating the functional regions of rhuZP3 using the CHO system for the expression of mutant forms of human ZP3 (similar studies have been performed in the mouse - see 47). In addition, we are developing a purification procedure to obtain homogenous rhuZP3 for further detailed biochemical studies. It is likely that using these tools a greater understanding of human gamete recognition will be achieved in the near future.

Acknowledgements:
The authors would like to thank Prof. J. Dean for the provision of the human ZP3, Prof. R. Mattes for providing the argU expression plasmid, pUBS520 and Prof. A. Sacco for supplying the anti-porcine ZP3 anti-serum. Dr Ergon Pinarbassi and Alan Whitmarsh produced rhuZP3. Professor Lippes provided human oviductal fluid (hOF). The hOF experiments were performed by JJ Zhu and the AR experiments by M Woolnough, C McCann and S Clements. The Krebs Institute is a designated B.B.R.C. Centre for Biomolecular Sciences. The experiments in this study were supported by : The University of Sheffield and Infertility Research Trust.

REFERENCES

1. Wassarman P.M. Mouse gamete adhesion molecules. Biol. Reprod. 1992; 146: 86-191.
2. Hasegawa A, Koyama K, Okazaki Y, Sugimoto M, Isojima S Amino acid sequence of a porcine zona pellucida glycoprotein ZP4 determined by peptide mapping and cDNA cloning. J Reprod Fertil 1994, 100, 245-255
3. Araki Y., Orgebin-Crist M.C., Tulsiani D.R.P. Qualitative chracterisation of oligosaccharide chains present on the rat zona pellucida glycoconjugates. Biol Reprod 1992, 46, 912-919
4. Schwoebel E., Prasad S., Timmons T. M., Cook R., Kimura H., Niu E., Cheung P., Skinner S., Avery S. E., Wilkins B., Dunbar B. S. Isolation and characterisation of a full length cDNA encoding the 55 kDa rabbit zona pellucida protein. J. Biol. Chem. 1991,266: 7214-7219.
5. Kinloch R.A., Mortillo S.A., Stewart C.L., Wassarman P.M. Embryonal carcinoma cells transfected with ZP3 genes differentially glycosylate similar polypeptides and secrete active mouse sperm receptor. J Cell Biol. 1991; 115:655-664.
6. Beebe S.J., Leyton L., Burks P., Ishikanau A., Fuerst T., Dean J., Saling P.M. Recombinant mouse ZP3 inhibits sperm binding and induces the acrosome reaction. Devl. Biol.1992; 151:, 48-54.
7. Prasad SV, Mujtaba S, Lee VH & Dunbar BS. Immunogenicity enhancement of recombinant rabbit 55-kilodalton zona pellucida protein expressed using the baccilovirus expression system. Biol Reprod 1995, 52, 1167-1178
8. Yurewicz E.C., Pack B.A., Sacco A.G. Porcine oocyte zona pellucida Mr 55,000 glycoproteins identification of O glysosylated domains Mol. Reprod. Dev. 1992; 33:, 182-188.
9. Taya T, Yamasaki N Tsubamato H, Hasegawa A, Koyama K. Cloning of a cDNA coding for the porcince zona pellucida glycoprotein ZP1 and its genomic organisation. Biochem Bioph Res Co 1995,207, 790-799
10. Storey B.T. Sperm capacitation and the acrosome reaction. P Natl Acad Sci USA 637, 459-473
11. Tulsiani D.R.P., Nahdas S.K., Cornwall G.A., Orgebin-Crist M.C. Evidence for the presence of high-mannose/hybrid oligosaccharide chain(s) on the mouse ZP2 and ZP3. Biol.Reprod 1992, 46: 93-100
12. Miller D.J., Macek M.B., Shur B.D. Complementarity between sperm surface -β1,4-galactosyl-transferase and egg-coat ZP3 mediates sperm-egg binding. Nature 1992, 357:589-593
13. Florman H.M., Wassarman P.M. O-linked oligosaccharides of mouse egg ZP3 account for its sperm receptor activity. 1985, 41: 313-324.

14. Leyton L., Saling P.M. vidence that aggregation of mouse sperm receptors by ZP3 triggers the acrosome reaction. J. Cell Biol. 1989, 108: 148-157.
15. Ringuette M.J., Chamberlin M.E., Baur A.W., Sobieski D.A., Dean J. Molecular analysis of cDNA coding for ZP3, a sperm binding protein of the mouse zona pellucida. Dev. Biol.1988; 127: 287-295.
16. Chamberlin M.E., Dean J. Human homolog of the mouse sperm receptor. Proc. Natn. Acad. Sci. U.S.A. 1990,87: 6014-6018.
17. Liang L. F., Chamow S. M., Dean J. Oocyte specific expression of mouse ZP-2: Developmental regulation of the zona pellucida genes. Mol. Cell Biol. 1990, 108: 148-157.
18. Cross N.L., Morales P., Overstreet J.W., Hanson F.W. Induction of the acrosome reaction by human zonae pellucida. Biol. Reprod. 1988, 38: 235-244.
19. Bielfeld P., Zaneveld L.J.D, De Jonge C.J. The zona pellucida induced acrosome reaction of human spermatozoa is mediated by protein kinases. Fertil Steril 1994, 61, 536-541
20. De Jonge CJ. The diagnostic significance of the induced acrosome reaction Reproductive Medicine Review 1994, 3:159-178
21. Tesarik J. Mendoza C, Moos J, Fenichel P, Fehlmann M. Progesterone action through aggregation of a receptor on the sperm plasma membrane. FEBS letters 1992, 308:116-120
22. Fastelli C, Baldi E, Krausz C, Casano R, Failli P, Forte. Decreased responsiveness to progesterone of spermatozoa in oligozoospermic patients. J Androl 1993,14: 17-22
23. Tesarik J, Carreras A, Mendoza C. Differential sensitivity of progesterone- and zona pellucida-induced acrosome reactions to pertussis toxin. Mol Reprod Dev 1993;34:183-189.
24. Liu D.Y., Bourne H., Baker H.W.G. Fertilisation and pregnancy with acrosome intact sperm by intracytoplasmic sperm injection in patients with a disordered zona pellucida-induced acrosome reaction. Fertil Steril 1995, 64:116-121
25. Yanagimachi R. (1994) Mammalian fertilization. In Knobil,E. and Neill,J.D. (eds),*The Physiology of Reproduction*. Raven Press Ltd, New York, pp. 189-317.
26. Florman H.M., First N.L. The regulation of acrosomal exocytosis. I. Sperm capacitation is required for induction of acrosome reactions by bovine zona pellucida on vitro. Dev Biol 1988, 128: 453-463
27. Florman H.M., Babcock D.F. (1990) In: Elements of Mammalian Fertilisation. 1 Basic Concepts PM Wassarman (Ed) 105-132 CRC Press Boca Ratan FL.

28. Bielfeld P., Anderson R.A., Mack S.R., De Jonge C.J., Zaneveld L.J.D. Are capacitation or calcium ion influx required for the human sperm acrosome reaction ? Fertil. Steril 1994, 62:1255 - 1261.
29. Zhu J.J., Barratt C.L.R., Lippes J., Pacey A.A., Lenton E.A., Cooke I.D. Human Oviductal Fluid Prolongs Sperm Survival. Fertil. Steril. 1994, 61: 360-366.
30. Zhu J.J., Barratt C.L.R., Lippes J., Pacey A.A., Cooke I.D. The sequential effect of human cervical mucus, oviductal and follicular fluid on sperm function. Fertil.Steril. 1994, 61, 1129-1135.
31. Wagh P.V., Lippes J. Human oviductal fluid proteins. III. Identification and partial purification. Fertil. Steril. 1989, 51: 81-88.
32. Lippes J., Wagh P. Human oviductal fluid (HOF) protein. IV. Evidence for HOF proteins binding to human sperm. Fertil. Steril, 1989, 53: 89-94.
33. Guan K., Dixon J.E. Eukaryotic proteins expressed in E Coli : An improved thrombin cleavage and purification procedure of fusion proteins with glutathione - S - Transferase. Anal. Biochem. 1991, 192: 262-267
34. Nishimura Y., Morita P., Nishimura Y., Sugino Y. A rapid and highlyy efficient method for the preparation of competent *Eschericia Coli* cells. Nucl. Acid Res.1990; 18: 6169.
35. Harlow E., Lane D. (1988) Antibodies. A laboratory Manual. Cold Spring Harbor Laboratory. Cold Spring Harbor Press, New York.
36. Sambrook J., Fritsch E. F., Maniatis T. (1989) Cold Spring Harbour Laboratory, Cold Spring Harbour Press, New York.
37. Whitmarsh A., Barratt C.L.R., Moore H.D.M., Hornby D.P. Structural features of recombinant human zona pellucida proteins ZP2 and ZP3. Hum Reprod 1994 (Abstract) Supplement #134
38. Moore H.D.M., Smith C.A., Hartman T.D, Bye A.P. Visualisation and characterisation of the acrosome reaction of human spermatozoa by immunolocalisation with monoclonal antibodies. Gam. Res. 1987; 17: 245-259.
39. Lippes J., Enders R.G., Pragay D.A., Bartholomew W.R. The collection and analysis of human fallopian tube fluid. Contraception 1972, 5, 85-103.
40. Shabanowitz R.B. Mouse antibodies to human zona pellucida. Evidence that human ZP3 is strongly immunogenic and contains two distinct isomer chains. Biol. Reprod. 1990, 43: 260-270.
41. Van Duin M., Ploman J.E.M., De. Breet I.T.M., Van Ginneken K., Bunschoten H., Grootenhuis A., Brindle J., Aitken R.J. Recombinant human zona pellucida protein ZP3 produced by Chinese hamster ovary cells induces the human sperm acrosome reaction and promotes sperm-egg fusion. Biol. Reprod. 1994, 51 607-617.

42. Brewis IA Barratt CLR Hornby DPH, Moore HDM. The signal transduction pathway of the acrosome reaction in response to recombinant ZP3 involves phorphorylation of a receptor kinase and a rapid influx of Ca^{2+} into human spermatozoa. J Reprod Fertil, 1995 Abstract Series #6
43. Moore HDM Clayton RA Barratt CLR, Hornby DP. Induction of the acrosome reaction in capacitated human spermatozoa with recombinant human ZP3 is associated with a 95kDa phosphotyrosine epitope and is inhibited with a specific monoclonal antibody. J Reprod Fertil 1995, Abstract Series #7
44. Lee M.A., Check JH, Kopf GS. A guanine nucleotide-binding regulatory proein in human sperm mediates acrosomal exocytosis induced by the human zona pellucida. Mol Reprod Dev 1992, 31:78-86
45. Williams M., Hill C.J., Scudamore I., Dunphy B., Cooke I.D., Barratt C.L.R. Sperm numbers and distribution within the human fallopian tube around ovulation. Hum Reprod 1993, 8:2014-2026
46. Pacey AA, Hill CJ, Scudamore I, Warren MA, Barratt CLR, Cooke ID. The interaction in vitro of human spermatozoa wuth epithelial cells from the human uterine tube. Hum Reprod 1995
47. Kinloch RA, Sakai Y, Wassarman PM. Mapping the mouse ZP3 combining sites for sperm by exon swapping and site-directed mutagenesis Proc Natl Acad Sci USA 1995,92:263-267

Human sperm acrosome reaction. Eds P. Fénichel, J. Parinaud.
Colloque INSERM/John Libbey Eurotext Ltd © 1995. Vol. 236, pp. 123-132.

The role of proteases in the mammalian sperm acrosome reaction

Jan Tesarik

American Hospital of Paris, 63, boulevard Victor Hugo, 92202 Neuilly-sur-Seine, France

ABSTRACT

The acrosome reaction combines the characteristics of a receptor-mediated cellular response and of a membrane-fusion exocytotic event. This distinction is useful to interpret data about the role of proteases in this complex reaction. An acrosin-like serine protease of seminal vesicle origin is immobilized on the plasma membrane covering the sperm acrosome. This protease is activated by a high molecular weight glycoprotein of the cumulus oophorus and potentiates the acrosome reaction-inducing action of progesterone, probably by locally releasing high concentrations of free progesterone from corticosteroid-binding globulin with which this steroid is complexed in the cumulus oophorus and follicular fluid. Effects of this protease on the action of ZP3, the other physiological acrosome reaction inducer, and on the function of corresponding receptors at the sperm surface are possible, but experimental data are lacking. On the other hand, unlike some nonmammalian species, proteases do not appear to be involved in the membrane fusion processes in mammalian spermatozoa. Some known effects of protease inhibitors on the acrosome reaction are attributable to the implication of proteases in postfusion events.

La réaction acrosomique est à la fois une réponse cellulaire contrôlée par des récepteurs et un phénomène d'exocytose impliquant la fusion membranaire. Cette distinction est utile pour comprendre les données existantes sur le rôle des protéases dans ce processus complexe. Une sérine protéase analogue à l'acrosine mais sécrétée par les vésicules séminales se fixe sur la membrane plasmique couvrant l'acrosome du spermatozoïde. Après l'activation par une glycoprotéine de haut poids moléculaire du cumulus oophorus, elle augmente l'effet de la progestérone sur la réaction acrosomique, probablement en provoquant la libération locale de la progestérone de sa liaison avec des protéines de transport augmentant la concentration de progestérone libre. Il est aussi possible que cette protéase influence l'action de la ZP3, l'autre inducteur physiologique de la réaction acrosomique, et la fonction des récepteurs correspondants sur la surface du spermatozoïde, mais ces possibilités restent à démontrer. D'autre part, le mécanisme interne de la fusion membranaire pendant la réaction acrosomique chez les mammifères n'implique pas selon toute probabilité l'action de protéases. Certains effets des inhibiteurs de protéases sur la réaction acrosomique peuvent être expliqués par une interférence avec des phenomènes qui suivent la fusion membranaire.

INTRODUCTION

The acrosome reaction (AR) is an exocytotic membrane fusion event, indispensable for fertilization, which is triggered in the sperm cell by agonists associated with the oocyte. Proteases are known to be implicated in membrane fusion processes in many other cell types, such as myoblasts (1) mast cells and adrenal chromaffin cells (2), and proteolysis has been suggested to be a universal component of the membrane fusion mechanism (3, 4). In agreement with this presumption, proteases were also supposed to be involved in the sperm AR. Indeed, Farach et al. (5) have presented evidence suggesting a role of metalloendoproteases in the AR of sea urchin spermatozoa. However, data obtained with mammalian spermatozoa were contradictory. So, a proteolytic activity has been shown to be involved in the membrane fusion events of the hamster sperm AR (6, 7), whereas other studies, using mouse and guinea pig spermatozoa, suggested that a trypsin-like protease activity is only required for the dispersal of acrosomal matrix and not for the preceding membrane fusion events (8-12).

These apparent discrepancies may be related to the fact that the AR is not only a membrane fusion process but also a complex cell signaling event which is subject to various control mechanisms implying different ligand-receptor systems and signal transduction pathways. Because none of the above experimental studies performed with mammalian spermatozoa dealt with the physiological AR and all used different stimuli that acted at different levels of individual signalling pathways, the inconsistencies between data may have been caused by the fact that some of the stimuli acted upstream and others downstream of the protease-sensitive events.

In this chapter, I will review the elements of the mammalian sperm AR mechanism that are potential targets to protease action. This conceptual scheme will be used to interpret pertinent experimental data.

MECHANISM OF THE ACROSOME REACTION

Detailed descriptions of individual components of the AR mechanism can be found in the corresponding chapters of this book. Here I only will recall the necessary minimum to put a frame to the protease issue.

The AR combines the characteristics of a receptor-mediated cellular response and of a membrane fusion process. When looked at as the former, the AR is an example of a multiligand multireceptor response showing both convergences and divergences at several levels of the corresponding signalling pathways. Two physiological AR-inducing agonists have been characterized, progesterone (13) and a zona pellucida glycoprotein termed ZP3 (14). Both agonists act in concert so that progesterone, present in a high concentration (~10 μM) in the cumulus oophorus with which the fertilizing spermatozoon comes in contact first, potentiates the subsequent action of ZP3 (15, 16). Progesterone has been shown to induce an influx of extracellular calcium ions into spermatozoa (17, 18), to provoke transmembrane chloride fluxes sensitive to certain antagonists of neuronal g-aminobutyric acid receptor type A (19, 20) and to activate, presumably in a calcium-independent manner, a sperm protein tyrosine kinase (21, 22). Solubilized zona pellucida material has been shown to provoke calcium influx into spermatozoa (23) and to stimulate tyrosine phosphorylation of a ~94 kDa protein in mouse (24) and human (25) spermatozoa. Ligand-induced receptor aggregation is believed to be involved in this latter response (26). Moreover, progesterone also produces aggregation of a sperm surface receptor (27, 28) and stimulates tyrosine phosphorylation of a ~94 kDa protein which appears to be the same as that phosphorylated in response to the zona pellucida (21). The progesterone-induced opening of a plasma membrane calcium channel and the stimulation of protein tyrosine kinase occur independently of each other and appear to be mediated by different types of receptors (29).

The signalling pathways that transduce the ligand-generated message to effectors of the AR also involve G proteins, cAMP, phospholipases A and C, and possibly protein kinase C although the presence of this enzyme in spermatozoa is still controversial (reviewed in 30). The ways the individual signalling pathways interact with each other are understood poorly although the existence of such interactions has been demonstrated. Anyway, these postreceptors signalling events are not supposed to be exposed to protease regulation and will thus not be dealt with in this chapter.

Having passed the intracellular part of the way, the AR-inducing signal reemerges as it attains the components of the sperm plasma membrane whose modification entails membrane fusion. From this time point, the AR can be looked at as an ordinary membrane fusion event (Fig. 1).

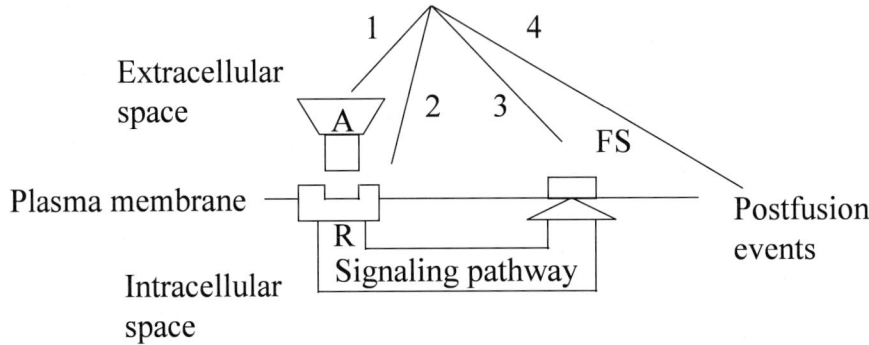

Figure 1. **Schematic representation of possible targets for protease action during the AR.** *The mechanism of the AR is illustrated in a simplified way so as to imply a single receptor (R) which, upon activation by agonist (A), transduces the message through a signalling pathway to a membrane fusion system (FS) responsible for exocytosis. The possible targets of protease action thus involve the agonist (1), the receptor (2), the membrane fusion system (3) and postfusion events (4) but exclude the intracellular loop of the signalling cascade.*

TARGETS FOR PROTEASE ACTION IN THE ACROSOME REACTION MECHANISM

From the above overview it is evident that proteases may intervene at the receptor level, by acting on the agonist, on the receptor or on both, and then again downstream of the intracellular loop of the signal transduction cascade, by modifying directly the membrane fusion process (Fig. 1).

Processing of receptor agonists

Progesterone that is present in the cumulus oophorus and follicular fluid is not free but is associated with a protein of ~50 kDa (13). This protein, isolated from the human cumulus oophorus, has been shown recently to be identical with corticosteroid-binding globulin (31). Progesterone is supposed to react with receptors of protein nature in the sperm plasma membrane. As a relatively small molecule, progesterone is unlikely to be able to bind durably two proteins at the same time. It is thus probable that progesterone must be released from corticosteroid-binding globulin to become fully active. This function would be best served by a protease immobilized at the sperm plasma membrane which would release high concentrations of free progesterone in the vicinity of the receptor. A protease showing the same immunoreactivity as acrosin has in fact been detected bound to the plasma membrane covering the acrosomal region of human spermatozoa (32, 33). A recent study has shown that this acrosin-like protease is probably not of acrosomal origin, although it resembles acrosin in structure and function, and that it is secreted by the seminal vesicles (34). As it is known that a high molecular weight glycoprotein of the cumulus extracellular matrix acts as a potent acrosin activator (35), the contact of spermatozoa with the cumulus matrix is likely to entail activation of the acrosin-like protease on the sperm surface. This protease, in its turn, can be expected to cleave corticosteroid-binding globulin in the cumulus matrix and thus release high local concentration of free progesterone (Fig. 2). However, the action of the acrosin-like protease is probably more complex because its activation also potentiates the action of free progesterone added to spermatozoa (35).

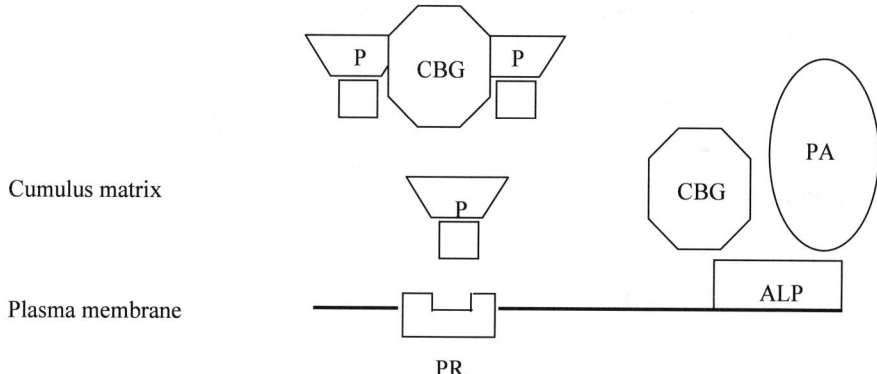

Figure 2. **Schematic representation of a probable mechanism by which a sperm-surface acrosin-like protease (ALP) potentiates the AR-inducing action of progesterone (P).** *A proacrosin activator (PA) from the cumulus extracellular matrix activates ALP which, in its turn, cleaves corticosteroid-binding globulin (CBG), the main P-binding protein of the cumulus matrix. This leads to a release of high concentrations of free P in the close vicinity of the sperm surface progesterone receptor (PR). Based on data from references 31-34.*

Little is known about the relationship between the proteolytic cleavage of ZP3 by sperm surface-associated proteases and the function of ZP3 as an AR-inducing agent. Previous studies have shown that the ZP3 peptide chain must be intact to exert its ligand activity (reviewed in 30). It remains to be elucidated whether and how proteases immobilized on the sperm plasma membrane modify the function of ZP3 subsequent to receptor binding.

Unmasking and processing of cell surface receptors
The removal of sperm surface components which occurs during sperm passage through the female genital tract or during in vitro incubation in appropriate culture media is known to be required for spermatozoa to achieve full functional capacity. It is supposed that this process leads to unmasking of functional epitopes that have previously been protected from premature activation by components of the surface coat. However, it is not clear whether proteolysis participates in any significant way in this unmasking process.

Limited proteolysis may also be part of the final processing of receptors, ion channels or membrane-associated enzymes on the sperm surface (36). Here again, experimental evidence is lacking but the matter surely deserves attention. It has been shown that the addition of external soluble proteases destroys easily progesterone-binding sites on the human sperm surface (28). Thus, if proteases do play a role in the receptor processing, their action must be highly selective and regulated.

Intracellular loop of the signal transduction pathway
The sperm cytoplasm is devoid of primary lysosomes and all proteolytic enzymes are packaged in the acrosome, an organelle functionally analogous to secretory granules of exocrine gland cells. The possibility of protease involvement in processes such as receptor recycling or postreceptor signal transduction events is thus highly improbable. Although a bovine sperm protease, recently identified as acrosin, has been shown to activate adenylyl cyclases of rat brain and human platelets (37), an implication of this activity in the mechanism of the AR has not been demonstrated.

Intrinsic mechanism of membrane fusion
Proteolysis of membrane proteins by metalloendoproteases has ben suggested to be required for membrane fusion (3, 4). Metalloendoproteases do appear to be involved in the AR of sea urchin spermatozoa (5). However, there are convincing data suggesting that this is not the case of mammalian spermatozoa (8-12, 38). However, some other data suggest the contrary (6, 7), and metalloendoproteases have been detected in hamster, pig and human spermatozoa (39).

Dispersion of acrosomal matrix

In addition to a battery of hydrolytic enzymes, the sperm acrosome contains matrix that is involved in the packaging of the acrosomal enzymes in a stable and spatially ordered fashion and in the regulation of their release and activation during the AR. Acrosin-binding proteins are the most extensively studied components of the acrosomal matrix (40-42). Owing to the presence of acrosomal matrix proteins, the solubilization of the acrosomal enzymes after the opening of the acrosome during the AR is slowed down, and the release of individual enzymes is sequential and gradual (40-42). The dispersion of the acrosomal matrix has been shown to be promoted by acrosomal proteases, particularly by acrosin (40-42), and this process can be efficiently inhibited by serine protease inhibitors (8-12) but not metalloendoprotease, acid protease and exopeptidase inhibitors (12).

Preparation of sperm plasma membrane for sperm-oocyte fusion

The development of the sperm ability to fuse with the oocyte is another phenomenon strictly linked to the AR (30). This process concerns the equatorial region of the sperm head where the plasma membrane remains intact after the completion of the AR and where the fusion with the oocyte plasma membrane is initiated. What exactly occurs to the plasma membrane covering the equatorial region during the acrosome reaction to render it fusogenic is not known. However, some data indicate that proteases, and acrosin in particular, are somehow involved in this process (43).

REFERENCES

1. Couch CB, Strittmatter WJ. Rat myoblast fusion requires metalloendoprotease activity. Cell 1983; 32:257-65.
2. Mundy DI, Strittmatter WJ. Requirement for metalloendoprotease in exocytosis: Evidence in mast cells and adrenal chromaffin cells. Cell 1985; 40:645-56.
3. Lucy JA. Do hydrophobic sequences cleaved from cellular polypeptides induce membrane fusion reactions in vivo? FEBS Lett 1984; 166:223-31.
4. Lennarz WJ, Strittmatter WJ. Cellular functions of metallo-endoproteases. Biochim Biophys Acta 1991; 1071:149-58.
5. Farach HA, Mundy DI, Strittmatter WJ, Lennarz WJ. Evidence for the involvement of metalloendoproteases in the acrosome reaction in sea urchin sperm. J Biol Chem 1987; 262:5483-7.
6. Dravland JE, Llanos MN, Munn RJ, Meizel S. Evidence for the involvement of a sperm trypsinlike enzyme in the membrane events of the hamster sperm acrosome reaction. J Exp Zool 1984; 232:117-28.

7. Meizel S. The importance of hydrolytic enzymes to an exocytotic event, the mammalian sperm acrosome reaction. Biol Rev 1984; 59:125-57.
8. Green DPL. The activation of proteolysis in the acrosome reaction of guinea-pig sperm. J Cell Sci 1978; 32:177-84.
9. Fraser LR. p-Aminobenzamidine, an acrosin inhibitor, inhibits mouse sperm penetration of the zona pellucida but not the acrosome reaction. J Reprod Fertil 1982; 65:185-94.
10. Perreault SD, Zirkin BR, Rogers BJ. Effect of trypsin inhibitors on acrosome reaction of guinea pig spermatozoa. Biol Reprod 1982; 26:343-51.
11. Huang TTF, Hardy D, Yanagimachi H, Teuscher C, Tung K, Wild G, Yanagimachi R. pH and proteinase control of acrosomal content stasis and release during the guinea pig acrosome reaction. Biol Reprod 1985; 32:451-62.
12. Flaherty SP, Swann NJ. Proteases are not involved in the membrane fusion events of the lysolecithin-mediated guinea pig sperm acrosome reaction. J Cell Sci 1993; 104:163-72.
13. Osman RA, Andria ML, Jones DA, Meizel S. Steroid induced exocytosis: the human sperm acrosome reaction. Biochem Biophys Res Commun 1989; 160:828-33.
14. Bleil JD, Wassarman PM. Sperm-egg interactions in the mouse: sequence of events and induction of the acrosome reaction by a zona pellucida glycoprotein. Dev Biol 1983; 95:317-24.
15. Roldan ERS, Murase T, Shi Q-X. Exocytosis in spermatozoa in response to progesterone and zona pellucida. Science 1994; 266:1578-81.
16. Melendrez CS, Meizel S, Berger T. Comparison of the ability of progesterone and heat solubilized porcine zona pellucida to initiate the porcine sperm acrosome reaction in vitro. Mol Reprod Dev 1994; 39:433-8.
17. Thomas P, Meizel S. Phosphatidylinositol 4,5-biphosphate hydrolysis in human sperm stimulated with follicular fluid or progesterone is dependent on Ca^{2+} influx. Biochem J 1989; 264:539-46.
18. Blackmore PF, Beebe SJ, Danforth DR, Alexander N. Progesterone and 17a-hydroxyprogesterone novel stimulators of calcium influx in human sperm. J Biol Chem 1990; 265:1376-80.
19. Wistrom CA, Meizel S. Evidence suggesting involvement of a unique human sperm steroid receptor/Cl$^-$ channel complex in the progesterone-initiated acrosome reaction. Dev Biol 1993; 159:679-90.
20. Blackmore PF, Im WB, Bleasdale JE. The cell surface progesterone receptor which stimulates calcium influx in human sperm is unlike the A

ring reduced steroid site on the GABAA receptor/chloride channel. Mol Cell Endocrinol 1994; 104:237-43.
21. Tesarik J, Moos J, Mendoza C. Stimulation of protein tyrosine phosphorylation by a progesterone receptor on the cell surface of human sperm. Endocrinology 1993; 133:328-35.
22. Luconi M, Bonaccorsi L, Krausz C, Gervasi G, Forti G, Baldi E. Stimulation of protein tyrosine phosphorylation by platelet-activating factor and progesterone in human spermatozoa. Mol Cell Endocrinol 1995; 108:35-42.
23. Florman HM, Tombes RM, First NL, Babcock DF. An adhesion-associated agonist from the zona pellucida activates G protein-promoted elevation of internal calcium and pH that mediate mammalian sperm acrosomal exocytosis. Dev Biol 1989; 135:133-6.
24. Leyton L, Saling P. 95 kd sperm proteins bind ZP3 and serve as tyrosine kinase substrates in response to zona binding. Cell 1989; 57:1123-30.
25. Naz RK, Ahmad K, Kumar R. Role of membrane phosphotyrosine proteins in human spermatozoal function. J Cell Sci 1991; 99:157-65.
26. Leyton L, Saling PM. Evidence that aggregation of mouse sperm receptors by ZP3 triggers the acrosome reaction. J Cell Biol 1989; 108:2163-8.
27. Tesarik J, Mendoza C, Moos J, Fénichel P, Fehlmann M. Progesterone action through aggregation of a receptor on the sperm plasma membrane. FEBS Lett 1992; 308:116-20.
28. Tesarik J, Mendoza C. Insights into the function of a sperm-surface progesterone receptor: Evidence of ligand-induced receptor aggregation and the implication of proteolysis. Exp Cell Res 1993; 205:111-7.
29. Mendoza C, Soler A, Tesarik J. Nongenomic steroid action: Independent targeting of a plasma membrane calcium channel and a tyrosine kinase. Biochem Biophys Res Commun 1995; in press.
30. Yanagimachi R. Mammalian fertilization. In: Knobil E, Neill JD, eds. The Physiology of Reproduction, Second Edition. New York: Raven Press, 1994:189-317.
31. Miska W, Fehl P, Henkel R. Biochemical and immunological characterization of the acrosome reaction-inducing substance (ARIS) of HFF. Biochem Biophys Res Commun 1994; 199:125-9.
32. Tesarik J, Drahorad J, Peknicova J. Subcellular immunochemical localization of acrosin in human spermatozoa during the acrosome reaction and zona pellucida penetration. Fertil Steril 1988; 50:133-41.
33. Tesarik J, Drahorad J, Testart J, Mendoza C. Acrosin activation follows its surface exposure and precedes membrane fusion in human sperm acrosome reaction. Development 1990; 110:391-400.

34. Cechova D, Jonakova V, Veselsky L, Töpfer-Petersen E. Serine protease activity in boar seminal vesicles and its immunological similarity to sperm acrosin. J Reprod Fertil 1994; 100:461-7.
35. Mendoza C, Moos J, Tesarik J. Progesterone action on the human sperm surface is potentiated by an egg-associated acrosin activator. FEBS Lett 1993; 326:149-52.
36. Moos J, Peknicova J, Tesarik J. Relationship between molecular conversions of acrosin and the progression of exocytosis in the calcium ionophore-induced acrosome reaction. Biochim Biophys Acta 1993; 1176:199-207.
37. Adeniran AJ, Shoshani I, Minuth M, Awad JA, Elce JS, Johnson RA. Purification, characterization, and N-terminal amino acid sequence of the adenylyl cyclase-activating protease from bovine sperm. Biol Reprod 1995; 52:490-9.
38. Diaz-Perez E, Thomas P, Meizel S. Evidence suggesting a role for human sperm metalloendoprotease activity in penetration of zona-free hamster eggs by human sperm. J Exp Zool 1988; 248:213-21.
39. Gottlieb W, Meizel S. Biochemical studies of metalloendoprotease activity in the spermatozoa of three mammalian species. J Androl 1987; 8:14-24.
40. Hardy DM, Oda MN, Friend DS, Huang TTF. A mechanism for differential release of acrosomal enzymes during the acrosome reaction. Biochem J 1991; 275:759-66.
41. Moos J, Peknicova J, Tesarik J. Protein-protein interactions controlling acrosin release and solubilization during the boar sperm acrosome reaction. Biol Reprod 1993; 49:408-15.
42. Baba T, Niida Y, Michikawa Y, Kashiwabara S, Kodaira K, Takenaka M, Kohno N, Gerton GL, Arai Y. An acrosomal protein, sp32, in mammalian sperm is a binding protein specific for two proacrosins and an acrosin intermediate. J Biol Chem 1994; 269:10133-40.
43. Takano H, Yanagimachi R, Urch UA. Evidence that acrosin activity is important for the development of fusibility of mammalian spermatozoa with the oolemma: inhibitor studies using the golden hamster. Zygote 1993; 1:79-91.

Role of the acrosome reaction in egg vestments and plasma membrane penetration

Patricio Morales and Miguel Llanos

P. Catholic University of Chile, Faculty of Biological Sciences, P.O. Box 114-D and INTA, University of Chile, P.O. Box 138-11, Santiago, Chile

Abstract

The current knowledge about egg vestments and membrane penetration indicates that the fertilizing human spermatozoon could traverse the cumulus oophorus using the hyaluronidase activity present in the protein PH20, located on the posterior head plasma membrane. Then, the fertilizing spermatozoon, with its acrosome intact, binds to the zona pellucida glycoprotein ZP3, and undergoes the acrosome reaction on the zona surface, stimulated by ZP3. We present evidences that human spermatozoa possess trypsin- and chymotrypsin-like activities involved in the zona-induced acrosome reaction. The acrosome reacted spermatozoon then penetrate the zona matrix by mean of a sequential process that may involve interaction with ZP2 and hydrolytic activity. As a result of the acrosome reaction, the plasma membrane over the equatorial segment acquires fusogenic activity. Once in the perivitelline space, the spermatozoon contacts the oocyte plasma membrane using some poorly known adhesion molecules present on the equatorial segment. Variations of this general pattern are presented and discussed.

Les connaissances actuelles sur les enveloppes de l'oeuf et la pénétration des membranes indiquent que le spermatozoïde humain fécondant pourrait traverser le cumulus oophorus à l'aide de l'activité hyaluronidase présente dans la protéine PH20, localisée sur la partie postérieure de la membrane plasmique de la tête du spermatozoïde. Ainsi le spermatozoïde fécondant, avec son acrosome intact, se lie à ZP3 (glycoprotéine de la zone pellucide) et effectue sa réaction acrosomique, induite par la ZP3 au contact de la zone pellucide. Nous démontrons ici que le spermatozoïde humain possède une activité trypsine et chymotrypsine-like impliquée dans l'induction de la réaction acrosomique par la zone pellucide. Le spermatozoïde pénètre la matrice zonale par l'intermédiaire d'un processus séquentiel qui pourrait impliquer l'interaction avec ZP2 et une activité hydrolitique. A l'issue de la réaction acrosomique, la cape post-acrosomique acquiert des propriétés fusiogéniques. Parvenu dans l'espace périvitellin, le spermatozoïde entre en contact avec la membrane plasmique ovocytaire à l'aide de molécules d'adhésion, encore mal connues, présentes sur le segment équatorial. Les variations de ce schéma général sont présentées et discutées.

INTRODUCTION

Mammalian sperm are not able to fertilize an oocyte upon ejaculation. First, they must undergo a scarcely understood process, termed capacitation, either in vivo or in vitro before gaining fertilizing ability. Since we lack a reliable marker for capacitation, it is considered that this process is completed when the spermatozoa are able to undergo an exocytotic event known as the acrosome reaction (AR). The AR has become then one of the best studied events in the process of fertilization. Fertilization is a very complex phenomenon, involving sequential interactions between the fertilizing spermatozoon and cumulus oophorus, zona pellucida and oolemma. The AR may be playing a key role in sperm penetration through these egg vestments. The aim of the present work is to summarize the current knowledge about the status of the acrosome during sperm and egg vestment interactions in humans.

SPERM INTERACTION WITH THE CUMULUS OOPHORUS

The cumulus oophorus is composed of cells and their matrix. The major component of the matrix is a polymerized hyaluronic acid that is conjugated with proteins. The matrix is secreted by cumulus cells during resumption of meiosis, causing a rapid expansion of the cumulus before ovulation (1). In electron micrographs, the matrix of the fully expanded cumulus appears as a fibrous network among cumulus cells (2).

Role of sperm capacitation.
Fertilization of human oocytes in vivo occurs before the dispersal of the cumulus cells (3). Therefore, the fertilizing spermatozoon must penetrate

through this egg vestment to reach the zona pellucida and then fuse with the oolemma. To do so, the sperm of most mammals must be already capacitated (4) and with its acrosome intact, since acrosome reacted sperm cannot penetrate the cumulus oophorus (5). In humans, however, this description may not be accurate, since White et al. (6) reported that sperm washed briefly after ejaculation, without the benefit of a formal capacitation period, readily penetrated the cumulus oophorus. However, they admitted the possibility that a small percentage of the sperm could have been capacitated before insemination. The requirement for sperm capacitation for cumulus penetration is still unsolved in humans.

Role of the AR.
The next question that arises is how do the sperm pass through the cumulus to reach the surface of the ZP? Does the AR occur while the sperm are traversing the cumulus? Are the acrosomal enzymes involved in this process? The mechanism by which acrosomal enzymes are released from spermatozoa is thought to be by fenestration of the membranes during the AR. If acrosomal enzymes are essential for sperm passage through the cumulus, we would expect that all the spermatozoa within the cumulus would have reacting or reacted acrosomes. The literature on this subject is scarce and ambiguous. Acrosome reacted and acrosome intact sperm were seen in the cumulus and entering the zona of eggs fixed at different periods after in vitro insemination (7, 8). Chen and Sathananthan (7) found that only 10-30% of human sperm reaching the zona of cumulus-invested oocytes had acrosome reacted to some degree 1 hr after insemination, and that at 2-3 hr 30-60% were undergoing the AR within the cumulus as well as on the zona surface. On the other hand, Soupart and Strong (9) and Tsuiki et al. (10) found only sperm with reacting or reacted acrosomes in the cumulus or corona cells. In the work of Soupart and Strong (9) the eggs were observed 24 hr after insemination; Tsuiki et al. (10) did not report the time after insemination at which the eggs were observed. It is quite possible that the sperm observed within the cumulus matrix by the latest groups of investigators (9, 10) may have been there for many hours and underwent the AR as a consequence of sperm senescence. Regarding the ability of the cumulus to induce the AR in vitro, there are contradicting reports. While some indicated that there was a positive effect (see references in 11) other indicated that the cumulus did not have any effect on the AR rate (see references in 6).

In vivo, all human sperm within the cumulus cells were acrosome reacted (12). The eggs observed were a pronuclear and a 2-cell stage recovered from the oviduct 35 and 37 h after intercourse and 80-83 hr after LH peak. The argument given above for sperm that may have remained within the cumulus matrix for an extended time is also valid in this case.

Role of acrosomal enzymes.

From the previous data is apparent that some sperm can penetrate to the ZP surface without undergoing the AR. It is not clear if acrosomal enzymes are required for such sperm to penetrate. If there are acrosome intact sperm in the cumulus, how did they manage to pass through the cumulus? There are several possibilities. For instance, enzymes such as hyaluronidase and acrosin may be bound to the outer surface of the sperm head plasma membrane (13, 14) or acrosomal enzymes may be released through "intact" acrosomal and plasma membranes (13, 15). Although the free passage of macromolecules through morphologically "intact" membranes seem highly unlikely, this possibility cannot be disregarded. Finally, the sperm may pass through the cumulus by purely mechanical means. Recent evidence provided by Gmachl et al. (16) and Lin et al. (17) supports the view that surface enzymes may assist the sperm during cumulus oophorus penetration. They have reported that PH-20 from several species, including humans, possess hyaluronidase activity (16, 17). PH-20 is a glycoprotein located at the posterior head of the plasma membrane of mouse, guinea pig, cynomolgus monkey, and human sperm (18, 17, 19). It migrates to the inner acrosomal membrane after the AR (19) where it is involved in the binding of acrosome reacted sperm to the ZP (20, 19). The finding of Lin et al. (17) provides the mechanism by which acrosome intact sperm would penetrate the cumulus oophorus. They suggested that the fertilizing spermatozoon penetrates the cumulus layer using the hyaluronidase activity of plasma membrane PH-20. Then, it reaches and binds to the zona where undergoes the AR (17).

SPERM INTERACTION WITH THE ZONA PELLUCIDA

The zona consists of several components, being the glycoproteins the most important. All zona glycoproteins have a polypeptide backbone that is differentially glycosylated thus providing molecules with a large charge heterogeneity. In humans as well as in other species, the zona is composed of three glycoproteins termed ZP1, ZP2 and ZP3 (21). Binding of sperm to the ZP is relatively species-specific, albeit zona components are highly conserved among mammals. It is not clear yet if the species specificity involves the protein backbone or carbohydrate side chains.

After the sperm have traversed the cumulus oophorus, they reach the ZP. The sequence of events currently accepted to be involved in sperm-zona interaction are: binding of acrosome intact sperm with the zona (primary binding), induction of the AR, binding of acrosome reacted sperm with the zona (secondary binding), and finally penetration of the acrosome reacted sperm through the zona matrix until reaching the perivitelline space and then fuse with the oocyte plasma membrane (22).

Primary sperm-zona binding.
In the mouse, the primary sperm-zona binding is mediated by the glycoprotein ZP3, via a class of 3.9 kDa O-linked oligosaccharide side chains (23). The cDNA sequence has been elucidated for ZP3 glycoproteins of the mouse, hamster, human, and marmoset. The interspecies homologies ranged from 67% to 91% (24-26). Thus, same function for this glycoprotein in different species is highly probable.

The candidates for being protein receptors for zona ligands on the sperm surface include: a) 1,4-ß-galactosyl transferase activity acting as a lectin rather than an enzyme (27); b) sp 56, isolated for its ability to bind ZP3 (28); c) a 95-kDa mouse sperm protein with sperm receptor kinase activity (29); d) 54-kDa lectin-like protein (30). Recently it was shown that the number of human spermatozoa bound to the zona is decreased in a group with low alpha-glucosidase activity (31).

Acrosome reaction.
After binding to the zona, some sperm may be stimulated to undergo the AR. In mouse, the polypeptide and the carbohydrate moieties of ZP3 are necessary for this event (32). A recombinant human ZP3, produced by chinese hamster ovary, is also able to induce the human sperm AR (33). Gi proteins (34) as well as protein kinases A, C and G (35) were suggested to be involved in signal transduction leading to zona-induced AR. The ZP-induced AR is related to the release of putative enzyme activities that might facilitate sperm passage through this egg coat and fusion with the oolemma (22). We still do not know if the human ZP-triggered AR involves calcium influx as it has been shown for bovine and mouse spermatozoa (36, 37).

Earlier reports have demonstrated that acrosome reacted sperm can initiate binding to the ZP (38). Are acrosome intact and acrosome reacted sperm equally able to bind to the ZP? In mouse, clearly only acrosome intact spermatozoa can bind to the ZP. However, in other species it has been observed that both acrosome intact and acrosome reacted spermatozoa are equally able to bind to the zona surface (39, 20). If human acrosome reacted sperm can initiate binding to the ZP, are they able to penetrate it and fertilize the egg? (see below).

Secondary sperm-zona binding.
Once the sperm have undergone the AR on the ZP, secondary binding takes place. This binding involves ZP2 and additional sperm macromolecules such as the proacrosin-acrosin system and PH-20 (40, 18). The sperm-ZP binding

has been related to the inmunocytochemical presence of proacrosin and acrosin, but not to the proteolytic activity of acrosin in human spermatozoa. Thus, egg recognition and protease activities may be independent functions of acrosin and its zymogen (41). It may be also that ZP2 binds to several types of receptors on the sperm surface, included those aforementioned and/or some others, yet not identified. Previously acrosome reacted sperm may initiate binding to the ZP using the mechanisms involved in secondary binding.

Sperm-zona penetration.
At present it is accepted that the AR is a requisite for zona penetration. Then, only acrosome reacted sperm can penetrate the zona and fuse with the oocyte plasma membrane. However, in the papers by Singer et al. (42) and Franken et al. (43) there are electron micrographs depicting acrosome intact, acrosome reacting and acrosome reacted human sperm embedded in the ZP. More experimental evidence is necessary to elucidate the meaning of these findings.

A model has been proposed for sperm-zona penetration, which seem to occur as a sequential event, first involving sperm secondary binding and then proteolytic cleavage of zona proteins. At present, however, is not entirely clear which sperm protease activity (ies) is (are) required for human zona penetration or even if they are necessary at all. In a previous report we showed that trypsin inhibitors blocked human sperm-zona penetration; however, the effect was due to an inhibition of the AR (44). In the work of Liu and Baker (45), sperm-zona penetration was blocked by treating the sperm with soybean trypsin inhibitor. They could not conclude, however, whether the blocking was due to inhibition of the lytic action of acrosin or to an inhibition of the AR. Oehninger et al. (46) reported that treatment of human sperm with progesterone enhanced hyperactivated motility and ZP penetration without changing the percentage of acrosome reacted sperm. Therefore, hyperactivated motility might be an additional important factor for zona penetration.

Are previously reacted sperm able to penetrate the ZP and fertilize?
It is not known how long mammalian spermatozoa maintain the ability to penetrate the ZP after completion of the AR. Barros et al. (47) indicated that hamster sperm, reacted before reaching the zona surface, lose ability to pass through the zona before they lose ability to swim or bind to it. Other reports, however, have shown that previously reacted guinea pig and rabbit sperm are able to penetrate homologous ZP (48, 39). These findings correlate with those of Barros et al. (49) who detected that acrosin on the inner acrosomal membrane of hamster sperm disappeared rather quickly after the AR, whereas that of the guinea pig and human sperm did not. Thus, sperm ability to penetrate the ZP after completion of the AR in a previous site may be

related to the presence of acrosin in its surface. The site (s), where the spermatozoa undergo the AR in vivo, has not been completely ascertained yet. The majority of the evidence suggests that in vivo the fertilizing spermatozoon initiates the AR after it binds to the ZP.

ROLE OF TRYPSIN- AND CHYMOTRYPSIN-LIKE ENZYMES IN SPERM-ZONA INTERACTION

TREATMENT	N° OF SPERM BOUND
Control for pAB (PBS, pH 7.3)	120 ± 25
pAB (1mM)	100 ± 30
Control for NPGB (DMSO) 0.1%)	91 ± 20
NPGB (10µM)	82 ± 18
Control for TPCK (DMSO 0.1%)	70 ± 9
TPCK (25µM)	94 ± 8
Control for ATEE (ethanol 0.1%)	80 ± 12
ATEE (1mM)	62 ± 9

Table 1. **Effect of trypsin and chymotrypsin inhibitors upon the number of sperm bound to the surface of the human zonae pellucida**[1]

[1] *Aliquots of 4.5 hr capacitated sperm were treated with trypsin or chymotrypsin inhibitors for 30 min. Control aliquots received the inhibitor solvents. Four human oocytes were then added to each aliquot and incubation continued another 30 min. The oocytes with adhered spermatozoa were fixed and the number of zona-bound spermatozoa was determined using phase contrast microscopy. pAB, p-aminobenzamidine; PBS, phosphate buffered saline; NPGB, p-nitrophenyl-p'-guanidino-benzoate; DMSO, dimethilsulfoxide; TPCK, N-tosyl-L-phenylalanine-chloromethyl ketone; ATEE, N-acetyl-L-tyrosine ethyl ester. There were no significant differences in the number of zona-bound sperm between each treated group and its control. (See text of references 44, and 50 for further explanation; reprinted with permission).*

Sperm-zona binding.
It has been reported that, before the morphologically visible human sperm AR begins, limited amounts of activated, immunoreactive acrosin (a trypsin-like enzyme) are mobilized to the sperm surface (15, 14). The enzyme was detected on the plasma membrane covering the acrosomal area, which made the authors suggest a role for acrosin in the primary human sperm-ZP binding (15, 14). Our own studies, using trypsin and chymotrypsin inhibitors, indicated that none of these enzymatic activities were involved in primary sperm-ZP binding (44, 50). Pretreatment with trypsin or chymotrypsin inhibitors did not have any effect on the number of sperm

bound to the human ZP (Table 1). Same observations were reported by Liu and Baker using soybean trypsin inhibitor (45).

TREATMENT	% OF ACROSOME REACTION	% OF ACROSOME REACTION INHIBITION
Control for pAB (PBS,PH 7.3)	37.2±3.9	0
pAB (1mM)	5.9±1.2	85±4
Control for NPGB (DMSO) 0.1%)	40.1±3.2	0
NPGB (10µM)	9.6 ± 1.8	76 ± 3
Control for TPCK (DMSO 0.1%)	27.4 ± 2.9	0
TPCK (80µM)	6.8 ± 0.6	74 ± 5
TPCK (80µM) and wash	6.3 ± 1.2	72 ± 3
Control for ATEE (ethanol 0.1%)	30.3 ± 2.4	0
ATEE (1mM)	2.1 ± 1.0	92. ± 3
ATEE (1mM) and wash	28.6 ± 2.1	3 ± 0.2

Table 2. **Inhibition of human zona pellucida induced acrosome reactions by trypsin and chymotrypsin inhibitors**
[1] *Aliquots of 4.5 hr capacitated sperm were treated with trypsin or chymotrypsin inhibitors for 30 min. Control aliquots received the inhibitor solvents. Four human oocytes were then added to each aliquot and incubation continued another 30 min. The oocytes with adhered spermatozoa were fixed and the acrosomal status of the zona-bound spermatozoa was determined as described previously. In some experiments, sperm suspensions treated with TPCK and ATEE were washed and resuspended in fresh media before adding the zonae. pAB, p-aminobenzamidine; PBS, phosphate buffered saline; NPGB, p-nitrophenyl-p'-guanidino-benzoate; DMSO, dimethilsulfoxide; TPCK, N-tosyl-L-phenylalanine-chloromethyl ketone; ATEE, N-acetyl-L-tyrosine ethyl ester (*) Significantly lower when compared to its respective control (P<0.005). (Reprinted with permission from references 44 and 50).*

Acrosome reaction.

We have reported that trypsin- and chymotrypsin-like activities are involved in the human sperm AR (44, 50). Both trypsin and chymotrypsin inhibitors were equally effective in blocking the ZP-induced AR (Table 2).

In addition, the inhibitory effect of ATEE, a chymotrypsin substrate, was reversed when the sperm were resuspended in fresh medium whereas the effect of TPCK, an irreversible inhibitor of chymotrypsin, was not. Our electron microscopy studies suggest that both enzymatic activities are involved in the membrane events of the AR (44, 50). Same results were reported using trypsin inhibitors and progesterone as the AR stimulus (51). Whether trypsin- and chymotrypsin-like activities are also involved in acrosomal matrix dispersal of human sperm is not known at present.

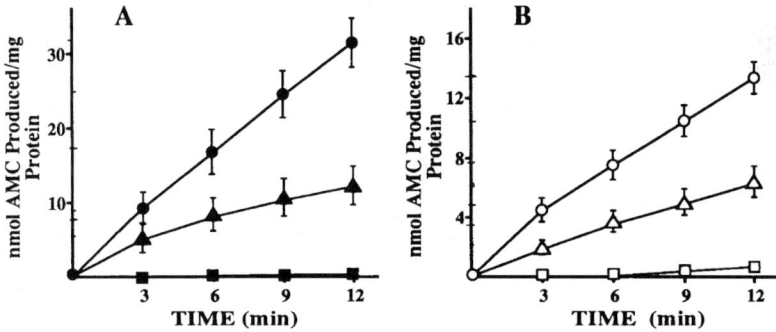

Figure 1. **Chymotrypsin-like activity in extracts of epididymal and ejaculated human spermatozoa:** *The assays were carried out with (A) or without calcium (B). The extracts were incubated with 80 µM TPCK (triangles), 1 mM chymostatin (squares) or PBS (circles). Enzymatic extracts of cauda epididymal and ejaculated sperm were obtained as described in Table 3. Chymotrypsin-like activity was assayed using the fluorogenic substrate Suc-Leu-Leu-Val-Tyr-AMC and monitored with excitation at 380 nm and emission at 460 in a spectrofluorometer. (Reprinted with permission from reference 50).*

Chymotrypsin-like activity was identified in crude extracts of human spermatozoa selected through a percoll gradient (Figure 1). The following evidence supports that the activity was indeed chymotrypsin-like: the activity was inhibited by chymotrypsin inhibitors and not affected by metalloendoprotease and aminopeptidase inhibitors. In addition, the activity was not affected in the absence of Ca^{+2}, a condition that precludes any calpain-like activity. The chymotrypsin-like activity has higher affinity for the substrate with the aminoacid Tyr before the AMC group (P1) than for the aminoacid Phe en P1 (Table 3). Recent evidence indicates that this activity is also present in human epididymal sperm, where they represent half of the activity found in ejaculated sperm. This difference may be due to contamination with seminal plasma activity or to an activation of the enzyme upon ejaculation.

SUBSTRATES	SPECIFIC ACTIVITY (nmol AMC mg Prot^{-1} min^{-1})	
	EPIDIDYMAL	EJACULATED
Suc-Leu-Leu-Val-Tyr-AMC	1.2 ± 0.3 (50%)	2.41 ± 0.04 (100%)
Suc-Ala-Ala-Pro-Phe-AMC	0.7 ± 0.5 (29%)	0.99 ± 0.6 (41%)
Suc-Ala-Ala-Phe-AMC	0.12 ± 0.4 (5%)	0.29 ± 0.6 (12%)
Suc-Leu-Tyr-AMC	0.05 ± 0.2 (2%)	0.08 ± 0.2 (3%)

Table 3. **Chymotrypsin-like activity in extracts of epididymal and ejaculated human spermatozoa1:**[1] *Cauda epididymal and ejaculated sperm, passed through a Percoll gradient, were resuspended in 1 mM benzamidine, 50 mM Hepes, 10% glycerol, pH 7.4 and then sonicated with three 20-watt bursts for 10 sec each, followed by centrifugation at 14,000 xg for 30 sec. The supernatant was used as the enzyme stock preparation. All these procedures were performed at 4 °C. Chymotrypsin-like activity was assayed using fluorogenic substrates and monitored with excitation at 380 nm and emission at 460 in a spectrofluorometer. The activity of ejaculated sperm toward Suc-Leu-Leu-Val-Tyr-AMC was considered 100%. Suc, Succinyl; AMC, 7-Amido-4-Methyl-Coumarin. (See text of reference 50 for further methodological details)*

Preliminary evidence suggests that the chymotrypsin-like activity resides in a band of Å220-kDa, when the electrophoresis was run under non-denaturating conditions (Figure 2). We do not know whether this band represents a single protein or a combination of several oligomers, with at least one of them possessing chymotrypsin-like activity, as has been described for marine invertebrates (52).

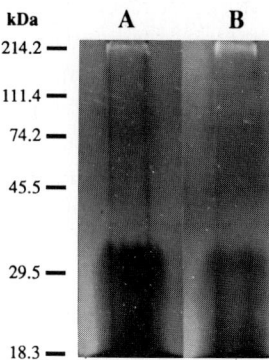

Figure 2. **Substrate-sodium dodecyl sulfate-polyacrylamide gel electrophoresis**. *Gels were prepared according to Laemmli (Nature 1970, 277:680). Enzymatic extracts of ejaculated sperm were obtained as described in Table 3 and then diluted in sample buffer without reducing agents. The diluted samples were not boiled before loading onto the gels. After electrophoresis the gel was incubated in 50 mM Tris buffer, pH 7.5, containing 2% casein for 30 min at 5 °C, and then the temperature was raised to 25 °C for 15 hr. The protein was fixed and stained in Coomassie blue for 2 hr and then washed (Garcia-Carreño et al., 1993, Anal. Biochem. 214:65). Extracts were incubated with 80 µM TPCK (A) or 0.1% DMSO (B).*

SPERM-INTERACTION WITH THE OOLEMMA

The AR is necessary to render the equatorial segment of the spermatozoa competent for sperm-egg fusion (22). The mechanism by which the plasma membrane over the equatorial segment become fusogenic is not yet clear. The acrosomal content, released during the AR, may alter the plasma membranes over this segment (22). Acrosin may play a role in this process since trypsin inhibitors prevent acrosome reacting sperm from becoming fusogenic (53, 54). The inhibitors did not block fusion of acrosome reacted sperm once they had undergone the AR in normal inhibitor-free medium (53, 54). Acrosin may activate latent fusion proteins in the equatorial segment region or remove steric and/or charge barriers to membrane apposition (54). Other factors implied in the development of sperm ability to fuse with the egg plasma membrane include metalloendoprotease (55), calpain II (56) and plasminogen activator/plasmin (57).

There are several candidates for the sperm components which mediate fusion with the egg plasma membrane. In mouse, both galactosyltransferase and a 40-kDa protein on the plasma membrane over the equatorial segment have been implied in sperm-egg fusion (58, 59). In rat, a

37-kDa protein on the equatorial segment of acrosome reacted sperm was described (60). In human, acrosin adsorbed on the plasma membrane over the equatorial segment and the postacrosomal region of acrosome reacted human sperm has been reported to be involved in sperm-egg fusion (14). In addition, a 43 kDa protein on the surface of acrosome reacted sperm may mediate this process (61). Other membrane adhesion molecules on the sperm surface implied for sperm-egg fusion in humans include fibronectin (62) and the complement Clq (63).

CONCLUDING REMARKS

There are still many unanswered questions regarding human sperm interaction with the egg coats. The requirement for sperm capacitation as well as the acrosomal status for sperm traveling through the cumulus oophorus need to be studied further. Do human sperm use the hyaluronidase activity of PH20 to penetrate the cumulus? If previously reacted human sperm can initiate binding to the ZP, Are they able to penetrate it and fertilize? Is it possible that acrosome intact sperm may penetrate the zona, or at least part of it? Would the hyaluronidase activity of PH20 help the sperm accomplish this task? Are acrosomal proteases involved in human sperm penetration through the ZP? Investigation of these and other related questions is a future goal. Certainly, more in vivo work will be necessary to gain further insight in this field and reach more definite conclusions.

This work was supported by grants Fondecyt 688/93 and European Economic Community N° CI1-CT92-0022.

REFERENCES

1. Tesarik J, Kopecny V. Late preovulatory suynthesis of proteoglycans by the human oocyte and cumulus cells and their secretion into the oocyte-cumulus-complex extracellular matrices. Histochem 1986; 85:523-528.
2. Yudin AI, Cherr GM, Katz DF. Structure of the cumulus matrix and zona pellucida in the golden hamster: a new view of sperm interaction with oocyte-associated extracellular matrices. Cell Tissue Res 1988; 251:555-564.
3. Pereda J, Coppo M. Ultrastructure of a two-cell human embryo fertilized in vivo. J IVF and ET 1984; 1:131.

4. Austin CR. Capacitation and the release of hyaluronidase from spermatozoa. J Reprod Fert 1960; 3:310-311.
5. Talbot P. Sperm penetration through oocyte investment in mammals. Amer J Anat 1985; 174:331-346.
6. White DR, Phillips D, Bedford J. Factors affecting the acrosome reaction in human spermatozoa. J Reprod Fert 1990; 90:71-80.
7. Chen C, Sathananthan AH. Early penetration of human sperm through the vestments of human eggs in vitro. Arch Androl 1986; 16:183-197.
8. Sathananthan AH, Trounson AO, Wood C, Leeton JF. Ultrastructural observations of the penetration of human sperm into the zona pellucida of the human egg in vitro. J Androl 1982; 3:356-364.
9. Soupart P, P.A. S. Ultrastructural observations on human oocytes fertilized in vitro. Fertil Steril 1974; 25:11-44.
10. Tsuiki A, Hoshiai H, Takahashi K, Suzuki M, Hoshi K. Sperm-egg interactions observed by scanning electron microscopy. Arch Androl 1986; 16:35-47.
11. Sullivan R, Duchesne C, Famhy N, Morin N, Dionne P. Protein synthesis and acrosome reaction-inducing activity of human cumulus cells. Hum Reprod 1990; 5:830-4.
12. Pereda J, Coppo M. An electron microscopy study of sperm penetration into the human egg investments. Anat Embryol 1985; 173:247-252.
13. Joyce C, Jeyendran RS, Zaneveld LJD. Release extraction and stability of hyaluronidase associated with human spermatozoa. Comparisons with the rabbit. J Androl 1985; 6:152-161.
14. Tesarik J, Drahorad J, Testar J, Mendoza C. Acrosin activation follows its surface exposure and precedes membrane fusion in human sperm acrosome reaction. Development 1990; 110:391-400.
15. Tesarik J, Drahorad J, Peknicova J. Subcellular immunochemical localization of acrosin in human spermatozoa during the acrosome reaction and zona pellucida penetration. Fertil Steril 1988; 50:133-141.
16. Gmachl M, Sagan S, Ketter S, Kreil G. The human sperm protein PH-20 has hyaluronidase activity. FEBS Let 1993; 336:545-548.
17. Lin Y, Mahan K, Lathrop WF, Myles DG, Primakoff P. A hyaluronidase activity of the sperm plasma membrane protein PH-20 enables sperm to penetrate the cumulus cell layer surrounding the egg. J Cell Biol 1994; 125:1157-63.
18. Lathrop WF, P CE, Myles DG, Primakoff P. cDNA cloning reveals the molecular structure of a sperm surface protein, PH-20, involved in sperm-egg adhesion and the wide distribution of its gene among mammals. J Cell Biol 1990; 111:2939-2949.

19. Primakoff P, Hyatt H, Myles DG. A role for the migrating sperm surface antigen PH-20 in guinea pig sperm binding to the egg zona pellucida. J Cell Biol 1985; 101:2239-2244.
20. Myles DG, Hyatt H, Primakoff P. Binding of both acrosome-intact and acrosome-reacted guinea pig sperm to the zona pellucida during in vitro fertilization. Dev Biol 1987; 121:559-567.
21. Shabanowitz RB, O'Rand MG. Characterization of the human zona pellucida from fertilized and unfertilized eggs. J Reprod Fert 1988; 82:151-161.
22. Yanagimachi R. Mammalian Fertilization. In: Knobil E, Neill JD, eds. The Physiology of Reproduction. New York: Raven Press; 1994:189-317.
23. Rosiere TK, Wassarman PM. Identification of a region mouse zona pellucida glycoprotein mZP3 that possesses sperm receptor activity. Dev Biol 1992; 154:309-317.
24. Chamberlin ME, Dean J. Human homology of the mouse sperm receptor. Proc Natl Acad Sci USA 1990; 87:6014-6018.
25. Ringuette MJ, Chamberlin ME, Baur AW, Sobieski DA, Dear J. Molecular analysis of cDNA coding for ZP3, a sperm binding protein of the mouse zona pellucida. Dev Biol 1988; 127:287-295.
26. Thillai-Koothan P, van Duin M, Aitken R. Clonign, sequencing, and oocyte specific expression of the marmoset sperm receptor protein, ZP3. Zygote 1993; 1:93-101.
27. Miller DJ, Maceck MB, Shur BD. Complementarity between sperm surface B-1,4-galactosyltransferase and egg-coat ZP3 mediates sperm-egg binding. Nature 1992; 357:589.
28. Bleil JD, Wassarman PM. Identification of a ZP3-binding protein on acrosome-intact mouse sperm by photoaffinity crosslinking. Proc Natl Acad Sci USA 1990; 87:5563-5567.
29. Leyton L, LeGuen P, Bunch D, Saling PM. Regulation of mouse gamete interaction by a sperm tyrosine kinase. Proc Natl Acad Sci USA 1992; 89:11692-11695.
30. Abdullah M, Widgren EE, O'Rand MG. A mammalian sperm lectin related to rat hepatocyte lectin-2/3. Molec Cell Biochem 1991; 103:155-161.
31. Ben-Ali H, Guerin JF, Pinatel MC, Mathieu C, Boulieu D, Tritar B. Relationship between semen characteristics, alpha-glucosidase and the capacity of the spermatzoa to bind to the human zona pellucida. Int J Androl 1994; 17:121-126.
32. Wassarman PM, Florman HM, Greve JM. Receptor-mediated sperm-egg interactions in mammals. In: Metz CB, Monroy A, eds. Biology of Fertilization. New York: Academic Press; 1985:341-360.

33. Vanduin M, Polman JEM, Debreet I, Vanginneken K, Bunschoten VH, Grootenhuis A, Brindle J, Aitken RJ. Recombinant human zona pellucida protein ZP3 produced by chinese hamster ovary cells induces the human sperm acrosome reaction and promotes sperm-egg fusion. Biol Reprod 1994; 51:607-617.
34. Lee MA, Check JH, Kopf GS. A guanine nucletide-binding regulatory protein in human sperm mediates acrosomal exocytosis induced by the human zona pellucida. Mol Reprod Dev 1992; 31:78-86.
35. Bielfeld P, Faridi A, Zaneveld LJD, De Jonge CJ. The zona pellucida induced acrosome reaction of human spermatozoa is mediated by protein kinases. Fertil Steril 1994; 61:536-541.
36. Florman HM, Tombes RM, First NL, Babcock DF. An adhesion-associated agonist from the zona pellucida activates G-protein promoted elevation in Ca^{2+} and pH that mediate mammalian sperm acrosomal exocytosis. Dev Biol 1989; 135:133-146.
37. Lee MA, Storey BT. Influx of Ca^{++} is the primary reaction mediating the first stage of the zona induced acrosome reaction in mouse spermatozoa. Biol Reprod ; 1988; 38 (Suppl 1):93.
38. Morales P, Cross NL, Overstreet JW, Hanson FW. Acrosome intact and acrosome reacted human sperm can initiate binding to the zona pellucida. Dev Biol 1989; 133:385-392.
39. Kuzan FB, Fleming AD, Seidel GE. Successful fertilization in vitro of fresh intact oocytes by periviteline (acrosome-reacted) spermatozoa of the rabbit. Fertil Steril 1984; 41:766-770.
40. Jones R. Unusual fucoidin-binding properties of chymotrypsinogen and trypsinogen. Biochim Biophy Acta 1990; 1037:227-232.
41. Francavilla S, Gabriele A, Romano R, Gianaroli L, Ferraretti AP, Francavilla F. Sperm-zona pellucida binding of human sperm is correlated with the immunocytochemical presence of proacrosin and acrosin in the sperm head but not with the proteolytic activity of acrosin. Fertil Steril 1994; 62:1226-1233.
42. Singer SL, Lambert H, Overstreet JW, Hanson FW, Yanagimachi R. The kinetics of human sperm binding to the human zona pellucida and zona-free hamster oocyte in vitro. Gamete Res 1985; 12:29-39.
43. Franken DR, Oosthuizen WT, Cooper S, Kruger TF, Burkman LJ, Coddington CC, Hodgen GD. Electron microscopic evidence on the acrosomal status of bound sperm and their penetration into human hemizonae pellucida after storage in a buffered salt solution. Andrologia 1991; 23:205-8.
44. Llanos M, Vigil P, Salgado AM, Morales P. Inhibition of the acrosome reaction by trypsin inhibitors and prevention of penetration of spermatozoa through the human zona pellucida. J Reprod Fert 1993; 97:173-8.

45. Liu DY, Baker HWG. Inhibition of acrosin activity with a trypsin inhibitor blocks human sperm penetration of the zona pellucida. Biol Reprod 1993; 48:340-8.
46. Oehninger S, Sueldo C, Lanzendorf S, Mahony M, Burkman LJ, Alexander NJ, Hodgen GD. A sequential analysis of the effect of progesterone on specific sperm functions crucial to fertilization in vitro in infertile patients. Hum Reprod 1994; 9:1322-1327.
47. Barros C, Jedlicki A, Bize I, Aguirre E. Relationship between the lenght of sperm preincubation and zona penetration in the golden hamster: a scaning electron microscopy study. Gamete Res 1984; 9:31-43.
48. Huang TTF, Fleming AD, Yanagimachi R. Only acrosome-reacted spermatozoa can bind to and penetrate zona pellucida: a study using the guinea pig. J Exp Zool 1981; 217:287-290.
49. Barros C, Capote C, Perez C, Crosby JA, Becker MI, De Ioannes A. Immunodetection of acrosin during the acrosome reaction of hamster, guinea-pig and human spermatozoa. Biol Res 1992; 25:31-40.
50. Morales P, Socias T, Cortez J, Llanos MN. Evidences for the presence of a chymotrypsin-like activity in human spermatozoa with a role in the acrosome reaction. Mol Reprod Dev 1994; 38:222-230.
51. Pillai MC, Meizel S. Trypsin inhibitors prevent the progesterone-initiated increase in intracellular calcium required for the human spem acrosome reaction. J Exp Zool 1991; 258:384-393.
52. Matsumura K, Aketa K. Proteasome (multicatalytic proteinase) of sea urchin sperm and its possible participation in the acrosome reaction. Mol Reprod Dev 1991; 29:189-199.
53. Dravland JE, Meizel S. The effect of inhibitors of trypsin and phospholipase A2 on the penetration of zona pellucida-free hamster eggs by acrosome-reacted hamster sperm. J Androl 1982; 3:388-395.
54. Takano H, Yanagimachi R, Urch U. Evidence that acrosin activity is important for the developemnt of fusibility of mammalian spermatozoa with oolemma: inhibitors studies using the golden hamster. Zygotes 1993; 1:79-91.
55. Díaz-Pérez E, Meizel S. Importance of mammalian sperm metalloendoprotease activity during the acrosome reaction to subsequent sperm-egg fusion: Inhibitor studies with human sperm and zona-free hamster eggs. Mol Reprod Dev 1992; 31:122-130.
56. Berruti G. Evidence for Ca^{2+} mediated F-actin-phospholipid binding of human sperm capacitation II. Cell Biol Int Rep 1991; 15:917-927.
57. Huarte J, Belin D, Bosco D, Sappino AP, Vasalli JD. Plasminogen activator and mouse spermatozoa: urokinase synthesis in the male genital tract and binding of the enzyme to the sperm cell surface. J Cell Biol 1987; 104:1281-1289.

58. Lopez LC, Shur BD. Redistribution of mouse sperm surface galactosyltransferase after the acrosome reaction. J Cell Biol 1987; 105:1663-1670.
59. Saling PM, Irons G, Waibel R. Mouse sperm antigens that participate in fertilization. I. Inhibition of sperm fusion with the egg plasma membrane using monoclonal antibodies. Biol Reprod 1985; 33:515-526.
60. Rochwerger L, Cohen DJ, Cuasnicu PS. Mammalian sper-egg fusion: the rat egg has complementary sites for a sperm protein that mediates gamete fusion. Mol Reprod Dev 1992; 31:34-41.
61. Okabe M, Matzno S, Magira M, Minura T, Kawai Y, Mayumi T. A human sperm antigen possibly involved in binding and/or fusion with zona-free hamster egg. Fertil Steril 1990; 54:1121-1126.
62. Fusi FM, Bronson RA. Evidence for the presence of an integrin cell adhesion receptor on the oolemma of unfertilized human oocytes. Mol Reprod Dev 1992; 31:215-222.
63. Fusi FM, Bronson RA, Hong Y, Ghebrehiwei B. Complement component Clq and its receptors are involved in the intreaction of human sperm with zona-free hamster eggs. Mol Reprod Dev 1991; 29:180-188.

Initiation of human sperm acrosome reaction by progesterone

Stanley Meizel

Department of Cell Biology and Human Anatomy, School of Medicine, University of California, Davis, California 95616-8643, USA

ABSTRACT

The mammalian sperm acrosome reaction (AR), an essential fertilization event, is a specialized form of exocytosis involving the sperm head membranes. Progesterone, a putative physiological initiator of the AR, can initiate the AR in human and other mammalian sperm in vitro by interaction with one or more plasma membrane receptors. This review will emphasize studies from my laboratory relating to: 1) the role of progesterone in mediating intracellular changes in human sperm Ca^{2+} and Cl^- required for the AR; 2) the type of progesterone receptor/ion channel(s) involved (particularly one resembling a $GABA_A$ receptor/Cl^- channel).

La réaction acrosomique chez les mammifères, étape essentielle de la fécondation, est une forme particulière d'exocytose impliquant les membranes de la tête du spermatozoïde. La progestérone, un inducteur physiologique potentiel de le réaction acrosomique, est capable d'induire in vitro la réaction acrosomique, chez l'humain ainsi que chez d'autres mammifères, par interaction avec un ou plusieurs récepteurs de la membrane plasmique. Cette revue mettra en valeur des études réalisées dans mon laboratoire sur: 1) le rôle de la progestérone dans les changements en Ca^{2+} et Cl^- intracellulaires nécessaires à la RA. 2) Le type de récepteurs à la progestérone/ canaux ioniques impliqués (et particulièrement un ressemblant au récepteur $GABA_A$/ canal Cl^-).

INTRODUCTION

The mammalian sperm acrosome reaction (AR), a modified exocytotic event involving fusion followed by vesiculation of sperm head membranes, is essential to penetration of the zona pellucida (a glycoprotein egg envelope) and to sperm egg-fusion (1). Mammalian sperm usually respond to AR initiators only after spending a period of hours either in the female reproductive tract or under certain in vitro incubation conditions. During this time, which varies greatly according to species and/or incubation media composition, the sperm undergo incompletely understood cellular modifications collectively termed capacitation (1).

Some studies had argued that the morphological events of the human AR were different than those of other mammals (reviewed in (2)). However, studies from this laboratory have shown that the human AR (including the progesterone-initiated AR) is similar to that of other mammals, with the outer acrosomal membrane and overlying plasma membrane fusing and the fused membranes undergoing fenestration and vesiculation (2,3).

While a glycoprotein of the zona pellucida is generally believed to be the in vivo initiator of the AR in a fertilizing sperm (4), human and other mammalian sperm can also undergo the AR in the cumulus oophorus, a mass of ovarian follicular cells surrounding the ovulated zona-enclosed egg (reviewed in (3,5)).

Moreover, progesterone secreted by the cumulus oophorus (ovarian follicular cells still surrounding the ovulated egg) can initiate the AR in vitro in the sperm of several mammals including the human (3, 6-9). My laboratory colleagues and I have hypothesized that progesterone acts by itself and/or in synergy with the zona to initiate the AR of fertilizing sperm in vivo (3).

In order for a sperm to become a fertilizing sperm if it has been acrosome-reacted by progesterone prior to zona-binding, it must subsequently bind to the zona and penetrate it. Guinea pig sperm but not mouse sperm that have undergone the AR prior to reaching the zona can bind to that egg envelope (4). Porcine sperm can evidently bind and penetrate under such conditions (10), and there are conflicting reports as to whether human sperm can do so (11, 12). However, evidence supporting a role for progesterone in the in vivo human sperm AR comes from reports suggesting a relationship between male infertility and an inability of sperm to respond to progesterone in vitro (13-15).

Although we were unable to demonstrate synergistic action between solubilized pig zona and progesterone in the in vitro pig AR (7), recent studies by Roldan and coworkers suggests that synergy between solubilized zona and progesterone can occur during the in vitro mouse sperm AR (8). In the latter studies it was important that progesterone be added to capacitated sperm a few minutes earlier than zona in order to act as a "primer". It should be noted that even in those studies of mouse sperm, a substantial number of AR occurred with progesterone alone.

The progesterone concentration in the cumulus has not been measured, but a rough estimate suggests that it could be present in µg/ml concentrations(3,6). We have been able to initiate the human sperm AR with concentrations of progesterone ranging from 1 µg/ml (approx., 3 µM) to as low as 250-100 ng/ml ((3) and unpublished studies). It should be noted that progesterone is the major AR initiator of human follicular fluid in vitro (6), and follicular fluid trapped in the cumulus extracellular matrix could also serve as a source of the steroid, at least until it is washed out by oviductal fluid. Moreover, the human sperm AR can occur in vitro in sperm exposed to human cumulus or to human cumulus spent culture medium (16, 17). In follicular fluid and cumulus spent medium, AR activity (later shown to be progesterone) was associated with a protein of 50,000 apparent molecular weight, and we hypothesized that this protein and/or similar binding-proteins might permit lower concentrations of progesterone to initiate the AR in vivo (discussed in (3)). Recent studies by other investigators suggest that cortisol-binding globulin may be one such a protein (18), although the concentration used in those studies, 225 nM was still relatively high.

PROGESTERONE, CA^{2+} AND THE ACROSOME REACTION

An extracellular Ca^{2+}-dependent increase in the concentration of free intracellular Ca^{2+} ($[Ca^{2+}]_i$) is required for initiation of the AR by physiological factors including progesterone(19-21). During progesterone-initiation of the human sperm AR, there is a several fold transient increase in $[Ca^{2+}]_i$ within seconds of steroid addition (detected by the fluorescent intracellular Ca^{2+} probe fura-2), and, interestingly, what appears to be a similar increase also occurs in uncapacitated, non acrosome-reacting human sperm (3,20,22). The latter result suggests capacitation involves more than just increased $[Ca^{2+}]_i$ We have recently begun to use fluorescence ratio-imaging to study the progesterone-mediated increase in human sperm $[Ca^{2+}]_i$. Our preliminary studies demonstrated that the progesterone-mediated increase in human sperm $[Ca^{2+}]_i$ begins in the mid-head region, rapidly (<1 sec) spreading anteriorly over the rest of the head (23).

The type of Ca^{2+} channel involved in the Ca^{2+} influx required for the progesterone-initiated AR is not yet known. There have been conflicting reports concerning the effects of various Ca^{2+} channel blockers (see (24) for references).

Foresta and coworkers reported that Na^+ is not required for the progesterone-initiated human sperm AR and that the progesterone-mediated increase in $[Ca^{2+}]_i$ is higher in the absence of Na^+ (25). They also suggested that Na^+ and Ca^{2+} entered through the same sperm channel. However, other studies by Foresta and coworkers (26) then led them to suggest that progesterone might activate two channels, a calcium and a sodium channel.. Results from my lab disagree with their conclusions concerning Na^+, Ca^{2+} and the AR. Indeed, we found that the absence of Na^+ inhibits the progesterone-mediated increase in human sperm $[Ca^{2+}]_i$ and AR (27). The importance of Na^+ to progesterone-mediated sperm Ca^{2+} increases is currently under investigation in my lab.

Removal of extracellular Ca^{2+} appeared to completely eliminate the increase in sperm $[Ca^{2+}]_i$ (detected with fura-2) due to progesterone (20,22), but fura-2 may have been present at a high enough concentration in sperm to produce a Ca^{2+} buffering that could conceal a small rapid transient due to intracellular store mobilization (20), or washing and high chelator concentration may have removed any such store from the sperm. We have reported that thapsigargin (50-500 nM), a highly specific inhibitor of the endoplasmic reticulum Ca^{2+}-ATPase Ca^{2+}-pump (and thus a mobilizer of intracellular Ca^{2+}) in other cells (28), can initiate the AR in capacitated human sperm (29). Initiation of the AR by thapsigargin apparently requires an influx of Ca^{2+} since preincubation with the calcium channel blockers La^{3+} or Ni^{2+} completely inhibited AR initiation. Mobilization of an intracellular Ca^{2+} store by thapsigargin may lead to an influx of extracellular Ca^{2+} (i.e. the capacitative Ca^{2+}- entry hypothesis of Putney). Higher (1-10 μM) concentrations of thapsigargin were shown to increase human sperm $[Ca^{2+}]_i$ and 10 μM to potentiate the ability of progesterone to do so(30). It should be noted that 10 μM thapsigargin has Ca^{2+}-ionophore-like effects on protein free lipid vesicles(3 1).

In many other cells, the endoplasmic reticulum is the site of such a Ca^{2+}-store, but there is no obvious endoplasmic reticulum in the cytoplasm of mature sperm. Thapsigargin would not mobilize any mitochondrial stores. Hypothetical Ca^{2+} storage sites include the nucleus and the outer acrosomal membrane (29, 30). Interestingly, receptors for IP3, a physiological releaser of intracellular Ca^{2+} stores have been detected in the acrosomal region of rat sperm(32). The idea that progesterone partially exerts its effect in human sperm by mobilizing intracellular Ca^{2+} is complicated by the finding that production of IP3 (at least in uncapacitated human sperm also exhibiting a rapid Ca^{2+} transient) seems to first require a Ca^{2+} influx (20).

Trypsin-like activity in sperm may have a role in the progesterone-mediated increase in $[Ca^{2+}]_i$. Pre-incubation of capacitated human sperm with either of two inhibitors of trypsin-like enzymes, benzamidine hydrochloride, a competitive inhibitor and 4'-acetamidophenyl 4-guanidinobenzoate, an irreversible inhibitor (and also an inhibitor of other serine proteases), inhibited the progesterone-mediated AR by 68-85% (33). Transmission electron microscopic examination of the sperm after progesterone treatment confirmed that the inhibitors blocked the membrane fusion events of the AR. In contrast, the inhibitors did not inhibit the ionomycin initiated AR. Using fura-2, we further demonstrated that both of the trypsin inhibitors inhibited (by 61-84%) the progesterone-stimulated rise in $[Ca^{2+}]_i$ required for the AR membrane events, but did not affect $[Ca^{2+}]_i$ in unstimulated sperm (33). Since such inhibitors do not inhibit binding of progesterone to putative sperm receptors (34), the results suggest that some sperm trypsin-like activity is directly or indirectly involved in increasing sperm $[Ca^{2+}]_i$ during stimulation by progesterone. It has been hypothesized that sperm surface trypsin-like activity is important because it cleaves a progesterone binding protein, thus producing a "high local " progesterone concentration (18), or that proteolysis plays a role after progesterone binds to a receptor (34).

In some somatic cells, another steroid, testosterone rapidly increases Ca^{2+} fluxes of rat heart myocytes and mouse kidney cortex slices, apparently via a mechanism involving increased polyamine synthesis (35). Moreover, the ubiquitous polyamines putrescine, spermidine and spermine are found in mammalian sperm (reviewed in (36)). Therefore, we tested the effects of two highly specific "suicide" inhibitors of polyamine synthesis, DL-a(difluoromethyl)ornithine hydrochloride (DFMO), an inhibitor of putrescine synthesis and (S'-{[(Z)-4-amino-2butenyl]methylamino}-S'-deoxyadenosine (MDL 73811)), an inhibitor of S-adenosylmethionine decarboxylase (required for spermidine and spermine synthesis). DFMO inhibited the AR by 79%, but preincubation with putrescine, the precursor of spermidine and spermine) or spermidine reversed that inhibition. MDL 73811 inhibited the progesterone-initiated AR by 83%, and preincubation with spermidine, but not putrescine or spermine, reversed that inhibition. Preincubations with putrescine alone or with spermidine alone followed by addition of the progesterone or solvent did not initiate the AR. MDL 73811 and DFMO partially inhibited the rapid progesterone-initiated increase in $[Ca^{2+}]_i$ (assayed with fura-2), and those inhibitions were partially reversed by putrescine and spermidine respectively. Putrescine or spermidine alone did not increase $[Ca^{2+}]_i$, nor did preincubation with either polyamine followed by progesterone addition increase $[Ca^{2+}]_i$ more than progesterone alone. Neither inhibitor was able to inhibit the AR initiated by the calcium ionophore, ionomycin. All of those results suggest that the sperm polyamine biosynthesis leading to increased spermidine is necessary for the rapid increase in $[Ca^{2+}]_i$ and subsequent AR caused by progesterone. While our evidence suggests the importance of polyamine synthesis to the progesterone-initiated increases in sperm Ca^{2+} influx and AR, the mechanisms involved are not yet known. Polyamines can activate a number of mammalian cell enzymes and can enhance the ligand binding affinities of several brain receptors (see (36) for references).

SPERM PLASMA MEMBRANE PROGESTERONE RECEPTOR(S)

Progesterone acts at the sperm plasma membrane. Human sperm $[Ca^{2+}]_i$ and the AR are increased by progesterone covalently conjugated to serum albumin (a molecule that does not enter the sperm) or by apparent "receptor" aggregation resulting from addition of non-stimulatory levels of progesterone followed by antibody against progesterone (37,38,39).

A conjugate of FITC-labeled BSA-progesterone has been used to localize progesterone "receptor" sites in the sperm head plasma membrane of 30% or 10% of viable human sperm (38,40). In those FITC-conjugate studies, some competition studies to show binding specificity were evidently made but results were not shown. The low number of sperm that bound FITC-labeled BSA-progesterone may be due to the possibility that only capacitated sperm display the receptor (41). Interestingly, increased protein tyrosine phosphorylation occurs in a protein of 94,000 apparent molecular weight when human sperm are exposed to progesterone (42), and tyrosine phosphorylation is one of the signal-transduction mechanisms involved in some receptor-mediated events in other cells.

We have recently attempted to identify plasma membrane progesterone receptors in human sperm using a monoclonal antibody (MAb C262) against the C-terminal steroid binding domain of the mammalian intracellular progesterone receptor (43). In our preliminary studies, we found that a 5 min. incubation of capacitated human sperm with C262 greatly inhibited the progesterone-initiated sperm AR (77% maximum with the highest antibody concentration) but that incubation with H151 (a MAb against the human estrogen receptor) was not inhibitory. H151 did not inhibit the progesterone initiated AR. Western Blot analysis was carried out after uncapacitated sperm were extracted in SDS sample buffer in the presence of protease inhibitors. C262, but not H151, detected a sperm protein band of approximately 50,000 apparent MW. Indirect immunofluorescence localization of the human sperm progesterone receptor using fixed and unfixed uncapacitated or capacitated sperm displayed fluorescence at the equatorial segment region of the sperm head plasma membrane. Sperm incubated with the negative control MAb did not show any fluorescence. These studies support the involvement of sperm plasma membrane receptors in the progesterone-initiated AR and may have identified one such a receptor.

My laboratory has reported data strongly suggesting the involvement of a unique steroid receptor/Cl⁻ channel complex (resembling but not identical to a $GABA_A$ receptor/Cl⁻ channel complex) in the progesterone-initiated human AR (44). This work and relevant studies in other species will be discussed below, but it is relevant to point out here that the 50,000 apparent MW of the candidate receptor protein detected by MAb C262 is similar to that of the subunits of neuronal and sperm $GABA_A$ receptors and the its localization was the same as that previously found for the $GABA_A$ like receptor (44).

PROGESTERONE, CL⁻ AND THE ACROSOME REACTION

We have found that the progesterone-mediated AR was completely inhibited if capacitated human or porcine sperm were first resuspended in a Cl⁻ deficient medium (44, 45). In those studies, it was shown for the first time that mammalian sperm were not damaged by the Cl⁻ deficient medium since they remained motile and since the effects of treatment could be reversed by resuspension in Cl⁻. containing medium.

Anesthetic progesterone metabolites and a synthetic anesthetic progestin, all with an OH group in the 3 α-position of a reduced A ring are all known to directly activate the Cl⁻ channel of $GABA_A$ receptor/Cl⁻ channel complexes in neurons. Therefore, in our human sperm studies, 3α-OH isomers were compared to their non-anesthetic 3β-isomers and to progesterone for the ability to initiate the AR. We reported that three different 3α-OH steroids (but not their nonanesthetic 3β-0H isomers) could initiate the AR, but progesterone was a better AR initiator than its 3α-OH metabolites (44). Possible explanations for the latter result are discussed below. In that human sperm study, we also found that 10 μM GABA stimulated the AR slightly. Recently, Roldan and coworkers (8) found that lower GABA concentrations (e.g. 0.5 μM) produced better AR initiation in mouse sperm than higher concentrations. Progesterone can potentiate the effect of GABA on neuronal $GABA_A$ receptor/ Cl channels (46), but we were unable to potentiate the GABA initiation of the human AR by adding progesterone. However, using the lower GABA concentration, Roldan and coworkers were able to do so in mouse sperm (8,24). As suggested earlier (44), it is also possible that progesterone might potentiate the ability of oviductal GABA to initiate the AR.

The $GABA_A$ receptor/Cl⁻ channel blockers picrotoxin or pregnenolone sulfate and the $GABA_A$ receptor antagonist bicuculline, which may also be a Cl⁻ channel blocker (47) caused a large reduction in the progesterone-initiated human and porcine AR (44,45). Surprisingly, picrotoxin did not inhibit the mouse AR initiated by progesterone but bicuculline did (24). Indirect immunofluorescence, using a monoclonal antibody to the bovine cerebral cortex $GABA_A$ receptor a-subunit, localized immunoreactivity in live and fixed sperm as a fluorescent band in the sperm plasma membrane, overlying or near the narrow equatorial segment region of the acrosome. Immunoblotting using this antibody detected two major bands with apparent molecular weights of 50 kD (as reported in other cell types) and 75 kD (not reported in other cells). We concluded that there was a role for a unique sperm steroid receptor/Cl^- channel complex (resembling but not completely identical to a $GABA_A$ receptor/Cl^- channel complex) in the progesterone-initiated AR.

Progesterone can potentiate the response of neuronal $GABA_A$ receptor/Cl^- channels to GABA, and progesterone metabolites with 3α-0H groups, but not progesterone itself activate neuronal $GABA_A$ receptor/Cl^- channels in the absence of GABA (48). If a $GABA_A$ receptor/Cl^- channel was involved in the AR, why was progesterone the most effective steroid AR initiator in the our studies? There are several possible explanations. First, the putative sperm steroid receptor/Cl^- channel complex of the highly differentiated sperm may be unique in its interaction with different progestins. The specific amino acid sequences and configuration of subunits in a $GABA_A$ receptor/Cl^- channel complex has major effects on the types of pharmacological agents with which it interacts (49). For example, although benzodiazepines bind to most $GABA_A$ receptor/Cl^- channels and increase their frequency of opening, there is at least one such somatic cell receptor/channel complex that lacks the benzodiazepine binding site (50). Another possible explanation for the higher potency of progesterone compared to the three anesthetic progestins is that progesterone may not only interact with a putative sperm steroid receptor/Cl^- channel complex but also better than the others with a sperm plasma membrane steroid receptor coupled to a sperm Ca^{2+} channel. With respect to the former, some of the added progesterone might be converted to 3α-OH progesterone metabolites by sperm (although this would be less likely in the case of progesterone-BSA conjugates).

We have recently reported that the increase in $[Ca^{2+}]_i$ essential to the AR is independent of the AR Cl^- requirement because progesterone increased $[Ca^{2+}]_i$ to the same extent in a Cl^- deficient medium and a Cl^- containing medium but the AR only occurred in the latter (51). Also, in those studies pregnenolone sulfate inhibited the AR but increased $[Ca^{2+}]$ to the same extent as progesterone, and picrotoxin did not significantly inhibit the $[Ca^{2+}]$ increase due to progesterone. Other laboratories have also reported that antagonists of $GABA_A$ receptor/Cl^- channels have little effect on progesterone-mediated changes in human sperm $[Ca^{2+}]_i$ (52, 53). We have suggested that such results may be due to the presence of two plasma membrane progesterone receptors: one receptor initiating the increase in $[Ca^{2+}]_i$ and the other initiating an increased Cl^- flux (51). It is also possible that only one sperm membrane progesterone receptor exists and that receptor "cross-talk" between that single receptor and the receptor/Cl^- channel occurs. It is worth noting that Cl^- is also essential for the zona-initiated AR in hamster and porcine sperm (45, 54). Interestingly, a receptor channel resembling a neuronal glycine receptor/Cl^- channel rather a $GABA_A$ receptor/Cl^- channel appears to be involved in the zona-initiated AR (45).

Wistrom and Meizel had hypothesized that Cl^- influx and reversal of HCO_3^-/Cl^- exchange may be involved in progesterone initiation of the human sperm AR, with the increased HCO_3^- leading to a more alkaline intracellular pH and/or increased adenylate cyclase activity (44). In order to detect progesterone-mediated intracellular Cl^- changes in human sperm, we have used the fluorescent Cl^- probe MEQ (55). Sperm are loaded with nonpolar diH-MEQ, which is oxidized by the cell to less permeable polar MEQ. The fluorescence of MEQ is quenched by Cl^-. Our preliminary studies show that addition of progesterone to capacitated sperm results in a rapid decrease in intracellular Cl^- that is inhibited by picrotoxin (51). We interpret these results as an efflux of Cl (rather than the originally hypothesized influx) through the sperm steroid receptor/Cl- channel that resembles a $GABA_A$ receptor/Cl channel. Perhaps sperm membrane depolarization caused by progesterone (25, 56), is due to the efflux of Cl^- through the steroid receptor/Cl^- channel. A Na^+/HCO_3^- cotransporter that acts to increase intracellular HCO_3^- in a number of cell types can be activated by membrane depolarization (57), and increased activity of a putative sperm Na^+/HCO_3^- cotransporter might be one result of sperm Cl^- efflux. Higher intracellular HCO_3^- could help stimulate the AR by increasing intracellular pH and/or adenylate cyclase (4). In this regard, it is of interest that high HCO_3^- (25 mM) is required for optimal progesterone-initiated human AR (58).

SOME OF THE IMPORTANT QUESTIONS STILL TO BE ANSWERED CONCERNING PROGESTERONE, PROGESTERONE RECEPTORS AND AR-INITIATION

1. Is there more than one progesterone receptor, or is there cross-talk between one receptor for progesterone and some other essential receptor that does not actually bind the steroid?
2. Is one progesterone receptor a modified $GABA_A$ receptor?
3. Is there some subtle but important relationship between Cl^- efflux and Ca^{2+} influx in the progesterone-initiated AR?

4. Is there any interconversion of progesterone by sperm to 3α-OH steroids capable of activating GABA$_A$ receptor/Cl$^-$ channels?
5. What is the concentration of progesterone in the cumulus extracellular matrix at the time of fertilization?
6. Is there a synergistic interaction between progesterone and zona during the in vitro and vivo human AR?

Acknowledgments
This research was supported by the NIH and in part by the Labor Foundation .

REFERENCES

1. Yanagimachi R, Mammalian Fertilization. In: Knobil E, Neill JD, Eds., Physiology of Reproduction, New York, Raven Press, Ltd., 1994, pp. 189-317.
2. Yudin AI, Gottlieb W, Meizel S. Ultrastructural studies of the early events of the human sperm acrosome reaction as initiated by human follicular fluid. Gamete Res. 1988; 20: 11-24.
3. Meizel S, Pillai MC, Diaz-Perez E, Thomas P. Initiation of the human sperm acrosome reaction by components of human follicular fluid and cumulus secretions including steroids. In: Bavister BD, Cummins J, Roldan ERS, Eds., Fertilization in Mammals, Norwell Mass., Serono Symposia, USA, 1990, pp. 205-222.
4. Kopf GS, Gerton GL. The mammalian sperm acrosome and the acrosome reaction. In: Wasserman PM, Eds., Elements of Mammalian Fertilization, Boston, CRC Press, vol. 1,1991, pp. 153-203.
5. Meizel S. Molecules that initiate or help stimulate the acrosome reaction by their interaction with the mammalian sperm surface. Am. J. Anat. 1985; 174: 285-302.
6. Osman RA, Andria ML, Jones AD, Meizel S. Steroid induced exocytosis: the human sperm acrosome reaction. Biochem. Biophys. Res. Comm. 1989; 160: 828-833.
7. Melendrez CS, Meizel S, Berger T. Comparison of the ability of progesterone and heat solubilized porcine zona pellucida to initiate the porcine sperm acrosome reaction in vitro. Mol Reprod. Dev. 1994; 39: 433-438.
8. Roldan RS, Murase T, Shi Q-X. Exocytosis in spermatozoa in response to progesterone and zona pellucida. Science 1994; 266: 1578-1581 .

9. Meyers SA, Overstreet JW, Liu IKM, Drobnis EZ. Capacitation in vitro of stallion spermatozoa: comparison of progesteroneinduced acrosome reactions in fertile and subfertile males. J. Androl. 1995; In Press.
10. Yoshizawa M, Nagai T, Yonezawa N, Nakano M. Native zona pellucida is required for completion of the sperm acrosome reaction in porcine fertilization. Theriogenol. 1994; 41: 1307-1 313.
11. Morales P, Cross NL, Overstreet JW, Hanson FW. Acrosome intact and acrosome-reacted human sperm can initiate binding to the zona pellucida. Dev. Biol. 1989; 133: 385-392.
12. Liu DY, Baker HWG. Inducing the human acrosome reaction with a calcium ionophore A23187 decreases sperm-zona pellucida binding with oocytes that failed to fertilize in vitro. J. Reprod. Fertil. 1990; 89: 127-134.
13. Tesarik J, Mendoza C. Defective function of a nongenomic progesterone receptor as a sole sperm anomaly in infertile patients. Fertil. Steril. 1992; 58: 793-797.
14. Falsetti C, Baldi E, Krausz C, Casano R, Failli P, Forti G. Decreased responsiveness to progesterone of spermatozoa in oligozoospermic patients. J. Androl. 1993;14: 17-22.
15. Oehninger S, Blackmore P, Morshedi M, Sueldo C, Acosta AA, Alexander NJ. Defective calcium influx and acrosome reaction (spontaneous and progesterone-induced) in spermatozoa of infertile men with severe teratozoospermia. Fertil. Steril. 1994; 61: 349-354.
16. Tesarik J. Comparison of acrosome reaction-inducing activities of human cumulus oophorus, follicular fluid and ionophore A23187 in human sperm populations of proven fertility in vitro. J. Reprod. Fertil. 1985; 74: 383-388.
17. Siiteri JE, Dandekar P, Meizel S. Human sperm acrosome reaction-initiating activity associated with the human cumulus oophorus and mural granulosa cells. J. Exp. Zool. 1988; 246: 71-80.
18. Miska W, Fehl P, Henkel R. Biochemical and immunological characterization of the acrosome reaction-inducing substance (ARIS) of HFF. Biochem. Biophys. Res Comm. 1994; 199: 125-129.
19. Thomas P, Meizel S. An influx of extracellular calcium is required for initiation of the human sperm acrosome reaction induced by human follicular fluid. Gamete Res. 1988; 20: 397-411
20. Thomas P, Meizel S. Phosphatidylinositol 4,5-bisphosphate hydrolysis in human sperm stimulated with follicular fluid or progesterone is dependent upon Ca^{2+} influx. Biochem. J. 1989; 264: 539-546.

21. Florman HM, Corron ME, Kim TD-H, Babcock DF. Activation of voltage-dependent calcium channels of mammalian sperm is required for zona pellucida-induced acrosomal exocytosis. Dev. Biol. 1992; 152: 304-314.
22. Blackmore PF, Beebe SJ, Danforth DR, Alexander N. Progsterone and 17α-hydroxyprogesterone: novel stimulators of calcium influx in human sperm. J. Biol. Chem. 1990; 265: 1376-1380.
23. Meizel S, Turner KO, Nuccitelli R. Localization of progesterone-mediated calcium influx and detection of progesterone-mediated chloride efflux in human sperm. Mol Biol. Cell, 1994; 5, Supplement: 345a.
24. Shi Q-X, Roldan ERS. Evidence that a $GABA_A$-like receptor is involved in progesterone-induced acrosomal exocytosis in mouse spermatozoa. Biol. Reprod. 1995; 52: 373-381.
25. Foresta C, Rossato M, Di Virgilio F. Ion fluxes through the progesterone-activated channel of the sperm plasma membrane. Biochem. J. 1993; 294: 279-283.
26. Foresta C, Rossato M, Di Virgilio F. Differential modulation by protein kinase C of progesterone-activated responses in human sperm. Biochem. Biophys. Res. Comm. 1995; 206: 408-413.
27. Garcia MA, Meizel S. Effects of sodium ion on the progesterone-initiated calcium influx and acrosome reaction in human sperm. Biol. Reprod. 1994; 50, Supplement 1: 105.
28. Lytton J, Westlin M, Hanley MR. Thapsigargin inhibits the sarcoplasmic or endoplasmic reticulum Ca-ATPase family of calcium pumps. J. Biol. Chem. 1991; 266: 17067-17071.
29. Meizel S, Turner KO. Initiation of the human sperm acrosome reaction by thapsigargin. J. Exp. Zool. 1993; 267: 350-355.
30. Blackmore PF. Thapsigargin elevates and potentiates the ability of progesterone to increase intracellular free calcium in human sperm: possible role of perinuclear calcium. Cell Calcium 1993; 14: 53-60.
31. Favero TG, Abramson JJ. Thapsigargin-induced Ca^{2+} release from sarcoplasmic reticulum and asolectin vesicles. Cell Calcium 1994; 15: 183-189.
32. Walensky LD, Snyder SH. Identification and localization of the inositol trisphosphate receptor in mammalian sperm. Mol Biol. Cell 1994; 5 (supplement): 346a.
33. Pillai MC, Meizel S. Trypsin inhibitors prevent the progesterone-initiated increase in intracellular calcium required for the human sperm acrosome reaction. J. Exp. Zool. 1991; 258: 384-393.
34. Tesarik J, Mendoza C. Insights into the function of a sperm surface progesterone receptor: evidence of ligand-induced receptor aggregation and the implication of proteolysis. Exp. Cell Res. 1993; 205: 111-117.

35. Koenig H, Fan C-C, Goldstone AD, Lu CY, Trout JJ. Polyamines mediate androgenic stimulation of calcium fluxes and membrane transport in rat heart myocytes. Circ. Res. 1989; 64: 415-426.
36. Meizel S, Turner KO. Effects of polyamine biosynthesis inhibitors on the progesterone-initiated increase in intracellular free Ca^{2+} and acrosome reactions in human sperm. Mol Reprod. Dev. 1993; 34: 457-465.
37. Meizel S, Turner KO. Progesterone acts at the plasma membrane of human sperm. Mol. Cell. Endocrinol 1991; 11: R 1 -RS.
38. Blackmore PF, Neulen J, Lattanzio F, Beebe SJ. Cell surfacebinding sites for progesterone mediate calcium uptake in human sperm. J. Biol. Chem. 1991; 266:18655-18659.
39. Tesarik J, Mendoza C, Moos J, Fenichel P, Fehlmann M. Progesterone action through aggregation of a receptor on the sperm plasma membrane. FEBS Letters. 1992;308: 116-120.
40. Tesarik J, Mendoza C, Moos J, Carreras A. Selective expression of a progesterone receptor on the human sperm surface. Fertil. Steril. 1992; 58: 784-792.
41. Mendoza C, Tesarik J. A plasma-membrane progesterone receptor in human sperm is switched on by increasing intracellular free calcium. FEBS Letters 1993; 330: 57-60.
42. Tesarik J, Moos J, Mendoza C. Stimulation of protein tyrosine phosphorylation by a progesterone receptor on the cell surface of human sperm. Endocrinology 1993; 133: 328-335.
43. Sabeur K, D.P. E, Meizel S. Plasma membrane progesterone receptor(s) in human sperm. Biol. Reprod. 1995; Supplement, (SSR abstracts): In Press.
44. Wistrom CA, Meizel S. Evidence suggesting involvement of a unique human sperm steroid receptor/Cl^- channel complex in the progesterone-initiated acrosome reaction. Dev. Biol. 1993; 159: 679-690.
45. Melendrez CS, Meizel S. Different Chloride channels are involved in the progesterone- and zona-initiated porcine sperm acrosome reaction. Mol Biol Cell 1994; 5, Supplement (ASCB abstracts): 345a.
46. Wu F-S, Gibbs TT, Farb DH. Inverse modulation of γ-aminobutyric acid- and glycine-induced currents by progesterone. Mol. Pharmacol. 1990; 37: 597-602.
47. Aprison MH, Lipkowitz KB. On the GABA receptor: a molecular modeling approach. J. Neurosci. Res. 1989; 23: 129-135.
48. Callachan BH, Cottrell GA, Hather NY, Lambert JJ, Nooney JM, Peters JA. Modulation of the $GABA_A$ receptor by progesterone metabolites. Proc. B. Soc. Lond. 1987; 231: 359.

49. Burt DR, Kamatchi GL. $GABA_A$ receptor subtypes: from pharmacology to molecular biology.FASEB J. 1991; 5: 2916-2
50. Anderson SMP, De Souza RJ, Cross AJ. The human neuroblastoma cell line, IMR-32 possesses a $GABA_A$ receptor lacking the benzodiazepine modulatory site. Neuropharm. 1993; 32: 455-460.
51. Tumer KO, Garcia MA, Meizel S.Progesterone-initiation of the human sperm acrosome reaction: the obligatory increase in intracellular calcium is independent of the chloride requirement. Mol. Cell. Endocrinol. 1994; 101: 221-225.
52. Baldi E, Casano R, Falsetti C, Krausz C, Maggi M, Forti G. Intracellular calcium accumulation and responsiveness to progesterone in capacitating human sperm. J. Androl. 1991; 12:
53. Blackmore PF, Im WB, Bleasdale JE. The cell surface progesterone receptor which stimulates calcium influx in human sperm is unlike the A ring reduced steroid site on the GABA receptor/chloride channel. Mol Cell Endocrinol. 1994; 104: 237-243.
54. Yoshimatsu N, Yanagimachi R. Effects of cations and other medium components on the zona-induced acrosome reaction of hamster spermatozoa. Dev. Growth Differ. 1988; 30: 65 1 -659.
55. Biwersi J, Verkman AS. Cell-permeable fluorescent indicator for cytosolic chloride. Biochem. 1991; 30: 7879-7883.
56. Calzada L, Salazar EL, Macias H. Hyperpolarization/ Depolarization on human sperm. Archiv. Androl. 1991; 26: 71-78.
57. Boron WF, Boulpaep EL.The electrogenic Na/HCO_3 cotransporter. Kidney Inter. 1989; 36: 392-402.
58. Sabeur K, Meizel S.Importance of bicarbonate to the progesterone-initiated human sperm acrosome reaction. J. Androl 1995; in Press.

Human sperm acrosome reaction. Eds P. Fénichel, J. Parinaud.
Colloque INSERM/John Libbey Eurotext Ltd © 1995. Vol. 236, pp. 165-177

Effect of steroids on calcium fluxes in human sperm

Peter F. Blackmore [a], Jed F. Fisher [b], Charles H. Spilman [c], Wha Bin Im [d] and John E. Bleasdale [c]

[a] *Department of Pharmacology, Eastern Virginia Medical School, P.O. Box 1980, Norfolk VA 23501, USA,* [b] *Department of Medicinal Chemistry,* [c] *Endocrine Pharmacology and Metabolism,* [d] *Department of CNS Disease Research, The Upjohn Company, Kalamazoo, MI 49001, USA*

Abstract

The characteristics of the cell surface progesterone receptor responsible for stimulating Ca^{2+} influx in human sperm was examined utilizing 160 steroid analogs. Several compounds were more effective than progesterone eg. 2α-methyl 17β-methoxy 5α-androstan-3-one. Some testosterone analogs eg. 2α,7α,17α-trimethyl testosterone were shown to be antagonists of progesterone. The progesterone receptor on sperm that was responsible for stimulating Ca^{2+} influx was unlike the $GABA_A/Cl^-$ channel since the A-ring reduced 3α-hydroxy pregnane steroids, which bind to the $GABA_A/Cl^-$ channel, were poor stimulators of sperm Ca^{2+} influx. Some synthetic progestins eg. cyproterone acetate and megestrol acetate were antagonists of progesterone in sperm. Several simple substitutions on the steroid ring structure were found to be either beneficial or detrimental to activity. It was concluded that the active steroids make close contact to the sperm progesterone receptor across the β-face of the steroid C and D rings (C-11, C-12, C-17). The proper placement of the C-21 methyl is important for activity. In contrast to the sperm receptor, progesterone interacts with the genomic receptor via the α-face of the molecule.

Les caractéristiques du récepteur membranaire à la progestérone, responsable de la stimulation de l'influx de Ca^{2+} dans le sperme humain, ont été examinées en utilisant 160 analogues de stéroïdes. Quelques-uns se sont *avérés plus efficaces que la progestérone comme le 2α,17β-methoxy 5α-androstan-3-1. Quelques analogues de la testostérone, tels que la 2α,7α,17α-trimethyl testosterone, se sont comportés comme des antagonistes de la progestérone. Le récepteur spermatique à la progestérone, responsable de la stimulation de l'influx de Ca^{2+}, est différent du canal $GABA_A/Cl^-$. En effet les 3α hydroxypregnanes à noyau A réduit qui se lient au canal $GABA_A/Cl^-$ sont de faibles stimulants de l'influx calcique du spermatozoïde. Quelques progestogènes synthétiques comme l'acétate de cyprotérone et l'acétate de megestrol sont des antagonistes de la progestérone au niveau du spermatozoïde. Plusieurs substitutions, simples, sur le noyau stérol ont été trouvées comme étant soit bénéfiques soit délétères sur l'activité. Au total les stéroïdes actifs entrent en contact avec le récepteur spermatique à la progestérone par la face β des noyaux C et D du stéroïde (C-11, C-12, C-17). La localisation adéquate du méthyl en C21 est capitale pour l'activité. Contrairement au récepteur spermatique, la progestérone entre en contact avec le récepteur génomique via la face α de la molécule.*

INTRODUCTION

There are now many studies showing that steroids can elicit a variety of rapid biological responses independent of their well characterized effects at the level of the genome. Some of these rapid effects have recently been reviewed. For example: progesterone (1,2), aldosterone (3), and vitamin D (4). The steroids β-estradiol, testosterone and glucocorticoids also exhibit many non-genomic effects in a variety of tissues eg. (5-7). These rapid biological effects of steroids, have often been shown to be mediated by cell surface (plasma membrane) receptors and they have been referred to as "non-genomic effects of steroids".

One of the most widely studied non-genomic steroid effect is that of progesterone to stimulate Ca^{2+} influx the acrosome reaction (AR) in human sperm (8,9). Earlier studies showed that human follicular fluid was able to elicit the AR in human sperm. An active component of follicular fluid which elicited the AR was demonstrated to be progesterone (10,11). These findings have prompted an extensive investigation into the signaling events that are stimulated by progesterone. The effect of progesterone to elicit the AR has also been observed in stallion, monkey (Blackmore, unpublished findings), hamster and mouse sperm (12).

One of the first molecules that sperm encounter in the female reproductive tract is progesterone, which is produced by the cumulus cells.

Since sperm posses a cell surface receptor for progesterone (see below), it is therefore of some significance in reproductive physiology. The influx of calcium that is stimulated by progesterone (described below) can stimulate the AR and may also be involved in capacitation (13,14). Both of these processes are calcium dependent, and if they don't occur then fertilization can't proceed. Sperm binding to a component of the zona pellucida, a glycoprotein called ZP_3, can also stimulate the AR (15).

We have shown that infertile patients with a high incidence of abnormal sperm forms (teratozoospermia) have a low incidence of spontaneous and progesterone induced AR, parallel abnormalities on progesterone induced changes on $[Ca^{2+}]_i$ were also observed (16). These results suggest that in teratozoospermia there is a defective non-genomic progesterone receptor/signal transduction system. Other studies have shown a defective sperm surface progesterone receptor system in some cases of male infertility (17).

PROGESTERONE SIGNAL TRANSDUCTION IN HUMAN SPERM

Since progesterone was shown to stimulate the AR in capacitated human sperm, studies were initiated to evaluate the ability of progesterone to stimulate Ca^{2+} influx. For these experiments, intracellular free calcium ($[Ca^{2+}]_i$) was measured in human sperm utilizing the fluorescent calcium indicator fura 2 (8,9,11). Studies showed that progesterone produced a very rapid (within several seconds) increase in $[Ca^{2+}]_i$. The increase in $[Ca^{2+}]_i$ was transient, although it still remained above basal values for many minutes. The effect of progesterone to elevate $[Ca^{2+}]_i$ was dose dependent, with small effects being observed with 1-10 nM and maximum effects seen with 1-10μM progesterone (8). The other naturally occurring steroid that was active on sperm was 17α-hydroxy progesterone. It had a similar time course and dose response to progesterone (8). It was known that 17α-hydroxy progesterone was a very weak stimulator of the genomic progesterone receptor. Several other steroids were examined , and were found to be very weak stimulators on $[Ca^{2+}]_i$ (8,9). These initial studies suggested that the receptor for progesterone on human sperm was unique, since it was specifically stimulated by progesterone and 17α-hydroxy progesterone and not testosterone and β-estradiol (8,9).

The source of the calcium responsible for the increase in $[Ca^{2+}]_i$ was examined next. It was well accepted that when hormones stimulate an increase in $[Ca^{2+}]_i$ (in most cells) it was mediated by intracellular mobilization from the endoplasmic reticulum, followed by influx of calcium from the extracellular fluid (18). When human sperm were suspended in medium devoid of free calcium (i.e. in the presence of the calcium chelator EGTA), progesterone was unable to elicit any increase in $[Ca^{2+}]_i$ (8). This finding was unique, since it showed that progesterone was unable to mobilize intracellular calcium stores but was only able to stimulate inflow of calcium from the extracellular space (18). Subsequent studies confirmed that human sperm did not posses any significant endoplasmic reticulum calcium stores (19). However the possible involvement of perinuclear calcium stores contributing to the increase in $[Ca^{2+}]_i$, induced by progesterone, was implied (19). The involvement of perinuclear calcium pools and remnants of the endoplasmic reticulum contributing to the increase in $[Ca^{2+}]_i$ need further investigation.

It appeared however that progesterone was able to stimulate calcium influx in human sperm and not mobilize any significant amounts of calcium from intracellular calcium stores (8). Other studies showed that progesterone was able to stimulate the influx of the calcium surrogate manganese into sperm (8), as measured by the quenching of intracellular fura 2 by manganese.

Having established that the predominant effect of progesterone was to stimulate calcium influx in human sperm, the next question asked was: where was the subcellular location of the progesterone receptor in sperm? Since progesterone is able to enter cells by passive diffusion, we performed experiments in which the progesterone molecule was confined extracellularly by coupling it to a high molecular weight molecule, bovine serum albumin (BSA) (9). The progesterone conjugate was able to stimulate calcium influx as effectively, although less potently as free progesterone (9,20,21). This result demonstrated that progesterone could be confined to the extracellular space and was able to elicit a full calcium influx response. Since the covalent coupling was *via* the 3 carbon on the A-ring, one may surmise that this position was unessential for activity (see below).

To confirm that the BSA conjugated progesterone was binding to a cell surface progesterone receptor, we visualized the binding to sperm by utilizing a fluorescent conjugate of the BSA-progesterone complex (20). It was demonstrated that the binding of the progesterone conjugate was to the head of human sperm (20). We have obtained more direct confirmation of the existence of a progesterone binding protein in human sperm and seminal plasma utilizing radioligand studies (22). The progesterone binding protein has an apparent molecular weight of 90-100 kDa (determined by SDS-PAGE). The protein also forms polymers in sucrose gradients (22). The k_d for progesterone binding was approx. 10 nM with optimal binding being observed at pH 7. The binding site was selective for progesterone and 17α-hydroxy progesterone, with β-estradiol and testosterone having lower affinity (22).

Thus the model proposed for progesterone stimulating the influx of calcium in human sperm was that progesterone bound to a receptor located on the extracellular surface of the sperm head . By some yet to be determined mechanism this binding prompted an influx of calcium into the head of the sperm. There is some evidence for the participation of proteases (23), tyrosine phosphorylation (24), pH (25), sodium ions (26) and polyamines (27) in the progesterone induced increase in $[Ca^{2+}]_i$ and the AR. Other second messenger systems have not been critically evaluated yet, such as the role played by inositol phosphates and G proteins (1,2). It appears however that the increase in inositol trisphosphate is secondary to the progesterone induced increase in $[Ca^{2+}]_i$ (11).

An area that has received some attention recently is that of the role played by $GABA_A/Cl^-$ channels in progesterone induced AR (12,28,29,30). These studies suggest that there may be two progesterone binding entities in human sperm (29,30). One binding protein is responsible for initiating Ca^{2+} influx, whereas the other one may be similar to the $GABA_A/Cl^-$ channel and mediate chloride fluxes (29,30). The $GABA_A/Cl^-$ channel is known to posses a steroid binding site for the A-ring reduced 3α- hydroxy pregnane steroids (eg. alfaxalone, allopregnanolone, pregnanolone)(31). Evidence to support the notion that the progesterone receptor responsible for initiating Ca^{2+} influx was not the $GABA_A/Cl^-$ channel was the fact that steroids which were very active on the $GABA_A/Cl^-$ channel were very poor stimulators of Ca^{2+} influx(30). Also other known modulators of $GABA_A/Cl^-$ channels such as picrotoxin, diazepam, GABA and pentobarbital did not influence basal $[Ca^{2+}]_i$ or the Ca^{2+} transient induced by progesterone (30).

CHARACTERISTICS ON THE PROGESTERONE BINDING SITE ON HUMAN SPERM

When synthetic potent genomic progestins were added to human sperm there was no Ca^{2+} influx (9,32). Some of the progestins that were tested were megestrol, medroxyprogesterone acetate, norgestrel, northindrone and norethynodrel (9,32). This result strongly suggests that the progesterone binding site was very different to that on the intracellular genomic receptor. This result was confirmed when the very potent genomic antiprogestins RU486 and ZK98.299 were shown to be poor antagonists of progesterone mediated Ca^{2+} influx (9). Both RU486 and ZK98.299 are effective in the nM range when acting on the genomic receptor, however to obtain any significant inhibition of progesterone induced Ca^{2+} influx in sperm , µM concentrations had to be used, 100 µM concentrations did produce approx., 80% inhibition (9). The conclusion from these studies was that the steroid binding site on the surface of human sperm must be different to the genomic receptor, although progesterone itself is effective on both receptors.

We next expanded the number of progesterone analogs and examined their effects to promote Ca^{2+} influx and to bind to the rabbit genomic progesterone receptor (32,33,34) Table I. It was evident from the data that there was no correlation between the two parameters examined (r = -0.28). For example many of the analogs were very strong stimulators on Ca^{2+} influx but were weak at binding to the uterine receptor (e.g. 2α-methyl progesterone) and some analogs had high affinity for the uterine receptor but were weak at stimulating Ca^{2+} influx (e.g. 19-nor-17,21-dimethyl progesterone). It appears that several modifications to the progesterone analogs are fatal to activity on sperm. For example the presence of the 17α acetate in megestrol acetate, medroxyprogesterone acetate and cyproterone acetate reduced activity drastically. Removal of the acetate in these analogs now produced good agonist activity on sperm (Table I).

A variety of substituents in the 2α- configuration e.g. chloro, nitrile, methyl and fluro, produced analogs that were 5- to 10- times more potent than progesterone. The increased potency of 2-substituted analogs was only seen when the substituent was in the α- configuration. While 2α- methyl progesterone was approx. 10-fold more potent than progesterone, 2β- methyl- progesterone was approx. 5-times less potent and 60% as effective as progesterone. Some other substitutions in the A-ring also increased Ca^{2+} influx e.g. 1,2-dehydro progesterone (114%) and 4β-methyl progesterone (142%) (32).

Because many of the potent synthetic progestins have substitutions at the 6-position of the pregnane nucleus (eg. megestrol acetate, cyproterone acetate and medroxyprogesterone acetate), the influence of 6-substitutions on Ca^{2+} influx were examined. A fluorine on C-6 in either the α or β configuration increased progesterone effectiveness (117 and 147% respectively) . A 6-methoxy group reduced effectiveness by 56%. The introduction of a 8,9-double bond increased activity of progesterone (129%). The presence of an hydroxyl group at C-11 in the β-configuration (but not α) increased effectiveness (but not potency) of progesterone at increasing Ca^{2+} influx (140%). A 2α- methyl together with an 11β-hydroxyl group increased effectiveness (180%) and potency by approx. 10-fold. The presence of the bulky 11α-cyclopentane-propionate on progesterone increased Ca^{2+} influx (32).

ANALOG	[Ca2+]i	UTERINE BINDING
Progesterone (P4)	100	100
9,11-dehydro-P4	139	79
1,2-dehydro-P4	144	23
8,9-dehydro-P4	129	29
14,15-dehydro-P4	66	88
4,5-dehydro-P4	117	9
11α-hydroxy-P4	30	4
11β-hydroxy-P4	183	42
11α-acetate-P4	9	<1
17α-hydroxy-P4	96	3
17α-hydroxy acetate-P4	10	89
17α-hydroxy caproate-P4	21	34
17α-hydroxy formate-P4	55	21
2α-fluoro-P4	144	51
2α-methyl-P4	117	17
4β-methyl-P4	142	17
6α-methyl-P4	85	72
21-fluoro-P4	149	65
19-nor-P4	95	156
19-nor-17,21-dimethyl-P4	1	162
norethindrone acetate	49	59
norethindrone	8	100
megestrol acetate	5	89
megestrol	79	*
norethynodrel	12	20
medroxy P4 acetate	14	70
medroxy P4	75	6
norgestrel	1	78
promegestrone (R5020)	10	163
cyproterone acetate	0	*
cyproterone	60	*

Table I. :Comparison of selected progesterone analogs for the capacity to increase $[Ca^{2+}]_i$ in human sperm and to bind to rabbit uterine cytosolic progesterone receptors. The binding affinities of cyproterone acetate and cyproterone for the rabbit uterine progesterone receptor relative to progesterone (100%) have been reported to be: cyproterone acetate (85%) >> cyproterone (35). (* not determined.)

The D-ring modifications that most influenced Ca^{2+} influx were all at C-17. 17α- hydroxy progesterone is inactive as a genomic progestin, but is as effective as progesterone at stimulating Ca^{2+} influx in sperm (8). Other α-hydroxy substitutions e.g. 11α-progesterone also had reduced binding to the uterine receptor (Table I), and it has been proposed that α-hydroxyls in general disrupt binding to the cytosolic genomic progesterone receptor, because the α face is involved in binding (36). In contrast, several α-hydroxy derivatives of progesterone eg. 14α- hydroxy (140%), 6α-hydroxy (60%), and 2α-hydroxy (82%) as well as 17α-hydroxy (96%) were effective at stimulating Ca^{2+} influx in sperm. This may imply that the α face of the progesterone analogs are not involved with binding to the cell surface progesterone receptor on sperm (see below for further evidence). Esterification of the 17α-hydroxy group with formate, acetate, propionate or caproate produced analogs with reduced Ca^{2+} influx activity relative to progesterone of 55, 10, 0, and 21% respectively. The 17α- hydroxy- nitrite analog of progesterone produced a Ca^{2+} influx of (100%) and 17α-tetrahydropyran-2-yloxy-progesterone (containing a very bulky substituent) was more effective than progesterone (133%) (32).

Modifications at C-20 and C-21 also had pronounced effects on Ca^{2+} influx. 21-Fluoro-progesterone had a Ca^{2+} influx value of 149% which was reduced to 89% by the introduction of a second 21-fluro group. Replacement of C-20 and C-21 of progesterone with a methoxy group was a common feature of a series of compounds (now an androstane ring structure) that were much more effective (but not more potent) than progesterone at stimulating progesterone influx. The following androstane analogs produced larger Ca^{2+} influx than progesterone: 2α-ethyl 17β-methoxy 5α-androstane 3-one (282%), 2α-nitrile 3-oxo 17β-methoxy 5α-androstane (243%), 2α- methoxy 17β- methoxy 5α- androstane 3-one (229%), 2α- methyl 17β- methoxy androst 4-en 3-one (163%) and 2α-nitrile 17β-methoxy 3-oxo androst 4-ene (160%). Representative of this group of androstane derivatives are 2α-methyl 17β-methoxy 5α-androstane 3-one and 2α-methyl androst 4-en-3-one which were found not to bind to the uterine cytosolic progesterone receptor (<1%). Interestingly, when the 2α-ethyl group of the most active androstane analog (above) (282%) was replaced with 2-ethylidene, the Ca^{2+} influx was drastically reduced to 25% of that observed with progesterone.

Replacement of the acetyl group on C-17 of progesterone with a hydroxyl group produces testosterone. A series of testosterone analogs were tested for Ca^{2+} influx, and while many were found to be ineffective at increasing $[Ca^{2+}]_i$ in sperm, several analogs inhibited the ability of progesterone to increase $[Ca^{2+}]_i$. Two analogs were found to be very effective antagonists of progesterone, they were 2α, 7α, 17α- trimethyl testosterone and 9(11) dehydro 2α, 17α-dimethyl testosterone. Both analogs at a concentration of 10 μM inhibited 10 μM progesterone by approx. 90% (32). A notable feature of both testosterone antagonists was that they both contained 2α-methyl groups. The presence of a 2α-methyl on progesterone increased its effectiveness as an agonist (Table I).

The potent genomic progestins norethynodrel, cyproterone acetate, norethindrone and megestrol acetate were examined for their ability to stimulate Ca^{2+} influx. These progestins had very little effect on $[Ca^{2+}]_i$ in sperm (9,32). However some of these progestins were able to inhibit the ability of progesterone to increase $[Ca^{2+}]_i$ in human sperm (32). One of the most potent inhibitors of progesterone was cyproterone acetate. Cyproterone acetate contains a 1,2α-methylene group, which may facilitate binding to the cell surface progesterone receptor, just like several of the other 2α substituents on progesterone. The lack of agonist activity of cyproterone acetate would appear to be due to some other modification of the molecule, such as the 17α-acetoxy (hydroxy acetate) group (Table I), because the free alcohol of cyproterone acetate, namely cyproterone (SH 881), has good agonist activity to increase $[Ca^{2+}]_i$ in sperm (Table I). A prediction from these findings would be that an analog that contains an 17α-acetoxy group, together with a 2α-methyl group it would be an antagonist. The progesterone analog 2α-methyl 9α-fluoro 11β-hydroxy 17α-acetoxy progesterone (at a concentration of 1 μM) antagonized a 10 μM concentration of progesterone to elevate $[Ca^{2+}]_i$ in human sperm by approx. 70% (32).

The unimportance of the progesterone A-ring ketone C-3 was evident by the full activity (103%) of 4,5α-dihydro 3β-ol derivative of progesterone. Neither the double bond nor the 3- ketone is required for activity. The full agonist activity (96%) activity of the 4,5β-dihydro 3α-ol derivative of progesterone was surprising. The 5β-configuration imparts a *cis* configuration of the steroid A,B-rings, which results in a downward projection of the A-ring rather than an outward projection. Both C-2 and C-3 of the 4,5β -dihydro 3α-ol derivative occupy different regions within the receptor when compared to C-2 and C-3 of the 4,5α-dihydro 3β-ol derivative. The presence of a trifluromethyl 1 *H* -pyrazole fused to the steroid A-ring possesses modest activity (34%), thus confirming the observation that the 3-ketone is not necessary for agonist activity and that there is open space at the receptor along the steroid C-2,3 A-ring edge. Thus the C-3 ketone of progesterone can't contribute to receptor recognition, and the C-2α derivatives most likely contribute primarily to potency rather than efficacy (32).

9α- Bromo 11β-fluro progesterone retains full efficacy (94%) (32). A fluro atom, as found in 11β-hydroxy 9α-fluro progesterone (93%) and 2α-methyl 11β-hydroxy 9α-fluro progesterone (95%), is sterically a small but strongly dipole active substituent. The 9α-bromo group of 9α- bromo 11β-fluro progesterone is an extremely large group, projecting downward in the center of the α-face of the steroid A,B- rings. Thus the tolerance of 9α-bromo and 9α-fluro groups strongly suggest that the A,B- ring α-face of the steroid is not important for recognition by the sperm cell surface progesterone receptor, since these groups shield the A,B-ring α-face. It is concluded that, in contrast to the genomic progesterone receptor for which structure- activity data show that binding of the steroid is *via* the α-face (35,36,37) the sperm receptor binds to the steroid β-face.

The very poor activity of the 6α- methyl 11-keto progesterone (6%) contrasts strikingly to the good agonist activity of 6α- methyl progesterone (85%). Molecular modeling of these two steroids shows a negligible structural difference between the two steroids. The effect of the 11-keto found in 6α-methyl 11-keto progesterone is localized to a very small difference at C-12 , the C-19 methyl and the D-ring conformation. The conclusion is that the overall steroid C,D-ring conformation is critical for agonist recognition.

CONCLUDING COMMENTS

The human cell-surface receptor can be activated by progesterone derivatives to cause an increase in $[Ca^{2+}]_i$. The structure-activity relationships for agonists vary markedly from those shown previously for the genomic intracellular receptor. For the sperm receptor the data suggests that full agonist activity occurs when the steroid is bound and positions its C-21 methyl correctly. Binding of the steroid does not appear to involve recognition of the A-ring of the steroid. However certain 2α-substitutions improve binding. Also recognition of the A,B-ring α-face, C-18 methyl, the B,C,D-ring (C-6,C-7,C-14,C-15) appear not to be involved in recognition. The data however suggests a close contact between the steroid and the receptor across the C,D-ring "upper" edge (C-11, C-12, C-17). The data also show that progesterone binds to the sperm cell surface receptor *via* the steroid β-face as opposed to the α-face as in the case of the intracellular genomic receptor. It may be feasible to construct steroids which interact specifically with the sperm cell surface receptor (and perhaps cell surface progesterone receptors in other cells) without interacting with the genomic progesterone receptor.

REFERENCES

1. Blackmore PF. Rapid non-genomic actions of progesterone stimulate Ca^{2+} influx and the acrosome reaction in human sperm. Cell. Signal. 1993; 5: 531-38.
2. Revelli A, Modotti M, Piffaretti-Yanez A, Massobrio M, Balerna M. Steroid receptors in human sperm. Hum.Reprod. 1994; 9:760-66.
3. Wehling M. The cell membrane as a target of mineralocorticoid action. Steroids 1995; 60: 153-6.
4. Baran DT. Non-genomic actions of the steroid hormone $1\alpha,25$-dihydroxyvitamin D_3 J.Cell. Biochem. 1994; 56: 303-6.
5. Sze PY, Iqbal Z. Glucocorticoid action on depolarization- dependent calcium influx in brain synaptosomes. Neuroendocrinology 1994; 59: 457-65.
6. Ravi J, Mantzoros CS, Prabhu AS, Ram JL, Sowers JR. In vitro relaxation of phenylephrine- and angiotensin II- contracted aortic rings by β-estradiol. Am.J.Hypertens. 1994; 7: 1065-9.
7. Lieberherr M, Grosse B. Androgens increase intracellular calcium concentration and inositol 1,4,5-triphosphate and diacylglycerol formation via a pertussis toxin-sensitive G-protein. J.Biol.Chem. 1994; 269: 7217-23.
8. Blackmore PF, Beebe SJ, Danforth DR, Alexander N. Progesterone and 17α-hydroxyprogesterone. Novel stimulators of calcium influx in human sperm. J.Biol.Chem. 1990; 265: 1376-80.
9. Blackmore PF, Neulen J, Lattanzio FA, Beebe SJ. Cell surface receptors for progesterone mediate calcium uptake in human sperm. J.Biol. Chem. 1991; 266: 18655-9.
10. Osman RA, Andria ML, Jones AD, Meizel S. Steroid induced exocytosis: the human sperm acrosome reaction. Biochem Biophys. Res. Commun. 1989; 160: 823-33.
11. Thomas P, Meizel S. Phosphatidylinositol 4,5-bisphosphate hydrolysis in human sperm stimulated with follicular fluid or progesterone is dependent upon Ca^{2+} influx. Biochem. J. 1989; 264: 539-46
12. Roldan ERS, Murase T, Shi Q-X. Exocytosis in spermatozoa in response to progesterone and zona pellucida. Science 1994; 266: 1578-81.
13. Ward CR, Kopf GS. Molecular events mediating sperm activation. Dev. Biol. 1993; 158: 9-34.
14. Zaneveld LJD, De Jonge CJ, Anderson RA, Mack SR. Human sperm capacitation and the acrosome reaction. Hum. Reprod. 1991; 6: 1265-74.
15. Wasserman PM. Zona pellucida glycoproteins. Ann. Rev. Biochem. 1988; 57: 415-42.

16. Oehninger S, Blackmore PF, Morshedi M, Sueldo C, Acosta AA, Alexander NJ. Defective calcium influx and acrosome reaction (spontaneous and progesterone induced) in spermatozoa of infertile men with severe tetratozoospermia. Fertil. Steril. 1994; 61: 349-54.
17. Tesarik J, Mendoza C. Defective function of a nongenomic progesterone receptor as a sole sperm anomoly in infertile patients. Fertil. Steril. 1992; 56: 793-7.
18. Felder CC, Singer-Lahat D, Mathes C. Voltage-independent calcium channels: regulation by receptors and intracellular calcium stores. Biochem.Pharmacol. 1994; 48: 1997-2004.
19. Blackmore PF. Thapsigargin elevates and potentiates the ability of progesterone to increase intracellular free calcium in human sperm: possible role of perinuclear calcium. Cell Calcium 1993; 14: 53-60.
20. Blackmore PF, Lattanzio FA. Localization of progesterone receptors on the head of human sperm. Biochem.Biophys.Res.Commun. 1991; 181: 331-6.
21. Meizel S, Turner KO. Progesterone acts at the plasma membrane of human sperm. Mol.Cell. Endocrinol. 1991; 11: R1-R5.
22. Neulen J, Ishikawa K, Blackmore PF, Beebe SJ. Identification and characterization of a novel progesterone binding protein in human semen. Endocrine J. 1993; 1: 397-404.
23. Pillai MC, Meizel S. Trypsin inhibitors prevent the progesterone-initiated increase in intracellular calcium required for the sperm acrosome reaction. J.Exp.Zool. 1991; 258: 348-93.
24. Tesarik J, Moos J, Mendosa C. Stimulation of protein tyrosine phosphorylation by a progesterone receptor on the cell surface of human sperm. Endocrinology 1993; 133: 328-35.
25. Blackmore PF, Lattanzio FA. Studies on the mechanism by which progesterone induces calcium influx in human sperm. J.Cell Biol. 1991; 1153: 144a.
26. Foresta C, Rossato M, DiVirgilio F. Ion fluxes through the progesterone-activated channel of the sperm plasma membrane. Biochem. J. 1993; 294: 279-283.
27. Meizel S, Turner KO. Effects of polyamine biosynthesis inhibitors on the progesterone- initiated increase in intracellular free Ca^{2+} and acrosome reaction in human sperm. Mol.Reprod.Dev. 1993; 34: 457-65.
28. Wistrom CA, Meizel S. Evidence suggesting involvement of a unique human sperm steroid receptor / Cl^- channel complex in the progesterone-initiated acrosome reaction. Dev. Biol. 1993; 159: 679-90.
29. Turner KO, Garcia MA, Meizel S. Progesterone initiation of the human acrosome reaction: the obligatory increase in intracellular calcium is

independent of the chloride requirement. Mol.Cell Endocrinol. 1994; 101: 221-5.
30. Blackmore PF, Im WB, Bleasdale JE. The cell surface progesterone receptor which stimulates calcium influx in human sperm is unlike the A ring reduced steroid site on the $GABA_A$ receptor /chloride channel. Mol. Cell. Endocrinol. 1994; 104: 237-43.
31. McEwen BS. Non- genomic and genomic effects of steroids on neural activity. Trends Pharmacol. Sci. 1991; 12: 141-7.
32. Blackmore PF, Fisher JF, Spilman CH, Bleasdale JH. Unusual steroid specificity of the novel cell surface progesterone receptor on human sperm. J. Biol. Chem. 1995; submitted for publication.
33. Spilman CH, Wilks JW. Progesterone receptor binding characteristics following freezer storage of uterine cytosol. J.Steroid Biochem. 1980; 13: 1249-51.
34. Korenman SG. Radio-ligand binding assay of specific estrogen using a soluble uterine macromolecule. J.Clin.Endocrinol.Metab. 1968; 28: 127-30.
35. Seth NM, Bhaduri AP. Progesterone receptor binding of steroidal and nonsteroidal compounds. Prog. Drug Res. 1986; 30: 151-88.
36. McGuire JL, Bariso CD, Shroff AP. Interaction between steroids and a uterine progestogen specific binding macromolecule. Biochemistry 1974; 13: 319-22.
37. Lee DL, Kollman PA, Marsh FJ, Wolff ME. Quantitative relationships between steroid structure and binding to putative progesterone receptors. J. Med. Chem. 1977; 20: 1139-46.

Chapter III
Chapitre III

Transduction pathways during acrosome reaction
Les voies de transduction du signal au cours de la réaction acrosomique

Exo(cyto)tic ion channels in mammalian sperm

Harvey M. Florman, Jose R. Lemos, Christophe Arnoult,
Jon A. Oberdof and Yang Zeng

*Worcester Foundation for Experimental Biology, Shrewsbury,
Massachussets 01545, USA*

ABSTRACT

Contact between sperm and the egg's zona pellucida initiates acrosome reactions during mammalian fertilization. ZP3, the acrosome reaction-inducing glycoprotein of the zona pellucida, activates a non-selective cation conductance in sperm, leading to membrane depolarization. Agonist stimulation also elevates internal pH. These two effects act in concert to promote opening of a voltage-sensitive, Ca^{2+} selective ion channel. The resultant Ca^{2+} influx is the proximal signal for acrosomal secretion during fertilization.

Au cours de la fécondation chez les mammifères, le contact entre le spermatozoïde et la zone pellucide initie la réaction acrosomique. ZP3, la glycoprotéine de la zone pellucide induisant la réaction acrosomique, active un processus non sélectif de conductance de cations conduisant à une dépolarisation membranaire. La stimulation par des agonistes élève également le pH intracellulaire. Ces deux effets agissent de façon synchrone afin d'ouvrir un canal Ca^{2+} sélectif et voltage dépendant. L'influx de Ca^{2+} qui en résulte est le signal primaire de la réaction acrosomique durant la fécondation.

INTRODUCTION

Sperm of many animal species, including all mammals, have a single secretory vesicle, or acrosome, in their anterior head. Exocytotic release of acrosomal contents is an essential prerequisite to fertilization. Our current understanding of the role of Ca^{2+} as an internal mediator of acrosome reactions stems from several early studies. A role for Ca^{2+} in stimulus-secretion coupling was established by pioneering studies of Katz and Douglas in neurosecretory models (1). A similar function during acrosomal secretion was suggested by the demonstration that external Ca^{2+} is required for egg jelly-induced acrosome reactions of echinoderm sperm. Subsequent demonstration that spontaneous acrosome reactions of guinea pig sperm required external Ca^{2+} and are associated with enhanced $^{45}Ca^{2+}$ influx extended the mediatory role of Ca^{2+} to mammalian species. Finally, it was shown that acrosome reaction-inducing factors are associated with eggs of both non-mammalian and mammalian species (2-4).

The model that emerged from these early studies focused on an agonist-induced elevation of sperm internal Ca^{2+} ($Ca^{2+}i$) that activates distal effectors and produces secretion. Yet, an understanding of the mechanisms of agonist-induced Ca^{2+} entry was poorly understood. This was due to two factors. The reduced cytoplasmic volumes of sperm, platelets and other small cells complicated direct biochemical or biophysical examination of ion transport mechanisms. These difficulties were further complicated by functional heterogeneity of sperm populations with regard to motility, capacitation, or interaction with eggs (4). Thus, information regarding mechanisms of agonist-activated ion transport is perceived dimly. These difficulties were circumvented by two advances during the last decade. First, the development of membrane permeant, ion-selective fluorescent probes permitted the incorporation of these compounds into small cells where microinjection approaches were not feasible. Second, advances in low light-level photodetector systems (such as silicon-intensified target camera and charge-coupled devices) and the general availability of biologically-oriented image processing programs permitted quantitative study of small fluorescence changes within cells. Thus, the direct examination of egg-induced ion transport in single sperm became feasible. The following discussion addresses the mechanism of egg agonist-induced Ca^{2+} influx into mammalian sperm.

SPONTANEOUS AND INDUCED SECRETION

All secretory cells exhibit low spontaneous exocytosis rates in the absence of stimulatory signals. Spontaneous release was studied in the greatest detail at neuromuscular junctions, where secretion releases neurotransmitter and produces miniature end plate potentials (1, 5). Stimuli such as membrane depolarization of the synaptic bouton enhances release above this basal level. Similarly, acrosome reactions occur in populations of mammalian sperm in the absence of stimulatory signals. The rate of spontaneous acrosome reaction in populations varies among species. It is generally observed that this rate is further enhanced during capacitation in vitro (4). Stimulatory agonists act by increasing the frequency of acrosome reaction above this basal level.

The first agonist activity capable of initiating mammalian sperm acrosome reactions was identified in zona pellucida extracts. Time course studies reveal that initial rates of reaction in mouse sperm populations are increased 30-50 fold relative to basal rates following treatment with zona pellucida extracts. In addition, sperm that acrosome react at the surface of the zona pellucida fertilize eggs in vitro and inhibition of zona pellucida-induced acrosome reactions prevents fertilization in vitro. Taken together, these observations suggest that a zona pellucida component is a physiologically-relevant regulator of acrosome reactions (2,4). The molecular nature of this agonist is considered below (see Acrosome Reaction-Inducing Agonists).

In considering the mechanism of Ca^{2+} entry during acrosome reactions, one must discriminate between spontaneous and agonist-induced events. It is now accepted that $Ca^{2+}i$ is a common final effector of secretion in many model systems, including sperm. Elevation of $Ca^{2+}i$ above threshold values produces acrosome reactions irrespective of whether it results from a physiologically relevant cue such as an egg-associated agonist, from non-physiological Ca^{2+} leak into cells during incubation in vitro, or from a pharmacological manipulation such as treatment with Ca^{2+} ionophores (2, 4). The central issue is that spontaneous and ionophore-induced acrosome reactions provide insights into distal effectors that couple elevated $Ca^{2+}i$ with secretion, but do not address the mechanism of agonist-induced Ca^{2+} entry. Until recently, much of the available information regarding initiation of acrosome reactions was derived from studies of spontaneous exocytosis. In contrast, this discussion will focus specifically on the activation of Ca^{2+} transport during stimulation of sperm with agonists from the zona pellucida.

ACROSOME REACTION-INDUCING AGONISTS

Search for an acrosome reaction-inducing agonist in the extracellular matrix of the mammalian egg, or zona pellucida, followed observations that sperm undergo acrosome reactions after adhesion to the zona pellucida (4). In addition, it was known that an acrosome reaction-inducing activity could be extracted from isolated zonae pellucidae. Finally, it was realized at the same time that the jelly coat of the sea urchin egg contained an glycoconjugate agonist that initiates acrosomal secretion (2, 4).

The initial structural and functional studies of the zona pellucida were reported by Wassarman and colleagues (6). The zona pellucida is composed of three glycoproteins designated ZP1, ZP2, and ZP3. Several lines of evidence indicate that ZP3 is the acrosome reaction-inducing agonist of the zona pellucida. First, recombinant ZP3 expressed by tissue culture cells in the absence of other zona pellucida glycoproteins, induces acrosome reactions (7, 8). Second, ZP3 accounts for all of the agonist activity present in soluble extracts of the zona pellucida (6). Finally, the ZP3 gene also encodes sperm agonist activity in other mammalian species (9). It can be concluded that ZP3 is the sperm agonist in the zona pellucida.

Progesterone (0), ATP (11), and other factors present in the female reproductive tract may also initiate acrosome reactions under certain conditions. Yet, it is unclear whether the primary physiological role of these agents is to control secretion, to act synergistically with ZP3 (12), or to control other Ca^{2+}-dependent processes. Here, we focus on ZP3 signal transduction.

ZONA PELLUCIDA-INDUCED CA^{2+} MOBILIZATION

Bovine sperm initiate acrosome reactions following adhesion to the zona pellucida during fertilization in vivo and following incubation with soluble zona pellucida glycoproteins in vitro (2, 13). The role of $Ca^{2+}i$ in the secretion was examined using intracellular fura 2, a fluorescent Ca^{2+} indicator dye (14). Fura 2 is distributed throughout the sperm. Dye quenching and dye release studies indicate that >80% of internal dye is in a cytosolic compartment, 10-15% is associated with the midpiece, and the remaining dye resides within or at the surface of the acrosome (15, 16). Alterations of internal pH (pHi) during zona pellucida stimulation were also examined using the intracellular, pH indicator dyes, BCECF and carboxyfluorescein (15)

Dye responses indicate that resting $Ca^{2+}i$ (150-200 nM) and pHj (6.6-6.65) of capacitated sperm are uniform throughout the cell and stable during several minutes of observation. These dyes do not detect the spatial pHj gradients that have been reported between cellular compartments, although this may be due to inappropriate dye distribution within the sperm. Addition of solubilized zonae pellucidae or of bovine ZP3 produces a stereotypic response in sperm that consists of the following stages (Fig. 1; open symbols). i) A lag phase following agonist addition (mean = 1.75 min; range = 0.5-5 min) during which $Ca^{2+}i$ and pHi remain stable at resting values. This lag exceeds the determined mixing time of this system (< 10 sec) and apparently reflects a relatively slow signaling process. Similar lag periods are noted in certain other secretory systems (17). ii) A response phase lasting 2-5 min during which Ca^{2+}_i and pHi increase to peak values (Ca^{2+}_i = 300-400 nM; pHi = 6.8). iii) A plateau phase lasting 10-15 min during which Ca^{2+}_i and pHi values remain elevated.

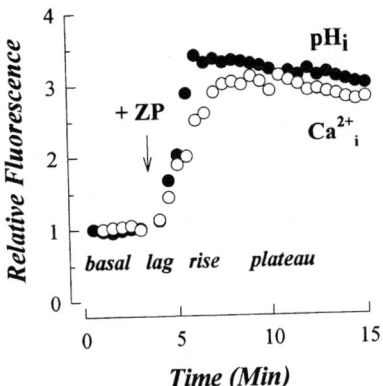

Figure 1: Zona pellucida stimulation elevates Ca^{2+}_i and pHi in capacitated sperm. Fluorescent indicators of Ca^{2+}_i (fura 2; open symbols) and pHj (BCECF; closed symbols) were generated in situ. Intracellular ion activities were determined in single sperm by image processing-enhanced fluorescence microscopy under basal conditions and following addition of solubilized zonae pellucidae (arrow). Experimental details have been published previously (15, 16, 18, 20).

Single cell analysis reveals extensive cell-to-cell heterogeneity regarding the length of the lag period, the rate of Ca^{2+}_i and pHi elevation during the response phase, and the final sustained levels achieved during plateau phase (15, 16, 18, 19). Two generalizations are drawn from this analysis. First, all sperm that undergo acrosome reactions exhibit the stereotypic response, whereas this pattern is not observed in cells that fail to acrosome react. Second, acrosome reactions always occur during the plateau phase; that is, they follow peak Ca^{2+}_i and pHi responses.

PATHWAYS OF ZONA PELLUCIDA INDUCES CA^{2+} ENTRY

What is the source of Ca^{2+} mobilized by zonae pellucidae and by ZP3? The steady state Ca^{2+}_i levels reported by indicator dyes such as fura 2 reflect a balance between Ca^{2+} flux across plasma and organelle membranes and Ca^{2+} buffering by cytosolic proteins (20, 21). The Ca^{2+} elevation and secretory responses of bovine sperm to a zona pellucida and to ZP3 stimuli are attenuated by Ca^{2+} entry blockers Co^{2+} and La^{3+} (18). This suggests that Ca^{2+}

influx from the extracellular environment is an essential component of the signaling cascade.

Several pathways for Ca^{2+} influx into somatic cells have been described, including entry through ligand- and voltage-gated ion channels and well as facilitated diffusion through various exchange pathways. Several lines of evidence indicate that the ZP3-activated signaling pathway utilizes a voltage-sensitive Ca^{2+} channel (16, 18). i) Sperm maintain an inwardly-negative membrane potential, as indicated by studies with potentiometric fluorescent probes that is partly determined by the K^+ diffusion potential (18, 22). Depolarization with elevated $[K^+]_o$ or with the Na^+/K^+ transporting ionophore, gramacidin D, in concert with alkalinization of pH; (see below) produces Ca^{2+} and acrosome reactions (16, 18). ii) Depolarization-induced $Ca^{2+}i$ and secretory responses are attenuated in concentration-dependent fashion by inhibitors of L-type voltage sensitive Ca^{2+} channels: PN200-110>nifedipine >nisoldipine>verapamil>diltiazem. Divalent metal cations also inhibit this response, although the observed selectivity ($Ni^{2+}>Cd^{2+}$) is reverse that anticipated at L-type channels. iii) Zona pellucida-initiated acrosome reactions and Ca^{2+}; elevations are also blocked by those same antagonists. iv) [^{3}H]PN200-110, the dihydropyridine antagonist of L-type Ca^{2+} channels, binds to a saturable, high-affinity class of binding sites on sperm plasma membrane vesicles (K_D = 0.3-0.5 nM; B_{MAX} = 4-8 fmol/mg protein). Specific binding was inhibited competitively by dihydropyridines, phenylalkylamines, benzodiazapines, and transition metal cations with the following rank order: PN200-110 > nifedipine > nisoldipine > verapamil > diltiazem > Ni^{2+} > Cd^{2+}. Bay K8644 however does not interact with the dihydropyridine binding site for [^{3}H]PN200-110 on sperm membranes.

Taken together, these observations suggest that the ZP3-activated Ca^{2+}_i regulatory mechanism of sperm has some of the anticipated properties of an L-type voltage-sensitive Ca^{2+} channel. This mechanism provides an essential component of the zona pellucida-induced Ca^{2+} elevation, although the relative contributions of intracellular and external sources of Ca^{2+} in this response have not been evaluated. Slow inactivation is a signature feature of the somatic L-type channel and is well suited for producing the sustained Ca^{2+}_i elevations observed during the plateau phase of ZP3 response. Yet, features of the sperm mechanism are inconsistent with an L-type channel, including the metal cation selectivity (Ni^{2+} >Cd^{2+}) and the absence of a Bay K8644 effect (1).

ROLE OF NON-SELECTIVE CATION CHANNELS IN CA^{2+} MOBILIZATION

Conductance through voltage-sensitive Ca^{2+} channels is regulated primarily by membrane potential, although the potential-dependent functions are modulated by phosphorylation state of channel subunits and, possibly, by direct interaction with G proteins (1). The effects of zona pellucida agonists on sperm membrane potential was examined using potentiometic fluorescent probes. Capacitated bovine sperm maintain an apparent plasma membrane potential of -30 to -40 mV, as determined by DiSC3(5) and DiSBAC2(3). (In the absence of direct electrophysiological calibration, dye responses must be considered "apparent membrane potentials.") This resting potential is determined partly, but not completely, by the K^+ permeability.

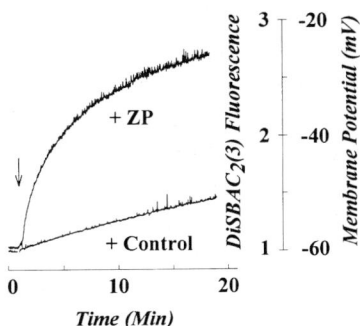

Figure 2 **Zona pellucida stimulation depolarizes sperm membrane potential.** *Membrane potential of capacitated sperm populations ($2.5x10^6$/ml) was deterrnined with the oxonol fluorescent probe, $DiSBAC_2(3)$. Calibrations were carried out with gramicidin D in K^+/N-methyl-D-glucamine+ media, such that the membrane potential is determined by the transmembrane K+ gradient. Data is displayed both as relative changes in $DiSBAC_2(3)$ fluorescence and as the calculated membrane potential. Fluorescence emission is collected under basal conditions and following addition (at arrow) of either solubilized zonae pellucidae (+ZP) or control glycoprotein (α_1-acid glycoprotein).*

Stimulation of sperm with zonae pellucidae/ZP3 depolarizes membrane potential (Fig. 2). The initial depolarization rates in different media permits an estimation of the permeability of the ZP3/zona pellucida-gated channel that mediates membrane potential alterations. This channel is permeant to monovalent (Na^+) and divalent (Ca^{2+}, Co^{2+}, Mn^{2+}, Ni^{2+}) cations, but not to Ch^+, Nmethyl-D-glucamine$^+$, or La^{3+}. In contrast, anions (Cl$^-$, $S0_4^{2-}$, aspartate$^-$, gluconate$^-$) do not support depolarization and apparently do not permeate this channel. Thus, ZP3 stimulation activates a depolarization mechanism with the characteristics of a poorly-selective cation channel.

Pretreatment of sperm with pertussis toxin or with PN200-110 prevents activation of the Ca^{2+}-selective channel by ZP3/zonae pellucidae. Under these circumstances agonist-evoked depolarizations are still observed. Previously, we discussed observations that the Ca^{2+} channel has the anticipated characteristics of a voltage-sensitive channel and that K^+-evoked depolarizations in the absence of ZP3 also open the channel (see above). Taken together, these results suggest that ZP3 activates a non-selective cation channel, producing a membrane depolarization that is essential for the opening of voltage-sensitive Ca^{2+} channels (Fig. 3).

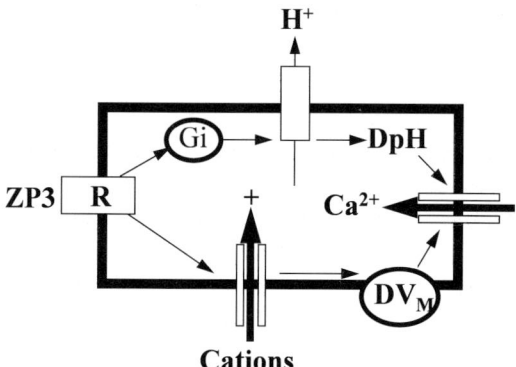

Figure 3 Model of ZP3 signal transduction. *Interaction of ZP3 with its cognate receptor (R) activates: i) a poorly-selective cation channel, leading to membrane depolarization (ΔVM); and ii) a G-protein dependent pHi regulator, leading to acid efflux and an elevation of pHi. These changes act in concert to control conductance through a voltage-sensitive Ca^{2+} channel. The resulting Ca^{2+} influx triggers acrosome reactions*

MODULATION OF CA^{2+} ELEVATION BY PH_I

ZP3 stimulation also alkalinizes pH_i (15). Figure 1 shows the stereotypic alterations in pH_j in single sperm cells (closed symbols). The time course of pH_j alterations is similar to that observed for $Ca^{2+}{}_i$. Yet, the zona pellucida-induced alterations of membrane potential, Ca^{2+}, and pH can be differentiated since: i) dihydropyridine treatment selectively attenuates Ca^{2+} influx while alkalinization is uneffected; and ii) pertussis toxin treatment blocks pHi responses but does not inhibit depolarization (16).

Several observations indicate that the pHi response is an essential modulator of the zona pellucida-activated Ca^{2+} elevation. Depolarization of sperm membrane potential by elevated $[K^+]_o$ or by gramicidin D fails to produce Ca^{2+}; elevations or acrosomal secretion in the absence of a simultaneous elevation of pH_i (18). pH_i can be systematically altered with permeant weak acids and weak bases. Under these conditions, the corresponding Ca^{2+}_i and secretory responses during comparable depolarizations is dependent upon pHi. Thus, elevated pHi does not evoke Ca^{2+} opening but is essential for the resulting Ca^{2+}_i response during depolarization.

MODEL OF ZP3-INDUCED CA^{2+} ELEVATION

These observations suggest a model in which ZP3 activates a bifurcated signaling pathway consisting of seperate limbs of depolarization and alkalinization. These responses, occurring in concert, provide the stimulus for Ca^{2+} channel opening (Fig. 3). Thus, the sperm Ca^{2+} channel functions as an integrator of a coincidence detection system, ensuring that Ca^{2+}_i elevations and acrosome reactions only occur when both signals are received. As sperm have only a single secretory vesicle, and as acrosome reacted sperm cannot efficiently penetrate the cumulus oophorus matrix or adhere to zonae pellucidae (2), it follows that these cells must have a mechanism of suppressing premature exocytosis.

REFERENCES

1. Hille, B. Ionic channels of excitable membranes. Sunderland, MA: Sinauer Assoc., 1992.
2. Florman, HM, Babcock, DF. Progress towards understanding the molecular basis of capacitation. In:Wassarman PM,ed. Elements of mammalian fertilization.Boca Raton, FL:CRC Press,1991: 105-132.
3. Ward, CR, Kopf, GS. Molecular events mediating gamete activation. Dev Biol 1993; 158: 9-34.
4. Yanagimachi, R .Mammalian fertilization. In: Knobil E, Neill JD, eds. The physiology of reproduction. NY: Raven Press, 1994: 189-317.
5. Stevens, CF. Quantal release of neurotransmitter and long-terrn potentiation. Neuron 1993; 10 (suppl): 55-63.
6. Wassarman, PM. Zona pellucida glycoproteins. Ann Rev Biochem 1988; 57: 415-442.
7. Kinloch, RA, Mortillo, S, Stewart, CL, Wassarman, PM. Embryonal carcinoma cells transfected with ZP3 genes differentially glycosylate similar polypeptides and secrete active mouse sperm receptor. JCellBiol 1991;115: 655-664.

8. Beebe, SJ, Leyton, L, Burks, D, Ishikawa, M, Fuerst, T, Dean, J, Saling, P. Recombinant mouse ZP3 inhibits sperm binding and induces the acrosome reaction. Dev Biol 1992; 151: 48-54.
9. Moller, CC, Bleil, JD, Kinloch, RA, Wassarman, PM. Structural and functional relationships between mouse and hamster zona pellucida glycoproteins. Dev Biol 1990; 137: 276-286.
10. Thomas, P, Meizel, P. Phosphatidylinositol 4,5-bisphosphate hydrolysis in human sperm stimulated with follicular fluid or progesterone is dependent upon Ca2+ influx. Biochem J 1989; 264: 539-546.
11. Foresta, C, Rossato, M, Di Virgilio, F. Extracellular ATP is a trigger for the acrosome reaction in human spermatozoa JBiol Chem 1992; 267: 19443-19447.
12. Roldan, ERS, Murase, T, Shi, Q-X. Exocytosis in spermatozoa in response to progesterone and zona pellucida Science 1994; 266: 1578-1581.
13. Florman, HM, First, NL. The regulation of acrosomal exocytosis. I. Sperm capacitation is required for induction of acrosome reactions by bovine zona pellucida in vitro. Dev Biol 1988; 128: 453-463.
14. Grynkiewicz, G, Poenie, M, Tsien, RY. A new generation of Ca^{2+} indicators with greatly improved fluorescence properties. JBiol Chem 1985; 260: 3440-3450.
15. Florman, HM, Tombes, RM, First, NL, Babcock, DF. An adhesion-associated agonist from the zona pellucida activates G protein-promoted elevations of internal Ca and pH that mediate mammaliansperm acrosomal exocytosis. Dev Biol 1989; 135: 133-146.
16. Florman, HM. Sequential focal and global elevations of sperm intracellular Ca^{2+} are initiated by the zona pellucida during acrosomal exocytosis. Dev Biol 1994;165: 152-164.
17. Mohr, FC, Fewtrell, C. IgE receptor-mediated depolarization of rat basophilic leukemia cells measured with the fluorescent probe bis-oxonal. JImmunol 1987; 138: 1564-1570.
18. Florman, HM, Corron, ME, Kim, TD-H, Babcock, D. Activation of voltage-dependent calcium channels of mammalian sperm is required for zona pellucida-induced acrosomal exocytosis. Dev Biol 1992; 152: 304-314.
19. Clark, EN, Corron, ME, Florman, HM. Caltrin, the calcium transport regulatory peptide of sperm, modulates acrosomal exocytosis in response to egg zonapellucida J Biol Chem 1993; 268: 5309-5316. 20) Carafoli, E. Membrane transport of calcium: an overview. Meth Enzymol 1988; 157: 3-11.

20. Konishi, M, Olson, A, Hollingworth, S, Baylor, SM. Myoplasmic binding of fura-2 investigated by steady-state fluorescence and absorbance measurements. Biophys J 1988; 54: 1089-1104.
21. Babcock, DF, Pfeiffer, DR. Independent elevation of cytosolic [Ca^{2+}] and pH of mamrnalian sperm by voltage-dependent and pH-sensitive mechanisms. JBiol Chem 1987; 262: 15041-15047.

Integration of tyrosine kinase and G protein-mediated signal transduction pathways in the regulation of mammalian sperm function

Gregory S. Kopf, Pablo E. Visconti, Jiri Moos, Hannah L. Galentino-Homer and Xioa Ping Ning

Division of Reproductive Biology, Department of Obstetrics and Gynaecology; University of Pensylvania, School of Medicine, Philadelphia, Pensyvannia 19104-6080, USA

ABSTRACT

Intercellular communication between gametes is essential to the unique event in the life cycle of an organism called fertilization. Achievement of successful fertilization results from requisite and reciprocal cell-induced sperm and egg activation events mediated by unique cellular and environmental cues associated with either the gametes or the reproductive tract/environment. In the case of the mammalian sperm, the interaction of this motile cell with the female reproductive tract/environment, as well as with the egg both at a distance and in close proximity, represent a series of integrated processes designed to deliver sperm with optimal fertilizing potential to the site of fertilization. The development of the fertilization-competent state occurs through a poorly understood process called capacitation, which may be integrated with changes in motility. Once capacitation has occurred, sperm have the ability to undergo acrosomal exocytosis in response to the egg's unique extracellular matrix, the zona pellucida (ZP). These two activation processes (capacitation and the ZP-induced acrosome reaction) appear to be regulated by intracellular signaling systems similar to those utilized by somatic cells. In the case of the ZP-induced acrosome reaction, several candidate sperm proteins have been implicated as binding proteins and/or receptors for the specific ZP ligand, but the nature/function of these candidates is controversial and still unresolved. It is postulated that ZP-induced acrosomal exocytosis displays some of the hallmarks of ligand-receptor-effector processes seen in other cell types, in which signal transduction may be effected through the activation of G protein-coupled effectors. In contrast, signal transduction processes regulating events associated with the capacitated state may be intrinsically controlled by maturational processes lying within the sperm plasma membrane. Such a signal transduction process appears to involve the integration of both protein kinase A (PKA) and tyrosine kinase/phosphatase signaling pathways in a manner that, to date, is unique to sperm. An understanding of signal transduction in mammalian sperm will ultimately yield information regarding the nature of the receptors to which these signal transduction pathways are coupled, the "intrinsic" nature of how sperm capacitation is initiated, and the intracellular effectors that ultimately regulate sperm function. Moreover, an understanding of these regulatory pathways will be essential for the future development of clinical approaches designed to enhance or preclude fertilization.

La communication intercellulaire entre les gamètes est essentielle à la fécondation, événement unique dans la vie d'un organisme. La fécondation résulte d'une activation spermatozoïde/ovocyte indispensable et réciproque médiée par des facteurs environnementaux et cellulaires uniques entre les gamètes ou bien avec le tractus génital. Chez les mammifères, l'interaction de cette cellule mobile avec le tractus/environnement génital femelle, ainsi qu'avec l'oeuf aussi bien à distance que à proximité immédiate, représente un grand nombre de processus destinés à rendre le spermatozoïde le plus fécondant possible lorsqu'il se trouve sur le site de fécondation. L'état de compétence fécondante s'acquiert au cours de la capacitation, phénomène mal connu, qui pourrait être intégré dans des modifications de la mobilité. A l'issue de la capacitation, le spermatozoïde est capable d'accomplir sa réaction acrosomique en réponse à l'unique matrice extracellulaire de l'oeuf, la zone pellucide (ZP). Ces deux mécanismes d'activation (la capacitation et la réaction acrosomique) sont régulés par des signaux intracellulaires semblables à ceux des cellules somatiques. Dans le cas de la réaction acrosomique induite par la ZP, de nombreuses protéines spermatiques ont été impliquées en tant que protéines de liaison et / ou récepteurs du ligand ZP spécifique, mais la nature/fonction de ces diverses protéines reste encore controversée et non élucidée. On pense que la réaction acrosomique induite par la ZP joue un rôle prépondérant dans le processus ligand/récepteur/effecteur observé dans les autres types cellulaires, dans lesquels la transduction du signal semble se produire par l'activation des protéines G. Contrairement aux précédents les signaux de transduction associés à la capacitation sembleraient être contrôlés par des procédés de maturation liés à la membrane plasmique du spermatozoïde. Ce processus de transduction du signal semble impliquer selon un mécanisme propre au spermatozoïde à la fois la PKA et la voie des tyrosine kinase/phosphatase. La compréhension des mécanismes de transduction du signal dans le spermatozoïde de mammifères pourra définitivement apporter des renseignements sur la nature des récepteurs auxquels ces signaux sont couplés, sur la nature intrinsèque de l'initiation de la capacitation et enfin sur les effecteurs intracellulaires régulant la fonction spermatique. Enfin une compréhension de ces voies de régulation est nécessaire au développement d'approches cliniques destinées à activer ou à empêcher la fécondation.

DEFINITION, ENDPOINTS AND REGULATION OF SPERM CAPACITATION

Unlike sperm of many lower species, mammalian sperm do not possess the ability to fertilize an egg immediately upon ejaculation, although they are motile and appear to be morphologically mature. In vivo, ejaculated sperm require a finite period of residence in the female reproductive tract to become fertilization-competent. This time-dependent acquisition of fertilization competence has been defined as "capacitation" by both Chang (1,2) and Austin (3,4). Capacitation in vitro has also been accomplished in a number of different species using cauda epididymal and/or ejaculated sperm under a variety of different incubation conditions. Historically, capacitation was originally defined as the time interval of sperm incubation (either in vivo or in vitro) that is required to bring about this final functional maturation of the sperm (5). This loose definition takes into account all of the heretofore poorly understood biochemical processes that ultimately regulate this event (reviewed in 6). The definition of capacitation has also been modified over the years to include the acquisition of the ability of the acrosome-intact sperm to undergo the acrosome reaction in response to its interaction with the ZP (7,8).

Capacitation has been shown to be correlated with changes in sperm intracellular ion concentrations, plasma membrane fluidity, metabolism, and motility (6 and references therein). Although these changes have been known for many years to accompany the process of capacitation, the molecular basis underlying these events is poorly understood. Moreover, it is unclear which, if any, of these events is obligate for capacitation. It is clear that capacitation can be achieved in vitro in balanced salt solutions containing appropriate concentrations of electrolytes, metabolic energy sources and serum albumin (as the primary protein source); this composition in many instances approximates that of the oviduct fluid (6). It appears that certain components of such media play an important role in promoting the capacitation process. Work in a variety of species has suggested that the presence of serum albumin (9, 10), Ca^{2+} (11-14) and $NaHCO_3$ (15-17) are required for capacitation, although Fraser (18) has suggested that the albumin requirement is for the acrosome reaction and not capacitation. Albumin is believed to be responsible for the removal of cholesterol from the sperm plasma membrane (9, 10, 19-23), possibly accounting for the membrane fluidity changes that have been documented in many species during the capacitation process (6 and references therein). However, it must also be emphasized that since the strict endpoint of capacitation is the ability to fertilize an egg and that this property is dependent on many different sperm functions (i.e., normal motility, hyperactivated motility, ability to undergo an acrosome reaction) it is not clear which sperm function(s) are affected by these media constituents. For example, it is suggested that both Ca^{2+} and $NaHCO_3$ are required for the induction of the acrosome reaction by the ZP (6, 8,1 5), as well as hyperactivation (16).

SIGNAL TRANSDUCTION PROCESSES REGULATING SPERM CAPACITATION

The transmembrane and intracellular signaling events regulating sperm capacitation are, likewise, poorly understood. As stated above some of these events may be coupled to changes in ionic movements within the sperm during this time. Changes in sperm cyclic nucleotide metabolism and protein phosphorylation have been implicated in a variety of sperm functions, including the initiation and maintenance of motility (6, 24, 25), induction of the acrosome reaction (8, 24), and capacitation (26-28). Changes in tyrosine phosphorylation of specific sperm proteins have also been demonstrated to occur under conditions that support capacitation (29,30), although a correlation or cause-and-effect relationship between these two parameters has not been examined.

Using the mouse as an experimental paradigm, our laboratory has initiated studies towards understanding the molecular basis of capacitation (31, 32). We have demonstrated that incubation conditions conducive to capacitation of cauda epididymal mouse sperm *in vitro* promote the tyrosine phosphorylation of a subset of proteins of M_r 40,000 - 120,000. Moreover, bovine serum albumin (BSA), Ca^{2+} and $NaHCO_3$ in the medium are absolutely required for these phosphorylations as well as capacitation, which we assessed by three independent methods (B pattern of chlortetracycline fluorescence, the ZP-induced acrosome reaction, and the ability to fertilize ZP-intact eggs). Caput sperm, which do not possess the ability to undergo capacitation and fertilize eggs, do not display the changes in protein tyrosine phosphorylation under incubation conditions normally conducive to the capacitation of caudal epididymal sperm. These data suggest that protein tyrosine phosphorylation may represent an important pathway that may ultimately regulate events associated with capacitation.

Of potential relevance to the requirement of extracellular Ca^{2+} and $NaHCO_3$ for these protein tyrosine phosphorylations is the observation that these particular ions have been demonstrated to be involved in the regulation of mammalian sperm cAMP metabolism, and that changes in the concentration of this intracellular second messenger have been linked to both capacitation and the acrosome reaction. For example, it is known that Ca^{2+} dependent elevations of guinea pig sperm cAMP concentrations are dependent on the presence of extracellular $NaHCO_3$ and that the effects of $NaHCO_3$ on this process do not appear related to changes in intracellular pH (33). The effects of this cation and anion may be at the level of the adenylyl cyclase, since the mammalian sperm enzyme has been demonstrated to be regulated directly/indirectly by Ca^{2+}(34), calmodulin (35)), and $NaHCO_3$ (36-38). Since there appears to be a relationship between Ca^{2+}, $NaHCO_3$, adenylyl cyclase and cAMP in the capacitation process (see above), it was of interest to determine whether any of these regulatory molecules were, in some fashion, linked to the protein tyrosine phosphorylation changes observed during capacitation (32). As with other sperm adenylyl cyclases, the mouse sperm enzyme was demonstrated to be regulated by $NaHCO_3$. It was demonstrated that the capacitation-associated changes in protein tyrosine phosphorylation that are dependent on the presence of BSA, Ca^{2+} and HCO_3^- can be mimicked in the absence of each of these required media constituents by the addition of active, but not inactive, membrane-permeable cAMP analogues. Correlated with the stimulatory effects of these cAMP analogues on protein tyrosine phosphorylation is a stimulatory effect of these analogues on capacitation. Moreover, protein tyrosine phosphorylation is accelerated by active cAMP analogues in media that support capacitation. Since the primary intracellular target for cAMP action is PKA, we examined whether the effects of the cAMP analogues on protein tyrosine phosphorylation and capacitation were mediated at the level of PKA. It was demonstrated that two different inhibitors of PKA that function by inhibiting the enzyme in two completely independent ways (Rp-cAMPS and H-89) blocked both protein tyrosine phosphorylation and capacitation. In contrast, inhibitors of protein kinase C and Ca^{2+}/calmodulin dependent protein kinases were without effect. Taken together, these data suggest that the stimulatory effects of cAMP on protein tyrosine phosphorylation and capacitation appear to be at the level of PKA. Up-regulation of protein tyrosine phosphorylation by cAMP/PKA in sperm is, to our knowledge, the first demonstration of such an interrelationship between tyrosine kinase/phosphatase and PKA signaling pathways. Such a signaling pathway during capacitation may be universal since similar results are seen in both human (39) and bull (40) sperm.

It is of interest that the sperm appears to intrinsically control events leading to capacitation and that the controlling factor(s) related to this maturational process may lie within the plasma membrane. Destabilization of the plasma membrane by changes in membrane fluidity could ultimately set in motion a series of intrinsic pre-programmed membrane and intracellular events that ultimately regulate those sperm functions that are normally associated with the capacitated state (e.g., changes in sperm motility; ability to undergo a ZP-induced acrosome reaction). Our data would not only support the idea that protein tyrosine phosphorylation might represent a key set of signaling events that are entrained as part of the onset of the capacitated state but that there appears to be a regulatory hierarchy that involves PKA.

Fig. 1 provides a working model for how such changes at the level of the sperm plasma membrane might engage a cAMP-dependent pathway that leads to protein tyrosine phosphorylation and the concomitant endpoints of capacitation. In this model, serum albumin, by virtue of its ability to serve as an extracellular sink for sperm membrane cholesterol efflux (9, 10,1 9-22), could lead to alterations in membrane fluidity with resultant changes in the permeability of the sperm to Ca^{2+} (14, 41) and /or HCO_3^- (37). Changes in the permeability of the sperm towards these ions can then regulate intracellular cAMP concentrations through stimulatory effects on adenylyl cyclase. Adenylyl cyclase could be regulated either directly by Ca^{2+} (34) or via calmodulin (35, 42). Moreover, sperm cAMP concentrations could be additionally modulated by Ca^{2+} at the level of a Ca^{2+}/calmodulin-stimulated cyclic nucleotide phosphodiesterase. Adenylyl cyclase could, likewise, be regulated by HCO_3^-, as has been demonstrated in the mouse and in sperm from other species (36, 38,4 3). The resultant changes in cAMP would modulate the activities of PKA, of which there appears to be both types I and II present in mouse sperm (Visconti and Kopf, unpublished observations), and such changes in enzyme activity would lead ultimately to changes in protein tyrosine phosphorylation.

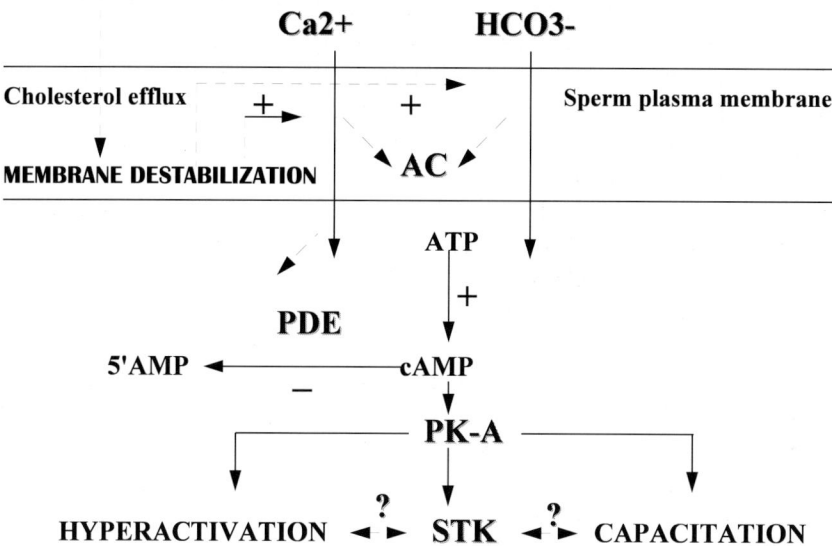

Figure 1. **Working model depicting the mechanism by which sperm surface changes that occur under conditions conductive to capacitation give rise to cAMP-dependent regulation of protein tyrosine phosphorylation and the capacitated state.** *Incubation of uncapacitated sperm under conditions conducive to capacitation gives rise to changes in the permeability of the sperm to Ca^{2+} and HCO_3^- via a change in membrane fluidity or membrane destabilization. These changes in membrane properties are thought to occur by the loss of cholesterol from the membrane; this loss may be accelerated by the presence of serum albumins, which can bind cholesterol. As a consequence of the increase in Ca^{2+} and HCO_3^- permeability, cAMP metabolism is altered. This could occur by the Ca^{2+} and/or HCO_3^- -induced activation of adenylyl cyclase (**AC**), resulting in an increase in intracellular cAMP. Ca^{2+} could also alter the hydrolysis of cAMP by stimulating the activity of a cyclic nucleotide phosphodiesterase(s) (**PDE**). The increase in cAMP then results in the activation of protein kinase A (**PK-A**) which leads to the activation of sperm tyrosine kinase(s) (**STK**) and/or inactivation of phosphoprotein phosphatases, the net result being an increase in protein tyrosine phosphorylation. As a consequence of an increase in protein tyrosine phosphorylation, events leading to capacitation and/or hyperactivation of motility are initiated. In this model capacitation and hyperactivation may or may not be coupled to one another. Arrows with dashed lines indicate hypothetical/uncharacterized pathways of regulation. Arrows with solid lines indicate characterized pathways of regulation observed in sperm. (+) indicates positive regulation; (-) indicates negative regulation.*

The endpoints of capacitation that such tyrosine phosphorylations might regulate are also unknown. Changes in sperm motility appear to accompany capacitation process (16, 44). Since it is known that cAMP plays an important regulatory role in the initiation of flagellar motility (24) and in alterations of the flagellar curvature (25), it is possible that such cAMP-dependent changes in protein tyrosine phosphorylation might be related to these motility changes. For example, it has been demonstrated that the initiation of flagellar motility in the sperm of the rainbow trout is accompanied by the tyrosine phosphorylation of a M_r 15,000 flagellar protein that occurs in a cAMP-dependent manner (45). This protein and the tyrosine kinase that regulates its phosphorylation have yet to be identified. It is also possible that changes in tyrosine kinase and/or phosphoprotein phosphatase activities and resultant protein tyrosine phosphorylations are involved in the regulation of ion channels (46 and references therein). It is interesting to note that the regulation of the voltage-gated cation channel in *Aplysia* bag neurons by tyrosine phosphorylation appears to be modulated in a cAMP-dependent manner (47).

Perhaps the most intriguing observations that have evolved from these studies are that the protein tyrosine phosphorylation state in mouse sperm appears to be regulated by cAMP through the action of PKA. To the best of our knowledge, these observations provide the first example of an up-regulation of protein tyrosine phosphorylation by cAMP/PKA, and suggests that there is cross-talk at some level between PKA and tyrosine kinase/phosphoprotein phosphatase signaling pathways in the sperm. Evidence exists for the down regulation of receptor tyrosine kinase actions by cAMP (48) but up-regulation has thus far not been demonstrated. Protein tyrosine phosphatase activity has been demonstrated to be both inhibited (49) and stimulated (50) by cAMP, effects of which could ultimately modulate the levels of protein tyrosine phosphorylation. The level at which cAMP/PKA functions to regulate the steady state levels of protein tyrosine phosphorylation in mouse sperm under conditions conducive to capacitation (i.e., tyrosine kinases; phosphoprotein phosphatases) will be the subject of intense scrutiny in our laboratory for the foreseeable future. Subsequent investigations into the mechanism by which cAMP/protein kinase regulates those tyrosine kinases/phosphoprotein phosphatases might yield new information about alternative modes of cross-talk between these two signaling pathways.

PROPERTIES OF THE ZONA PELLUCIDA

A major sperm activation event that occurs in mammalian sperm is the induction of the acrosome reaction, which is an exocytotic event. Since the acrosome reaction is an absolute prerequisite to successful fertilization in mammals, the regulation of this event is critical and there is ample evidence supporting the notion that this reaction proceeds in response to extracellular signals emanating from the egg, its associated cellular and acellular structures and the female reproductive tract. The acrosome reaction is essential for fertilization in mammals since it is required for the penetration of the ZP. There is a consensus from both *in vivo* and *in vitro* studies in numerous mammalian species that the ZP is a primary signal in mediating acrosome reactions that are associated with the fertilizing sperm (8). This exocytotic reaction occurs subsequent to the species-specific binding of sperm via the ZP.

Species-specific sperm-egg recognition and interaction, sperm activation (i.e., acrosomal exocytosis), and an egg-induced block to polyspermy in the mouse all appear to be mediated by the ZP (51). The ZP of the mouse egg is composed of three sulfated glycoproteins designated as ZP1, ZP2, and ZP3, and is truly an egg-associated product since it is synthesized and secreted throughout the period of oocyte growth (51, 52). The ZP isolated from all other mammals studied to date are composed of two to four glycoproteins, the number of which appears to be species-dependent (8, 51, 53). Considerable charge heterogeneity of the ZP glycoproteins exist in different species, which is presumably due to the degree of glycosylation and/or sulfation of the individual polypeptide chains. In the mouse, ZP1 (M_r=200,000) is a dimer connected by intermolecular disulfide bonds and appears to function to maintain the three dimensional structure of the ZP by crosslinking filaments composed of repeating structures of ZP2/ZP3 heterodimers. ZP2 (M_r=120,000 under nonreducing and reducing conditions) may mediate the binding of acrosome-reacted sperm to the ZP (51, 54). Upon fertilization, the egg effects a modification of ZP2 to a form called ZP2$_f$ (51) which is brought about by the action of a protease most likely secreted from the egg as a consequence of cortical granule exocytosis (55). ZP2$_f$ has a M_r=120,000 under nonreducing condition that shifts under reducing conditions to M_r=90,000 suggesting that the proteolysis of the ZP2 molecule results in the generation of fragments that are held together by disulfide bonds. The biological consequence of the conversion of ZP2 to ZP2$_f$ is that ZP2$_f$ no longer will bind to acrosome reacted sperm (54). ZP3 (M_r=83,000) accounts for both the sperm binding and the acrosome reaction-inducing activities of the ZP of unfertilized eggs (51). The sperm binding activity appears to be conferred by O-linked carbohydrate moieties and not by its polypeptide chain (51). Alpha-linked terminal galactose residues at the nonreducing termini of these O-linked oligosaccharide chains play a critical role in this binding activity (56). The acrosome reaction-inducing activity of ZP3, in contrast, appears to be conferred by both the carbohydrate and protein portions of the molecule, although the exact nature of the interaction between the protein and carbohydrate required for biological activity is not clear at this time. Fertilization is associated with a loss of both the sperm binding and acrosome reaction-inducing activities of the ZP3 molecule (51). The loss of these two important biological activities is associated with a minor biochemical modification of the ZP3 molecule since the electrophoretic mobility of ZP3 from fertilized eggs is similar to that of ZP3 from unfertilized eggs. It is probable that the loss of carbohydrate from ZP3 as a consequence of a specific cortical granule glycosidase(s) released following the cortical reaction accounts for this loss of activity (57).

Although the ZP of a number of other species have been characterized to various degrees at the biochemical level (e.g., pig, bull, rabbit, human, rhesus monkey, rat, cat, dog), little is known about the biological activities of the individual glycoproteins comprising these ZP (53). Some of these species, however, possess homologues to ZP3, consistent with the potential conservation of ZP3 and its function. For example, the human ZP3 homologue has been cloned and displays a high degree of sequence homology to the mouse (58). Ringuette et al. (59) have demonstrated conserved sequences in the genomic DNA of human, cow, rat, rabbit and pig using ZP3-specific probes, and genomic cloning of the hamster ZP3 gene reveals remarkable similarity in gene organization and in polypeptide structure to the mouse ZP3 gene and gene product, respectively (60). Characterization of the hamster ZP has demonstrated the presence of three major glycoproteins (61). Hamster ZP3 (M_r=56,000), and not ZP1 and ZP2, possesses sperm binding activity, and the intact hamster ZP possesses the ability to induce the acrosome reaction of hamster sperm (61). It is likely, therefore, that similar biological activities are associated with the homologous ZP1, ZP2 and ZP3 glycoproteins in other mammals.

INTERACTION OF SPERM WITH THE ZONA PELLUCIDA

The properties of ZP1, ZP2 and ZP3 from both unfertilized and fertilized eggs provide a framework with which to formulate a model to explain the interaction of sperm with the intact ZP. Since only acrosome-intact mouse sperm bind to the ZP (62), the existence of a specific binding protein/receptor(s) for ZP3 on the plasma membrane overlying the sperm acrosome that mediates sperm binding and the induction of acrosomal exocytosis has been proposed. Since acrosome reacted sperm do not interact with ZP3, secondary interactions of these sperm with the ZP would then occur through the interaction of a putative receptor(s) for ZP2 on the sperm inner acrosomal membrane. Upon penetration of the ZP by acrosome reacted sperm, these cells then traverse the perivitelline space and then bind and fuse with the plasma membrane of the egg. Subsequent to sperm-egg fusion, the egg undergoes the cortical granule reaction, which results in the release of cortical granule-associated enzymes (51). These enzymes convert ZP2 to $ZP2_f$ and modify ZP3, such that acrosome-intact sperm no longer bind to the ZP (via ZP3) and acrosome-reacted sperm that are bound to the ZP (via ZP2) no longer interact and penetrate the ZP since they are unable to establish secondary binding interactions with $ZP2_f$. Such egg-induced modifications of this extracellular matrix constitute the ZP block to polyspermy. Inherent in such a model is the highly specific and coordinated nature of the interactions of acrosome-intact and acrosome-reacted sperm with ZP3 and ZP2, respectively. Such interactions would presumably be mediated via specific sperm-associated binding proteins/receptors for these extracellular matrix glycoproteins.

The species-specificity of gamete adhesion, a prerequisite to acrosomal exocytosis, strongly implicates the existence of molecules on the sperm surface with novel domains that must interact with acrosome reaction inducing ligands of the ZP in a specific and potent manner to elicit biological responses. Presently, putative sperm-associated binding proteins/receptors for known molecules that induce the acrosome reaction have not been unequivocally identified in any species, although there appears to be more available information in the mouse than in other species. Identification of such binding proteins/receptors has been hampered by the lack of information pertaining to the precise identity of the active sperm adhesion and acrosome reaction inducing moieties of the ZP, as well as the seemingly complex nature of the interactions of such molecules with the sperm surface.

There are several lines of evidence which support that idea that sperm-ZP interaction in the mouse may occur through specific binding and/or receptor-mediated events. ZP3 possesses a number of properties which make it ideally suited as a ligand to mediate the initial steps of sperm-egg interaction proper (e.g., sperm binding) and subsequent sperm activation (e.g., induction of the acrosome reaction). Although conserved at the genomic level in a variety of species (59), ZP3 subserves very specific functions as a component of the egg-associated extracellular matrix (51). 1) ZP3 is synthesized only by the growing oocyte. 2) Little apparent amino acid sequence homology exists between ZP3 and any other known proteins or glycoproteins thus far examined (59). 3) The ordered crosslinking of ZP2/ZP3 heterodimers by ZP1 gives rise to structural domains that ensures that the ZP3 ligand is immobilized and functions only at short distances. 4) Both the sperm binding and acrosome reaction-inducing activities of ZP3 are observed in the nanomolar range (51). 5) Mouse sperm appear to possess complementary binding sites (receptors?) for ZP3 that are localized over the acrosomal cap region and are present in numbers (10,000 - 50,000 binding sites/cell) similar to that observed for receptor numbers in many hormonally-responsive cells (63-65).

These aforementioned properties of ZP3 are consistent with its role as the physiologically-relevant ligand that accounts for both the sperm binding and acrosomal exocytosis-inducing properties of the structurally-intact ZP. However, it should be emphasized that care must be exercised in construing the properties and mode of action of solubilized and purified ZP3 as being identical to those of an immobilized and crosslinked ZP3 associated with a three-dimensional extracellular matrix. This word of caution should apply to all studies using solubilized and purified ZP components, since the importance of spatial constraints in mediating these effects on sperm are not fully appreciated. Such constraints could certainly influence the interpretation of data pertaining to sperm-associated binding proteins/receptors for ZP3.

IDENTITY OF SPERM-ASSOCIATED BINDING PROTEINS / RECEPTORS FOR THE ZONA PELLUCIDA

Putative sperm-associated binding proteins/receptors for ZP3 have been described using a variety of experimental approaches. The binding of ^{125}I-ZP3 and gold-labeled ZP3 to mouse sperm by whole mount autoradiography and transmission electron microscopy, respectively, has demonstrated that binding is associated with the plasma membranes overlying the acrosomal and post-acrosomal regions of the sperm head of acrosome-intact sperm, as well as the post-acrosomal region of the sperm head of acrosome-reacted sperm (63,65). ^{125}I-ZP3 binding is competed by unlabeled ZP3, but not ZP2 (63), and ZP3 binding does not occur on somatic cells (63,65). These results suggest that specific sperm-associated binding sites for ZP3 exist in discrete and appropriate cellular domains of this highly differentiated cell. More recently, purified ZP3 or glycopeptides of ZP3 possessing sperm binding activity were shown to specifically crosslink to a M_r=56,000 protein of acrosome-intact mouse sperm (66). This protein interacts specifically with ZP3-, but not ZP2-, affinity columns, and the binding of the protein to the ZP3 column has characteristics of high affinity interactions. This experimental approach is promising with regard to establishing the molecular identity of putative binding proteins/receptors for ZP3 on the sperm surface. Further characterization of this protein has revealed that this protein (called sp56) is a peripheral membrane protein which is located on the outer surface of the sperm head plasma membrane, that region of the sperm that interacts with ZP3 (67). More recent cloning and analysis of this protein reveals that sp56 is a member of a superfamily of protein receptors, members of which include the alpha subunit of complement 4B-binding protein, and that its expression is restricted to round spermatids (68).

Leyton and Saling (29) demonstrated that anti-phosphotyrosine antibodies react with mouse sperm plasma membrane proteins of Mr=52,000, 75,000 and 95,000. Indirect immunofluorescence using these antibodies demonstrated positive immunoreactivity associated with the acrosomal region of the sperm head. ^{125}I-ZP3 binds to a M_r=95,000 sperm protein on nitrocellulose blots following electrophoretic transfer, and these investigators conclude that this protein is the same protein that reacts with the anti-phosphotyrosine antibodies. Recently, these investigators have demonstrated that the M_r=95,000 protein, when electroeluted from SDS gels and incubated with (γ -^{32}P)ATP, becomes phosphorylated (69). The phosphorylation of this protein is increased upon addition of solubilized ZP, and this phosphorylation is reduced upon the addition of tyrphostin RG-50864, an inhibitor of tyrosine kinases. This particular inhibitor was also demonstrated to inhibit the ZP-induced acrosome reaction. It is suggested that the M_r=95,000 protein may be a receptor for ZP3 that possesses tyrosine kinase activity.

Recent studies by Kalab et al (70), however, call into question the identity and function of this M_r=95,000 phosphotyrosine-containing protein. These investigators purified this protein and then subjected it to limited tryptic digestion and subsequent amino acid analysis. Three sequenced peptides revealed 100% amino acid identity to a mouse hepatoma hexokinase. The purified protein, which migrated at M_r=116,000 under reducing conditions (p95/116), reacted with an antiserum to the purified rat brain hexokinase, type 1, and comigrated on SDS-PAGE with the purified rat brain enzyme under both nonreducing and reducing conditions. Unlike p95/116, the rat brain enzyme was not a phosphotyrosine-containing protein. The p95/116 protein could be immunoprecipitated with the hexokinase antiserum or an O-phosphotyrosine antibody. Limited tryptic digestion of the purified p95/116 and the rat brain enzyme generated subsets of identical peptides that reacted with the hexokinase antiserum. However, p95/116 also contained phosphotyrosine-containing peptides that were not present in the rat brain hexokinase. When different mouse tissues were probed with the hexokinase antiserum all tissues, with the exception of liver, contained immunoreactive protein. In contrast, only sperm and testis possessed a phosphotyrosine-containing form of hexokinase. These data suggest that the germ cell component of the testis possesses a unique tyrosine-phosphorylated form of hexokinase. The role of this protein as a putative ZP3 receptor must, therefore, be carefully re-examined.

A sperm surface b-galactosyltransferase (Gal-transferase) activity has been postulated to mediate the binding of mouse sperm to the ZP by binding oligosaccharide residues on ZP3. This enzyme has been implicated in mediating cell-cell and cell-extracellular matrix interactions in other cells. Many of the experiments supporting the role of this enzyme in sperm-ZP interaction are based on indirect studies where inhibitors of, and antibodies to, the enzyme were shown to block sperm-ZP binding. Recently, however, Miller et al. (71) have demonstrated that the mouse sperm Gal-transferase can galactosylate ZP3, but not ZP1 and ZP2, *in vitro*. Following the acrosome reaction, the enzyme loses its ability to utilize ZP3 as a substrate, and the ZP from fertilized eggs loses its ability to serve as a substrate for galactosylation.

At first glance, the presence of multiple ZP3 binding protein/receptor candidates may be confusing since there is presently no overwhelming evidence to support one candidate over another. It is possible, however, that multiple binding proteins/receptors might function to mediate the dual biological functions of ZP3 (e.g., sperm binding and induction of the acrosome reaction), and that the interaction of these components with ZP3, as well as with one another, must occur in an ordered fashion on the sperm surface to first establish binding of sperm to ZP3 that then permits signal transduction to occur in order to initiate acrosomal exocytosis (see Fig. 2). The concept of multiple, interactive protein domains giving rise to ligand binding and signal transduction is not a novel concept in cell biology. In addition, these domains need not necessarily be identical. In the case of sperm-ZP3 interaction this possibility has originated from data pertaining to nature of the interaction between the ZP (or ZP3) and the sperm surface to mediate both sperm binding and the induction of the acrosome reaction. Several laboratories have established the fact that sperm binding to the ZP, and the ZP-induced acrosome reaction are two independent processes and that the ZP3-induced acrosome reaction in the mouse appears to consist of discrete and independently regulated events (8). Moreover, studies from a number of laboratories using different approaches have provided evidence that the interaction of ZP3 with the sperm surface may occur in a multivalent or cooperative fashion, and that multiple interactions followed by possible receptor aggregation may ultimately lead to signal transduction and acrosomal exocytosis (see references in 8). These observations would certainly be consistent with a model evoking multiple sperm protein domains that form a functional ZP3 receptor signal transduction complex that is capable of transducing intracellular signals to regulate the acrosome reaction (Fig. 2). It is possible that the ZP, itself an extracellular matrix, possesses the ability to aggregate receptors on the sperm surface, as this has been demonstrated in other systems.

ZONA PELLUCIDA-MEDIATED SIGNAL TRANSDUCTION

The mechanism by which specific regulators of sperm function effect signal transduction, or informational flow across the sperm plasma membrane, to modulate intracellular second messenger systems leading to appropriate cellular responses is only starting to be understood. The mouse remains the model system in which most is known about the signal transduction mechanisms modulating sperm function in response to ZP (or ZP3). As previously stated, the unique structure of ZP3, its biological potency, and the probable existence of complementary ZP3 receptor(s) on the sperm surface satisfy a number of criteria required to control specific cell-cell recognition events in a receptor-mediated fashion. As in many somatic cells, sperm guanine nucleotide-binding regulatory proteins (G proteins) play a critical role as signal transducing elements in mediating ZP3-mediated acrosomal exocytosis. Sperm from all species studied thus far (invertebrates; mammals) possess G proteins, as assessed by numerous criteria (72-75). Mammalian sperm contain G proteins of the G_i class, and mouse sperm contain all three subtypes of G_i, namely G_{i1}, G_{i2} and G_{i3} (74). These assignments have been made based on the ability of the a subunits of these heterotrimeric proteins to serve as substrates for pertussis toxin (PTX)-catalyzed ADP-ribosylation, the molecular weights of the a subunits, Cleveland digests of the a subunits, and immunoreactivity with anti-peptide antisera generated against conserved Gi_a domains (72, 74). Mouse sperm also contain G proteins that are not PTX substrates, namely G_z (74) and G_q (Visconti and Kopf, unpublished observations), but the functions of these proteins have not been examined. Unlike somatic cells, sperm do not appear to contain a G protein with properties similar to G_s (8). Immunocytochemical studies have demonstrated that G proteins in bovine (76), as well as mouse and guinea pig (74), sperm are present in the acrosomal region of these cells; these G proteins appear to be of the G_i class.

The physiological role of the sperm G_i proteins in the ZP-mediated acrosome reaction has been examined in the mouse, bull and human (77-80). Functional inactivation of the G_i proteins by PTX treatment of the cells does not affect the ability of the sperm to bind to interact with their homologous ZP, but inhibits the bound sperm from undergoing acrosomal exocytosis. The inhibitory effect of PTX on this event is strictly confined to acrosomal exocytosis induced by ZP3 (or ZP in the human and cow), whereas exocytosis that occurs spontaneously in a small population of cells, in response to a nonspecific agent such as the divalent cation ionophore A23187, or in response to progesterone is insensitive to this treatment (78, 80, 81). These data suggest that sperm G_i proteins may act as critical signal transducing elements downstream from initial sperm-ZP binding events to mediate acrosomal exocytosis by an extracellular matrix component, ZP3.

If the ZP (ZP3)-induced acrosome reaction is an example of stimulus-secretion-coupling that occurs in a receptor-mediated fashion, it would be predicted that receptor-G protein interaction subsequently leads to the generation of intracellular second messengers and/or the modulation of ionic changes within the sperm. Two criteria should be met in order to establish the signal transducing function of a G protein in such a system. First, occupation of putative ZP3 receptors should result in G protein activation in a manner described for other ligand-receptor-G protein interactions, Second, resultant G protein activation should then modulate the intracellular effector systems that are required for acrosomal exocytosis There is experimental evidence that supports both of these criteria.

Recently, it has been demonstrated that solubilized mouse egg ZP stimulate high affinity GTPase activity and specific GTPγ ^{35}S binding in both permeabilized, capacitated mouse sperm (82) and partially purified membranes obtained from these cells (83). These endpoints of G protein activation are stimulated by the ZP in a concentration dependent manner that is blocked by PTX pretreatment, suggesting that sperm G_i proteins are being activated under these conditions. The component of the intact ZP that stimulates G_i is ZP3, and not ZP1 or ZP2. Moreover, ZP from fertilized eggs have lost their ability to stimulate G_i, consistent with the loss of the biological activities of ZP3 following fertilization. Incubation of ZP with sperm membranes results in the preferential activation of G_{i1} and G_{i2}, as assessed by a reduction in PTX-catalyzed ^{32}P-ADP ribosylation in immunoprecipitates obtained following incubation of the membranes with $G_{i\alpha}$ subtype-specific antisera (84). These data suggest that the ZP-mediated stimulation of G_i involves the preferential stimulation of G_{i1} and G_{i2}. More recently, it has been demonstrated that a high speed (100,000 x g) supernatant fraction obtained following detergent-extraction of sperm membranes displays ZP-mediated G protein activation with properties similar to that seen in the intact membranes (85). These data suggest that a functional ZP-G protein signaling complex can be isolated in a soluble form, thus making it now possible to isolate and identify the components of such a complex. This complex should include the binding proteins/receptor(s) for ZP3.

As previously discussed, there are a number of candidates that have been suggested as putative ZP3 binding proteins/receptors. The activation of G proteins in sperm by ZP3 suggests the presence of functional G protein receptors that modulate ZP3 function. If one accepts the hypothesis that multiple interactive proteins could undergo aggregation and form a signaling complex to mediate the responses of sperm to ZP3, it is possible that a heretofore unidentified member of the G protein class of cell surface receptors may be involved in some aspect of ZP3-mediated signal transduction. A superfamily of such receptors has been identified which contains seven transmembrane-spanning domains and includes the muscarinic acetylcholine receptor, the a- and b-adrenergic receptors, and the dopamine receptor. In two recent reports, mRNAs corresponding to cDNAs encoding novel, putative G protein coupled receptors, which may be part of this family, have been found in pachytene spermatocytes and round spermatids (86, 87). To date, however, no ligand for these putative receptors has been identified, although the protein encoding one of these receptors (DTMT) (87) appears to exist in mature sperm (88). As mentioned above, work is ongoing in this laboratory to identify the signal transduction complex that forms in response to ZP3-sperm binding. Such studies will go a long way to identify such a putative G protein-coupled ZP3 receptor.

Alternatively, some of the ZP3 binding protein/receptor candidates described above might couple in some manner to G proteins. Although the amino acid sequence for the sp56 clone is now known (68), it is not yet known whether such a protein can interact with G proteins. There is considerable evidence to suggest that receptors possessing tyrosine kinase activity can interact either directly or indirectly with G proteins (89 and references therein), so it is possible that putative receptor tyrosine kinases could couple to G proteins to mediate signal transduction in sperm. Although the M_r=95,000 phosphotyrosine-containing protein has been identified as a unique form of hexokinase (70), its ability to function as a potential ZP3 receptor tyrosine kinase must be carefully re-evaluated.

INTRACELLULAR EFFECTORS REGULATING THE ZONA PELLUCIDA-INDUCED ACROSOME REACTION

Since there is substantial evidence that acrosomal exocytosis is a highly regulated process, initiated by ZP (or ZP3) whose effects are likely mediated by cell surface receptors and signal transducing G proteins, it is likely that intracellular regulation of acrosomal exocytosis is similar to other receptor-mediated exocytotic events. Such intracellular signals include changes in ionic conductance, changes in cyclic nucleotide metabolism and changes in phospholipid metabolism (Fig. 2) It would also be predicted that these intracellular effector systems would be modulated in a receptor-dependent fashion.

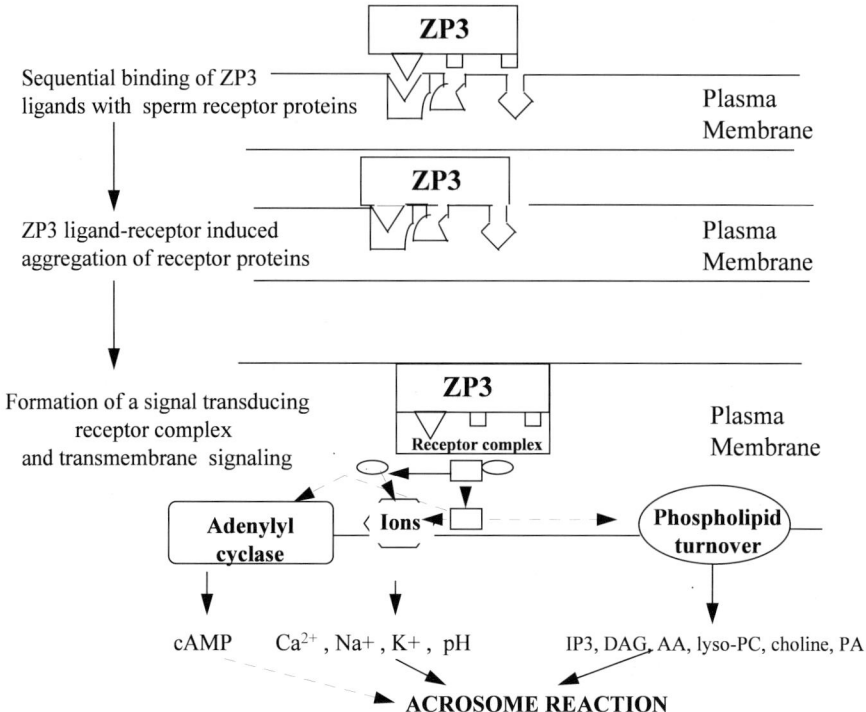

Figure 2. **Model for the interaction of the zona pellucida glycoprotein, ZP3, with the plasma membrane overlying the acrosome of mouse spermatozoa to mediate sperm binding and acrosomal exocytosis.** *In this model, the ZP3 molecule is composed of multiple "functional ligands" ( ) which interact with complementary cell surface receptors /binding proteins present in the sperm plasma membrane. These ZP3-associated ligands are shown as being different from one another in this model, but this does not necessarily have to be the case. Moreover, three ZP3-associated ligands are shown although the actual numbers of ligands involved are not known and are shown in this fashion for illustrative purposes only. The proper interaction of ZP3 with the sperm surface requires the sequential binding of these ligands with sperm-associated receptors. Once these interactions are established signal transduction is effected by the formation of a functional signal transducing complex which forms in response to ligand-receptor induced aggregation of receptor proteins. Acrosomal exocytosis is then initiated in response to changes in second messengers / ionic conductance that are regulated in response to receptor-mediated signal transduction. In this model a variety of effector systems are shown to be targets for the a and/or bg subunits of heterotrimeric G proteins, as indicated by the dashed arrows. cAMP (adenosine-3',5'-cyclic monophosphate); IP_3 (inositol 1,4,5-trisphosphate); AA (arachidonic acid); lyso-PC (lysophosphatidylcholine); PA (phosphatidic acid).*

The nature of the intracellular signal pathways activated in response to sperm-ZP (or ZP3) interaction are only starting to be investigated. Studies in both mouse and bull sperm have demonstrated that elevations in intracellular Ca^{2+} and intracellular pH represent some of the earliest responses of sperm incubated with ZP or ZP3 (79, 90, 91). Such studies were performed with Ca^{2+} and pH indicator dyes and have reported localized changes to the acrosomal region. In bovine sperm, the ZP-induced Ca^{2+} entry, as well as sperm membrane potential and the acrosome reaction, are dependent upon membrane depolarization, and the Ca^{2+} uptake and acrosome reaction are inhibited by antagonists of voltage-dependent Ca^{2+} channels (92). These data suggest that mammalian sperm, like marine invertebrate sperm, contain voltage-dependent Ca^{2+} channels that are activated in response to biological effectors of the acrosome reaction. PTX inhibits the ZP (and ZP3)-induced pH changes in mouse sperm (78), as well as the ZP-induced pH and Ca^{2+} changes in bull sperm (79), indicating that sperm G_i proteins may regulate such ionic changes. Incubation of bovine sperm under depolarizing conditions, which would activate such voltage-dependent Ca^{2+} channels, bypasses the inhibitory effects of PTX on the acrosome reaction, suggesting that G_i proteins might regulate such Ca^{2+} channels indirectly (92).

Alterations in phospholipid metabolism and/or cyclic nucleotide metabolism have also been suggested to play important intermediary roles in the sperm acrosome reaction (8). Biologically-active phorbol diesters and diacylglycerols alter the kinetics of the ZP-mediated acrosome reaction in mouse sperm, thus suggesting that this exocytotic event could be regulated in some manner by protein kinase C (93). The products of phospholipase C turnover (e.g., IP_3 and sn-1,2 diacylglycerol), as well as the role of other phospholipases (A_2 or D), have not yet been examined in sperm challenged with ZP or ZP3. Noland et al (94) have reported that solubilized ZP from mouse eggs cause transient elevations in sperm cyclic AMP concentrations that are dependent on the presence of extracellular Ca^{2+}. These cyclic AMP elevations precede and are correlated with the induction of the acrosome reaction by the ZP, suggesting that cyclic AMP may be a potential participant in the signaling pathway leading to acrosomal exocytosis. These ZP-induced cAMP changes appear to be mediated by the activation of the sperm adenylyl cyclase (95). It will be of interest to determine whether such intracellular signaling systems are coupled to sperm G_i proteins, since these second messenger systems are coupled in a receptor-mediated fashion to G proteins in other cell types.

Acknowledgments
I would like to acknowledge the members of my laboratory, whose hard work and dedication are greatly appreciated. This work is supported by the NIH

(HD06274, HD22732; HD28514). G.S.K., H.G.H. and X.N. are supported by the NIH; P.E.V. is supported by the Rockefeller Foundation; J.M. is supported by the Agency for International Development.

REFERENCES

1. Chang, MC. Fertilizing capacity of spermatozoa deposited into the fallopian tubes. Nature 1951; 168: 697-698.
2. Chang MC. Development of fertilizing capacity of rabbit spermatozoa in the uterus. Nature 1955; 175: 1036-1037.
3. Austin CR. Observations on the penetration of the sperm into the mammalian egg. Aust. J. Sci. Res 1951; [B] 4: 581-596.
4. Austin CR. The "capacitation" of the mammalian sperm. Nature 1952; 170: 326.
5. Chang MC. The meaning of sperm capacitation. J. Androl 1984; 5: 45-50.
6. Yanagimachi R. Mammalian fertilization. In: The Physiology of Reproduction, E. Knobil and J.D. Neill, eds., Raven Press, New York; 1994: pp. 189-317.
7. Florman HM, Babcock DF. Progress towards understanding the molecular basis of capacitation. In: Elements of Mammalian Fertilization, P.M. Wassarman, ed., CRC Press, Boca Ratan, FL,; 1991: pp. 105-132.
8. Kopf GS, Gerton GL. The mammalian sperm acrosome and the acrosome reaction. In: Elements of Mammalian Fertilization, P.M. Wassarman, ed., CRC Press, Boca Ratan, FL; 1991: pp. 153-203.
9. Go KJ, Wolf DP. Albumin-mediated changes in sperm sterol content during capacitation. Biol. Reprod 1985; 32: 145-153.
10. Langlais J, Roberts KD. A molecular membrane model of sperm capacitation and the acrosome reaction of mammalian spermatozoa. Gamete Res 1985; 12: 183-224.
11. Yanagimachi, R. Requirements of extracellular calcium ions for various stages of fertilization and fertilization-related phenomena in the hamster. Gamete Res 1982; 5: 323-344.
12. Coronel CE, Lardy HA. Characterization of Ca^{2+} uptake by guinea pig epididymal spermatozoa. Biol. Reprod 1987; 37: 1097-1107.
13. Fraser, L.R. Minimum and maximum extracellular Ca^{2+} requirements during mouse sperm capacitation and fertilization in vitro. J. Reprod. Fert 1987; 81: 77-89.
14. Ruknudin, A, Silver IA. Ca^{2+} uptake during capacitation of mouse spermatozoa and the effect of an anion transport inhibitor on Ca^{2+} uptake. Mol. Reprod. Dev 1990; 26: 63-68.

15. Lee MA, Storey BT. Bicarbonate is essential for fertilization of mouse eggs; Mouse sperm require it to undergo the acrosome reaction. Biol. Reprod 1986; 34: 349-356.
16. Neill JM, Olds-Clarke P. A computer-assisted assay for mouse sperm hyperactivation demonstrates that bicarbonate but not bovine serum albumin is required. Gamete Res 1987; 18: 121-140.
17. Boatman DE, Robbins RS. Bicarbonate: carbon-dioxide regulation of sperm capacitation, hyperactivated motility, and acrosome reactions. Biol. Reprod 1991; 44: 806-813.
18. Fraser LR. Albumin is required to support the acrosome reaction but not capacitation in mouse spermatozoa in vitro. J. Reprod. Fert 1985; 74: 185-196.
19. Davis BK. Inhibitory effect of synthetic phospholipid vesicles containing cholesterol on the fertilizing ability of rabbit spermatozoa. Proc. Soc. Exp. Biol. Med. 1976; 152: 257-261.
20. Davis BK. Interactions of lipids with the plasma membrane of sperm cells. I. The antifertilization action of cholesterol. Arch. Androl. 1980; 5: 249-254.
21. Davis BK, Byrne R, Hungund B. Studies on the mechanism of capacitation. II. evidence for lipid transfer between plasma membrane of rat sperm and serum albumin during capacitation in vitro. Biochem. Biophys. Acta. 1979; 558: 257-266.
22. Davis BK, Byrne R, Bedigian K. Studies on the mechanism of capacitation: albumin-mediated changes in plasma membrane lipids during in vitro incubation of rat sperm. Proc. Nat'l. Acad. Sci., U.S.A. 1979; 68; 257-266.
23. Suzuki F, Yanagimachi R. Changes in the distribution of intramembraneous particles and filipin-reactive membrane sterols during in vitro capacitation of golden hamster spermatozoa. Gamete Res. 1989; 23: 335-347.
24. Garbers DL, Kopf GS. The regulation of spermatozoa by calcium and cyclic nucleotides. Adv. Cyclic Nuc. Res. 1980; 13: 251-306.
25. Lindemann CB, Kanous KS. Regulation of mammalian sperm motility. Arch. Androl. 1989; 23: 1-22.
26. Berger T, Clegg ED. Adenylate cyclase activity in porcine sperm in response to female reproductive tract secretions. Gamete Res. 1983; 7: 169-177.
27. Stein DM, Fraser LR. Cyclic nucleotide metabolism in mouse epididymal spermatozoa during capacitation in vitro. Gamete Res. 1984; 10: 283-299.
28. Monks NJ, Stein DM, Fraser LR. Adenylate cyclase activity of mouse sperm during capacitation in vitro: effect of calcium and a GTP analogue. Int. J. Androl. 1986; 9: 67-76.

29. Leyton L, Saling P. 95 kd sperm proteins bind ZP3 and serve as tyrosine kinase substrates in response to zona binding. Cell 1989; 57: 1123-1130.
30. Duncan AE, Fraser LR. Cyclic AMP-dependent phosphorylation of epididymal mouse sperm proteins during capacitation in vitro: identification of an Mr 95,000 phosphotyrosine-containing protein. J. Reprod. Fert. 1993; 97: 287-299.
31. Visconti PE, Bailey J, Moore GD, Pan D, Olds-Clarke P, Kopf, GS. Capacitation in mouse spermatozoa. I. Correlation between the capacitation state and protein tyrosine phosphorylation. Development 1995; 121: 1129-1137.
32. Visconti PE, Moore GD, Bailey J, Connors SA, Leclerc P, Pan D, Olds-Clarke P, Kopf GS. Capacitation in mouse spermatozoa. II. Tyrosine phosphorylation and capacitation are regulated by a cAMP-dependent pathway. Development 1995; 121: 1139-1150.
33. Garbers DL, Tubb DJ, Hyne RV. requirement of bicarbonate for Ca^{2+}-induced elevations of cyclic AMP in guinea pig spermatozoa. J. Biol. Chem. 1982; 257: 8980-8984.
34. Hyne RV, Garbers DL. Regulation of guinea pig sperm adenylate cyclase by calcium. Biol. Reprod 1979;.21: 1135-1142.
35. Gross MK, Toscano DG, Toscano WA. Calmodulin-mediated adenylate cyclase from mammalian sperm. J. Biol. Chem. 1987; 262: 8672-8676.
36. Garty NB, Salomon Y. Stimulation of partially purified adenylate cyclase from bull sperm by bicarbonate. FEBS Lett. 1987; 218: 148-152.
37. Okamura N, Tajima Y, Sugita Y. Decrease in bicarbonate transport activities during epididymal maturation. Biochem. Biophys. Res. Commun. 1988; 157: 1280-1287.
38. Visconti PE, Muschietti JF, Flawia MM, Tezon J. Bicarbonate dependence of cAMP accumulation induced by phorbol esters in hamster spermatozoa. Biochim. Biophys. Acta 1990; 1054: 231-236.
39. Moos J, Carrera A, Tesarik J, Moss SB, Gerton GL, Kopf GS. Regulation, localization and identity of phosphotyrosine-containing proteins in human sperm Biol. Reprod.1995; 52 (Suppl.): 168.
40. Galantino-Homer H, Visconti PE, Kopf GS. Regualtion of protein tyrosine phosphorylation during bovine sperm capacitation by a cAMP-dependent pathway. Biol. Reprod. 1995; 52 (Suppl.): 60.
41. Singh JP, Babcock DF, Lardy HA. Increased calcium ion influx is a component of capacitation of spermatozoa. Biochem. J. 1978; 172: 549-556.
42. Kopf GS, Vacquier VD. Characterization of a calmodulin stimulated adenylate cyclase from abalone spermatozoa. J. Biol. Chem.1984; 259: 7590-7596.

43. Okamura N, Tajima Y, Soejima A, Masuda H, Sugita Y. Sodium bicarbonate in seminal plasma stimulates the motility of mammalian spermatozoa through direct activation of adenylate cyclase J. Biol. Chem. 1985; 260: 9699-9705.
44. Olds-Clarke P. Variation in the quality of sperm motility and its relationship to capacitation. In: "Fertilization in Mammals", B. Bavister, J. Cummins and E. Roldan, eds., Serono Symposia USA, Norwell, MA, 1990: pp. 91-99.
45. Hayashi H, Yamamoto K, Yonekawa H, Morisawa M. Involvement of tyrosine protein kinase in the initiation of flagellar movement in rainbow trout spermatozoa. J. Biol. Chem. 1987; 262: 16692-16698.
46. Siegelbaum SA. Ion channel control by tyrosine phosphorylation. Curr. Biol. 1994; 4: 242-245.
47. Wilson GF, Kaczmarek LK. Mode-switching of a voltage-gated cation channel is mediated by a protein kinase A-regulated tyrosine phosphatase. Nature 1993; 366: 433-438.
48. Wu J, Dent P, Jelinek T, Wolfman A, Weber MJ, Sturgill TW. Inhibition of the EGF-activated MAP kinase signaling pathway by adenosine 3',5'-monophosphate. Science 1993; 262: 1065-1069.
49. Begum N, Graham AL, Sussman KE, Draznin B. Role of cAMP in mediating effects of fasting on dephosphorylation of the insulin receptor. Amer. J. Physiol. 1992; 262: E142-E149.
50. Brautigan DL, Pinault FM. Activation of membrane protein-tyrosine phosphatase involving cAMP- and Ca^{2+}/phospholipid-dependent protein kinases. Proc. Nat'l. Acad. Sci. U.S.A. 1991; 88: 6696-6700.
51. Wassarman PM. Zona pellucida glycoproteins. Ann. Rev. Biochem. 1988; 57: 415-442.
52. Shimizu S, Tsuji M, Dean J In vitro biosynthesis of three sulfated glycoproteins of murine zonae pellucidae by oocytes grown in follicle culture. J. Biol. Chem. 1983; 258: 5858-5863
53. Dunbar BS, Prasad SV, Timmons TM Comparative structure and function of mammalian zonae pellucidae. In B.S. Dunbar and M.G. O'Rand (eds.) A Comparative Overview of Mammalian Fertilization, Plenum Press, Inc., New York, 1991; 7-114
54. Bleil JD, Greve JM, Wassarman PM Identification of a secondary sperm receptor in the mouse egg zona pellucida: Role in maintenance of binding of acrosome-reacted sperm to eggs. Dev. Biol. 1988; 128: 376-385
55. Moller CC, Wassarman PM Characterization of a proteinase that cleaves zona pellucida glycoprotein ZP2 following activation of mouse eggs. Dev. Biol. 1989; 132: 103-112
56. Bleil JD, Wassarman PM Galactose at the non-reducing terminus of O-linked oligosaccharides of mouse egg zona pellucida glycoprotein ZP3 is

essential for the glycoprotein's sperm receptor activity. Proc. Natl. Acad. Sci., U.S.A.1988; 85: 6778-6782
57. Miller DJ, Gong X, Decker G, Shur BD. Egg cortical granule N-acetylglucosaminidase is required for the mouse zona block to polyspermy. J Cell Biol 1993; 123:1431-1440.
58. Chamberlin ME, Dean J Human homolog of the mouse sperm receptor. Proc. Natl. Acad. Sci., U.S.A. 1990; 87: 6014-6018
59. Ringuette MJ, Chamberlin ME, Baur AW, Sobieski DA, Dean, J. Molecular analysis of cDNA coding for ZP3, a sperm binding protein of the mouse zona pellucida. Dev. Biol. 1988; 127: 287-295
60. Kinloch RA, Ruiz-Seiler B, Wassarman PM Genomic organization and polypeptide primary structure of zona pellucida glycoprotein hZP3, the hamster sperm receptor. Dev. Biol. 1990; 142: 414-421
61. Moller CC, Bleil JD, Kinloch RA, Wassarman PM Structural and functional relationships between mouse and hamster zona pellucida glycoproteins. Dev. Biol. 1990; 137: 276-286
62. Saling PM, Sowinski J, Storey BT An ultrastructural study of epididymal mouse spermatozoa binding to zonae pellucidae in vitro: Sequential relationship to the acrosome reaction. J. Exp. Zool. 1979; 209: 229-238.
63. Bleil JD, Wassarman PM Autoradiographic visualization of the mouse egg's sperm receptor bound to sperm. J. Cell Biol. 1986; 102: 1363-1371
64. Vazquez MH, Phillips DM, Wassarman PM Interaction of mouse sperm with purified sperm receptors covalently linked to silica beads. J. Cell Sci. 1989; 92: 713-722
65. Mortillo S, Wassarman PM Differential binding of gold-labeled zona pellucida glycoproteins mZP2 and mZP3 to mouse sperm membrane compartments. Development 1991; 113: 141-149
66. Bleil JD, Wassarman PM Identification of a ZP3-binding protein on acrosome-intact mouse sperm by photoaffinity crosslinking. Proc. Natl. Acad. Sci. U.S.A. 1990; 87: 5563-5567
67. Cheng A, Le T, Palacios M, Bookbinder LH, Wassarman PM, Suzuki F, Bleil JD Sperm-egg recognition in the mouse: characterization of sp56, a sperm protein having specific affinity for ZP3. J Cell Biol 1994; 125: 867-878.
68. Bookbinder LH, Cheng A, Bleil JD Tissue- and species-specific expression of sp56, a mouse sperm fertilization protein. Science 1995; 269: 86-89.
69. Leyton L, LeGuen P, Bunch D, Saling PM Regulation of mouse gamete interaction by a sperm tyrosine kinase. Proc. Natl. Acad. Sci.,U.S.A. 1992; 89: 11692-11695
70. Kalab P, Visconti P, Leclerc P, Kopf GS p95, the major phosphotyrosine-containing protein in mouse spermatozoa, is a form of hexokinase with unique properties. J. Biol. Chem. 1994; 269, 3810-3817.

71. Miller DJ, Macek MB, Shur BD Complementarity between sperm surface b-1,4-galactosyltransferase and egg-coat ZP3 mediates sperm-egg binding. Nature 1992; 357: 589-593
72. Kopf GS, Woolkalis MJ, Gerton GL Evidence for a guanine nucleotide-binding regulatory protein in invertebrate and mammalian sperm: Identification by islet-activating protein-catalyzed ADP-ribosylation and immunochemical methods. J. Biol. Chem. 1986; 261: 7327-7331
73. Bentley JK, Garbers DL, Domino SE, Noland TD, VanDop C Spermatozoa contain a guanine nucleotide binding protein ADP-ribosylated by pertussis toxin. Biochem. Biophys. Res. Commun. 1986; 138: 728-734
74. Glassner M, Jones J, Kligman I, Woolkalis MJ, Gerton GL, Kopf GS Immunocytochemical and biochemical characterization of guanine nucleotide-binding regulatory proteins in mammalian spermatozoa. Dev. Biol. 1991; 146: 438-450
75. Karnik NS, Newman S, Kopf GS, Gerton GL Developmental expression of G protein a subunits in mouse spermatogenic cells: Evidence that G_{ai} is associated with the developing acrosome. Dev. Biol. 1992; 152: 393-402
76. Garty NB, Galiani D, Aharonheim A, Ho YK, Phillips DM, Dekel N, Salomon Y G-proteins in mammalian gametes: an immunocytochemical study. J. Cell Sci. 1988; 91: 21-31
77. Endo Y, Lee MA, Kopf GS Evidence for the role of a guanine nucleotide-binding regulatory protein in the zona pellucida-induced mouse sperm acrosome reaction. Dev. Biol. 1987: 119: 210-216
78. Endo Y, Lee MA, Kopf GS Characterization of an islet activating protein-sensitive site in mouse sperm that is involved in the zona pellucida - induced acrosome reaction. Dev. Biol. 1988; 129: 12-24
79. Florman HM, Tombes RM, First NL, Babcock DF An adhesion-associated agonist from the zona pellucida activates G protein-promoted elevations of internal Ca^{2+} and pH that mediate mammalian sperm acrosomal exocytosis. Dev. Biol. 1989; 135: 133-146
80. Lee MA, Check JH, Kopf GS A guanine nucleotide-binding regulatory protein in human sperm mediates acrosomal exocytosis induced by the human zona pellucida. Mol. Reprod. Dev. 1992; 31: 78-86
81. Tesarik J, Carreras A, Mendoza C Differential sensitivity of progesterone- and zona pellucida-induced acrosome reactions to pertussis toxin. Mol. Reprod. Dev. 1992; 34: 183-189
82. Wilde MW, Ward CR, Kopf GS Activation of a G protein in mouse sperm by the zona pellucida, an egg-associated extracellular matrix. Mol. Reprod. Dev. 1992; 31: 297-306
83. Ward CR, Storey BT, Kopf GS Activation of a G_i protein in cell-free membrane preparations of mouse sperm by the zona pellucida and ZP3,

components of the egg's extracellular matrix. J. Biol. Chem. 1992; 267: 14061-14067
84. Ward CR, Storey BT, Kopf GS. Selective activation of G_{i1} and G_{i2} in mouse sperm by the zona pellucida, the egg's extracellular matrix., J. Biol. Chem 1994; 269: 13254-13258.
85. Ning XP, Ward CR, Kopf GS. Activation of a G_i protein in digitonin/cholate-solubilized membrane preparations of mouse sperm by the zona pellucida, an egg-specific extracellular matrix. Mol. Reprod. Dev. 1995; 40: 355-363.
86. Meyerhof W, Muller-Brechlin R, Richter D Molecular cloning of a novel putative G protein-coupled receptor expressed during rat spermiogenesis. FEBS Lett. 1991; 284: 155-160
87. Parmentier M, Libert F, Schurmans, Schiffman S, Lefort A, Eggerickx D, Ledent C, Mollereau C, Gerard C, Perret J, Grootegoed A, Vassart G Expression of members of the putative olfactory receptor gene family in mammalian germ cells. Nature 1992; 355: 453-455
88. Vanderhaeghen P, Schurmans S, Vassart G, Parmentier M. Olfactory receptors are displayed on dog mature sperm cells. J. Cell Biol. 1993; 123: 1441-1452.
89. Ward CR, Kopf GS Molecular events mediating sperm activation. Dev. Biol. 1993; 158: 1-26
90. Lee MA, Storey BT Evidence for plasma membrane impermeability to small ions in acrosome-intact mouse spermatozoa bound to mouse zonae pellucidae, using an aminoacridine fluorescent probe: time course of the zona-induced acrosome reaction monitored by both chlortetracycline and pH probe fluorescence. Biol. Reprod. 1985; 33: 235-246
91. Lee MA, Storey BT. Endpoint of first stage of zona pellucida-induced acrosome reaction in mouse spermatozoa characterized by acrosomal H^+ and Ca^{2+} permeability: Population and single cell kinetics. Gamete Res.1989; 24: 303-326
92. Florman HM, Corron ME, Kim TD, Babcock DF Activation of voltage-dependent calcium channels of mammalian sperm is required for zona pellucida-induced acrosomal exocytosis. Dev. Biol. 1992; 152: 304-314
93. Lee MA, Kopf GS, Storey BT Effects of phorbol esters and a diacylglycerol on the mouse sperm acrosome reaction induced by the zona pellucida. Biol. Reprod. 1987; 36: 617-627
94. Noland TD, Garbers DL, Kopf GS An elevation in cyclic AMP concentration precedes the zona pellucida-induced acrosome reaction of mouse spermatozoa. Biol. Reprod. 1988; 38: (Suppl.), 94
95. Leclerc P, Kopf GS. Mouse sperm adenylyl cyclase: General properties and regulation by the zona pellucida. Biol. Reprod. 1995; 52, 1227-1233.

Role of protein kinase C in human sperm acrosome reaction

Zvi Naor, Ronit Rotem and Moshe Kalina

Department of Biochemistry, George 5, Wise Faculty of Life Sciences and Department of Histology and Cell Biology, Sackler School of Medicine, Tel Aviv University, Ramat Aviv 69978, Israel

ABSTRACT

We found the presence of protein kinase C (PKC) in ejaculated human sperm by enzymatic activity assay and immunohistochemistry. The sperm head PKC is localized in the acrosome, equatorial segment and post-acrosomal region. In the flagellum, PKC is associated with the segmented column of the neck and is distributed along the mid-, principal- and end-pieces. Immunoreactive sites were observed in patches along the axoneme and outer dense fibers and were evenly distributed between these regions. The colocalization of PKC with various cytoskeletal elements suggests that the proteins involved are potential substrates for sperm PKC subspecies. Addition of the PKC activator 12-0-tetradecanoylphorbol-13-acetate (TPA) resulted in increased flagellar motility and acrosome reaction in a Ca^{2+}-independent fashion. On the other-hand, the Ca^{2+} ionophore, ionomycin, stimulated flagellar motility and acrosome reaction in a PKC-independent mechanism. We propose that PKC is involved in the regulation of motility and acrosome reaction in human sperm.

Nous avons mis en évidence, par mesure de l'activité enzymatique et par immunohistochimie, la présence de protéine kinase C dans le spermatozoïde humain. La PKC est localisée au niveau de la tête spermatique, dans l'acrosome, le segment équatorial et la région post-acrosomique. Dans le flagelle, la PKC est associée à la colonne segmentée du cou et est distribuée tout au long des pièces intermédiaire, principale et *terminale. Des sites immunoréactifs ont été observés en patch le long de l'axonème et des fibres denses externes, la répartition entre ces deux régions étant homogène. La colocalisation de la PKC avec différents éléments du cytosquelette suggère que les protéines impliquées sont des substrats potentiels pour les PKC du spermatozoïde. L'addition de 12-0-tetradecanoylphorbol-13-acétate (TPA), activateur de la PKC, se traduit par une augmentation, Ca^{2+} indépendante, de la mobilité flagellaire et de la réaction acrosomique. D'autre part, le ionophore calcique, la ionomycine, augmente selon un mécanisme indépendant de la PKC, la mobilité flagellaire et la réaction acrosomique. Nous pensons que la PKC est impliquée dans la régulation de la mobilité et de la réaction acrosomique du spermatozoïde humain.*

INTRODUCTION

Protein Kinase C (PKC) is a key regulatory element in signal transduction of hormones, neurotransmitters, growth factors and antigens (1-3). PKC plays a role in synaptic transmission, memory and learning, growth, metabolism, differentiation, contraction, exocytosis, ion channels regulation, gene expression and transformation. The enzyme is a family of related subtypes including: conventional PKCs (cPKC: α, βI, βII and γ) which are activated by Ca^{2+} and phospholipid; novel PKCs (nPKC: δ, ε, η and θ) and atypical PKCs (aPKC: ξ and λ) which are Ca^{2+}-independent, phospholipid activated subtypes. Differential expression and activation of the various PKC subtypes might be linked to the numerous functions mediated by PKC in various cells. Nevertheless, the biological role of the various PKC subtypes is not yet known.

Rat seminiferous tubules and Leydig cells (4,5) but not ram spermatozoa (6) showed PKC activity. Thus the lack of reports on mammalian spermatozoa PKC activity led us to investigate the presence and role of PKC in human sperm physiology.

Human sperm PKC activity is relatively low (2.5% of the specific activity of rat brain) and is found mainly in the particulate fraction (55%) (7, 8). Low activity of PKC was also found in bull and ram sperm but the enzyme was found mainly (80%) in the soluble fraction and only 20% in the particulate fraction of both species (9). The presence of PKC in mammalian sperm is in line with documentation on activation of phosphoinositide turnover and other signal transduction units (10-12 and references therein). Nevertheless, the nature of the ligand which activates sperm PKC is not yet known.

PKC AND HUMAN SPERM MOTILITY

PKC activators such as the tumor promoter phorbol ester 12-0-tetradecanoylphorbol-13-acetate (TPA) (Fig. 1) or the diacylglycerol analog l-oleoyl-2-acetylglycerol (OAG) were found to stimulate human sperm motility (7,8). Stimulation of sperm motility was also noticed upon the addition of the Ca^{2+} ionophore, ionomycin (8). Removal of Ca^{2+} abolished the effect of ionomycin but not that induced by TPA. On the other hand the use of PKC inhibitors resulted in inhibition of the TPA, but not the ionomycin response (8). We therefore suggested that separate pathways involving Ca^{2+} or PKC can mediate the stimulation of human sperm flagellar motility. Since cyclic AMP was also reported to be involved in sperm-motility, it seems that multiple and separate signal transduction cascades might be operating for different ligands which stimulate sperm motility.

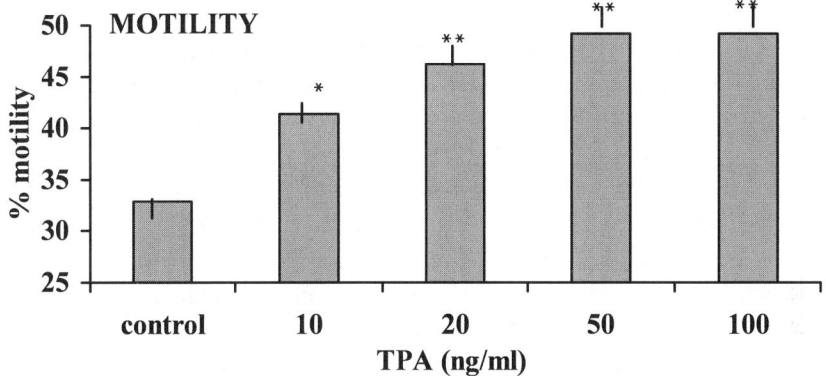

Figure. 1. **Effect of TPA on human sperm motility.** *Sperm was incubated with increasing concentrations of TPA for 30 min. in Ham's F-10 medium containing human serum albumin (0.5%). For further details see refs. 7,8.*

Further support to the notion that PKC is involved in human sperm motility emerged when regression analysis revealed an excellent correlation between motility and percent PKC stained cells from various donors (7).

PKC AND ACROSOME REACTION

Mammalian spermatozoa undergo the acrosome reaction during fertilization to penetrate the oocyte vestment. Fusion of the outer acrosomal membrane and the overlying plasma membrane culminates in the release of the acrosomal content. As an exocytotic response, the acrosome reaction is thought to be absolutely dependent on Ca^{2+} (13,14). The presence of PKC in mammalian sperm prompted us to examine its potential role in acrosome reaction and the Ca^{2+} requirements for the process.

Others have demonstrated ;stimulation of human and mouse spermatozoa acrosome reaction by TPA or diacylglycerol analogs (15,16). We found stimulation of acrosome reaction by TPA and OAG in human and bovine spermatozoa and the effect was dependent on prior capacitation (9,17). Comparative studies on the effect of TPA and the Ca^{2+} ionophore ionomycin upon human sperm acrosome reaction revealed separate mechanisms for the stimulants (17). Stimulation of acrosome reaction by TPA was inhibited by PKC inhibitors or down regulation of endogenous PKC activity, but not by Ca removal (17). On the other hand stimulation of human acrosome reaction by ionomycin was blocked by Ca^{2+} removal but not by PKC inhibitors or down-regulation. Thus separate mechanisms involving Ca^{2+} or PKC can mediate acrosome reaction in an independent fashion.

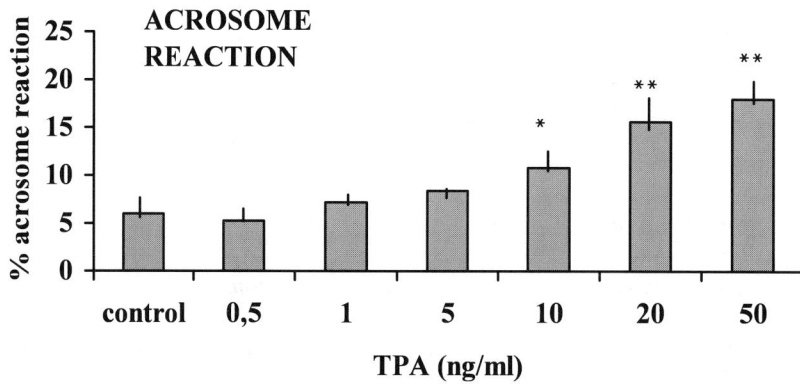

Figure. 2: **Effect of TPA on human sperm acrosome reaction**. *Sperm was preincubated for 18h in Ham's F-10 medium containing human serum albumin (0.5%) for capacitation. After a wash procedure, sperm was incubated with increasing concentrations of TPA for 60 min. in the above medium at 33°C. For further details see ref. 17.*

LOCALIZATION OF PKC IN HUMAN SPERM

PKC was found to be localized mainly in the equatorial segment of the human sperm on a distinct band (7). Staining was also found in the principal piece of the tail. In bull sperm PKC was found mainly in the post-acrosome region and the upper region of the acrosome (9). Less-staining of the post-acrosomal region was noticed in the ram sperm while the upper region of the acrosome was more strongly stained (9). Further analysis with type-specific antibodies revealed the presence of PKCα and PKCβII in the equatorial segment of the human sperm, raising the possibility that the two subspecies might be involved in mediating the acrosome reaction (17). Interestingly PKCα and PKCβII were implicated in exocytotic responses in pituitary and PC-12 cells (18,19) and the acrosome reaction is an exocytotic response.

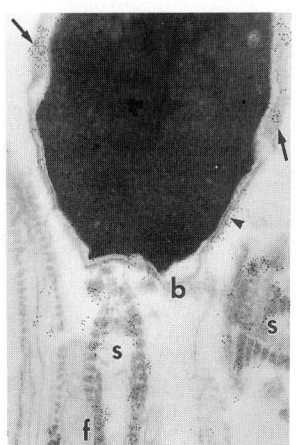 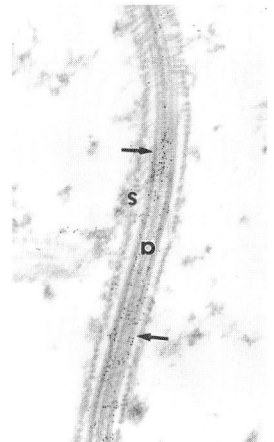

Figure. 3. **Localization of PKC in human sperm by immunogold labeling.** *Anti-PKC MAb and gold anti-mouse (8-nm) were used on araldite-embedded thin sections of glutaradelyde-fixed (unosmicated) human sperm. Left: PKC localization in the sperm head and neck. Gold particles can be observed-in the equatorial segment (arrows) and in the post-acrosomal dense laminae (arrowheads). In the sperm neck, labeling can be observed in the basal plate (b) and segmented columns (s); the outer dense fibers are also labeled (f). Right: Gold particles are seen in patches along the principal piece associated with the axoneme (a) and outer dense fibers (ar-rows), but not in the fibrous sheath (s)(20).*

We found that PKCβI and PKCε were present in the principal piece of the tail, suggesting involvement of the subtypes in mediating sperm motility (17). Compartmentalization of various PKC subtypes in the human sperm might enable phosphorylation of distinct substrates leading to selective activation of sperm functions.

Using the immunogold technique at the electron microscopical level, gold particles were found localized in patches along the acrosome and the tail as well as labeling of the equatorial segment and the postacrosomal dense laminae (Fig. 3) (20). The basal plate and the segmented columns of the sperm neck were also labeled. Gold particles were distributed between the elements of the axoneme and the outer dense fibers along the mid- and principal piece of the tail (20). The mitochondria in the midpiece and the fibrous sheath in the principal piece were not labeled.

Human sperm have a highly specialized cytoskeletal: organization (21). Localization of myosin in the neck, vimentin in the equatorial segment and actin and spectrin in the principal piece of the tail might be linked to the presence of PKC in these domains. Co-distribution of PKC and cytoskeletal elements might identify potential substrates for sperm PKC which are involved in motility and acrosome reaction.

CONCLUSION

PKC is present in mammalian sperm in distinct structures and seems to play a role in motility and acrosome reaction but the nature of the ligand activating the enzyme remains to be elucidated.

Acknowledgment
We thank Dr. Y. Nishizuka for the PKC antibodies.

REFERENCES

1. Nishizuka Y. The molecular heterogeneity of protein kinase and its implications for cellular regulation. Nature 198, 334: 661-5.
2. Kikkawa U, Ogita K, shearman MS, Ase K, Sekiguchi K, Naor Z, Ido M, Nishizuka Y, Saito N, Tanaka C, Ono Y, Fujii, Igarashi K. The heterogeneity and differential expression protein kinase C in nervous tissues. Phil Trans Roy 5 1988; 320: 313-24.
3. Nishizuka Y. Intracellular signaling by hydrolysis phospholipids and activation of protein Kinase C. Science 1992; 258: 607-14.
4. Kimura K, Kath N, Sakurada K, Kubo 5. Phospholipid-sensitive Ca^{2+}-dependent protein kinase system in testis: localization and endogenous substrates. Endocrinology 1984; 115: 2391-9
5. Nikula H, Naor Z, Parvinen M, Huhtaniemi I. Distribution activation of protein kinase C in the rat testis tissue. Cell Endocrinol 1987; 49: 39-49.
6. Roldan ERS, Harrison RAP. Absence of active protein kinase C in ram spermatozoa. Biochem. Biophys. Commun 1988; 155: 901-6.

7. Rotem R, Paz GF, Homonnai ZT, Kalina M, Naor Z. Protein Kinase C is present in human sperm: Possible role in flagellar motility. Proc Natl Acad Sci USA 1990; 87: 7305-
8. Rotem R, Paz GF, Homonnai ZT, Kalina M, Naor Z. Further studies on the involvement of protein Kinase C in human flagellar motility. Endocrinology 1990; 127: 2571-7.
9. Breitbart H, Lax J, Rotem R, Naor Z. Role-of protein Kinase C in the acrosome reaction of mammalian spermatozoa. Biochem J 1992; 281: 473-6.
10. Domino SE, Garbers DL. The tucose sulfate glycoconjugate that induces an acrosome reaction in spermatozoa stimulates inositol 1, 4, 5 trisphosphate accumulation. J Biol Chem 1988 ; 263: 690-5.
11. Kopf GS, Woolkalis MJ, Gerton GS. Evidence for guanine nucleotide binding regulatory protein in invertebrate and mammalian sperm. J Biol Chem 1986; 261: 7327-33.
12. Roldan ERS, Murate T , Shi Q-X . Exocytosis in spermatozoa in response to progesterone and Zona pellucida. Science 1994; 266: 1578-81.
13. Kopf GS, Wilde MW . S ignal transduction processes leading to acrosomal exocytosis in mammalian spermatozoa. Trends Endocrinol Metab 1990; 1: 362-8.
14. Yanagimachi R, Usui N. Calcium dependence of the acrosome reaction and activation of guinea pig spermatozoa. Exp Cell Res 1974; 89: 161-74
15. Lee MA, Kopf GS, Stoney BT. Effects of phorbol ester and diacylgycerol on the mouse sperm acrosome reaction induced by the Zona pellucida. Biol Reprod 1987; 36: 616-27.
16. De Jonge C, Han HL, Mack SR, Zaneveld JD. Effect of phorboldiesters synthetic diacylglcyerols and a protein kinase C inhibitor on the human sperm acrosome reaction. J Androl 1991; 12 (1): 62-70.
17. Rotem R, Paz GF, Homonnai ZT, Kalina M, Lax J, Breitbart H, Naor Z. Calcium-dependent induction of acrosome reaction'by protein kinase C in human sperm, Endocrinology 1992; 131: 22 3 5-4 3 .
18. Ben-Shlomo H, Naor Z. Preferential release of catecholamine from permeabilized PC12 cells by α- and, β-type protein kinase C subspecies. Biochem J 1991; 280: 65-9.
19. Naor Z, Dan-Cohen H, Hermon J, Limor R. Induction of exocytosis in permeabilized pituitary cells by α-and β-type protein Kinase C. Proc Natl Acad Sci USA 1989; 88: 4501-4.
20. Kalina M, Sacher R, Rotem R, Naor Z. Ultrastructural localization of protein Kinase C in human sperm. J Histochem Cytochem 1995; 43: 439-45.
21. Virtanem I, Badley A, Spaasivno R, Lehto V-P. Distinct cytoskeletal domains revealed in sperm cells. J Cell Biol 198.4; 899: 1083-8.

Human sperm acrosome reaction. Eds P. Fénichel, J. Parinaud.
Colloque INSERM/John Libbey Eurotext Ltd © 1995.Vol. 236, pp. 225-243

Role of phosphoinositides in the mammalian sperm acrosome reaction

Eduardo R.S. Roldan

Department of Development and Signalling, The Babraham Institute, Cambridge CB2 4AT, United Kingdom

Abstract

The phosphoinositides (PIs) play a central role during exocytosis in mammalian spermatozoa. Stimulation of capacitated mouse sperm with zona pellucida, progesterone or epidermal growth factor (EGF) results in the hydrolysis of both phosphatidylinositol 4-phosphate (PtdIns(4)P) and phosphatidylinositol(4,5) bisphosphate (PtdIns (4,5) P_2). Likewise, stimulation of human sperm with progesterone leads to PI hydrolysis. So far, there is no report indicating that zona pellucida would induce PI hydrolysis in human spermatozoa, although it could be predicted that this is a likely event. The breakdown of the PIs is essential for subsequent exocytosis and serves mainly to generate messenger diacylglycerol (DAG). The other product of PtdIns(4,5)P_2 hydrolysis, inositol(1,4,5) trisphosphate, does not appear to have any significant role, since it is produced after Ca^{2+} entry. DAG is involved in the activation of Ca^{2+}-dependent events which are instrumental in bringing about membrane fusion. First, the PI-derived DAG seems to be related to the regulation of phosphatidylcholine-specific phospholipase C, an enzyme which generates additional DAG. Second, DAG (both PI- and phosphatidylcholine-derived) is also involved in the activation of phospholipase A_2, a key enzyme that serves to generate metabolites important for the late steps of fusion.

Les phosphoinositides (PIs) jouent un rôle central au cours de l'exocytose de l'acrosome des spermatozoïdes des mammifères. La stimulation de spermatozoïdes de souris par des zones pellucides, de la progestérone ou de *l'EGF, induit l'hydrolyse du phosphatidylinositol 4 - phosphate (PtdIns(4) P) et du phosphatidylinositol (4,5) biphosphate (PtIns(4,5)P2). De plus, la stimulation des spermatozoïdes humains conduit également à l'hydrolyse des PI. Jusqu'ici, il n'y a aucune donnée indiquant que la zone pellucide induirait l'hydrolyse des PI dans les spermatozoïdes humains, bien que ceci soit probable. La chute des PIs est essentielle à l'exocytose ultérieure et sert essentiellement à générer du diacylglycerol (DAG). L' autre produit d'hydrolyse du PtdIns (4,5)P2, l'inositol (1,4,5) triphosphate, ne semble pas avoir un rôle significatif, puisqu'il est produit après l'entrée de Ca^{2+}. Le DAG est impliqué dans l'activation des mécanismes Ca^{2+} dépendants qui contribuent à mener à bien la fusion des membranes.. Premièrement, le DAG semble être lié à la régulation d'une phospholipase C spécifique de la phosphatidylcholine, une enzyme qui génère du DAG supplémentaire. Deuxièmement, le DAG (dérivé à la fois des PIs et de la phosphatidylcholine) est également impliqué dans l'activation de la phospholipase A2, une enzyme clef dont le rôle est de générer des métabolites importants pour les étapes tardives de la fusion.*

INTRODUCTION

At fertilization, mammalian spermatozoa undergo an exocytotic process in response to oocyte-associated agonists. This exocytotic process is characterized by a sequence of events: (a) agonist-receptor interaction, (b) the activation of a number of transducing mechanims and the generation of second messengers, and (c) the fusion of the outer acrosomal membrane with the overlying plasma membrane to release and/or expose the contents of the acrosomal granule.

There has been considerable controversy around the issue of whether there is just a single agonist responsible for the initiation of exocytosis in spermatozoa, or whether there are various agonists involved. The prevailing view is that the zona pellucida (ZP)[1], the egg's acellular coat, is the agonist responsible for the intiation of exocytosis (1,2). However, recent work has

---

[1] Abbreviations used: ZP: zona pellucida; PI: phosphoinositide; PtdIns: phosphatidylinositol; PtdIns(4)P: phosphatidylinositol 4-phosphate; PtdIns(4,5)P_2: phosphatidylinositol (4,5)bisphosphate; Ins(1,4,5)P_3: inositol (1,4,5)trisphosphate; DAG, diacylglycerol: PtdCho: phosphatidylcholine; PIC: phosphoinositidase C (PI-specific PLC); PLC: phospholipase C; PLD: phospholipase D; PLA$_2$: phospholipase A$_2$; EGF: epidermal growth factor; PTK: protein tyrosine kinase.

revealed that spermatozoa can undergo exocytosis in response to other natural agonists that are present in (or are secreted by) the egg cellular vestments, or at the site of fertilization (3,4). Thus, although it is probably true that the ZP is the main agonist of exocytosis, it is also important to realize that its action is primed or modulated by other agonists. This view implies that various receptors on the sperm surface would mediate the action of such agonists, and that a variety of signal transduction pathways could be activated in response to such stimulation. In addition, there is the possibility of interaction ('cross-talk') between several transducing pathways. Finally, one can ask the question 'why are there several agonists, and various signal transduction pathways, involved in this exocytotic process?' Spermatozoa are highly compartmentalized cells, and the sperm head (besides acting as carrier of the genetic material) appears to be involved solely in exocytosis of the acrosomal granule. The process is irreversible and, possibly, not related to any other in this cell compartment. Therefore, the need for various pathways of signal transduction might, at first glance, appear redundant.

This review will attempt to summarize knowledge of aspects of signal transduction and generation of second messengers during acrosomal exocytosis, paying special attention to pathways leading to phosphoinositide hydrolysis, and the events modulated by the resulting metabolites. A discussion of why are there various agonists, and redundant pathways, is perhaps premature, and will not be attempted here.

HYDROLYSIS OF PHOSPHOINOSITIDES IN RESPONSE TO AGONISTS OF ACROSOMAL EXOCYTOSIS

The phosphoinositides (PIs) phosphatidylinositol (PtdIns), phosphatidylinositol 4-phosphate (PtdIns(4)P) and phosphatidylinositol (4,5)bisphosphate (PtdIns(4,5)P_2) (Fig. 1) are minor components of the plasma membrane of eukaryotic cells, including spermatozoa (5,6). In spermatozoa, the PIs seem to be located on the inner aspect of the plasma membrane and the outer aspect of the outer acrosomal membrane (7). The PIs appear to turn over actively, even under resting conditions; this is clearly shown by the ability of sperm PIs to incorporate [^{32}P]P$_i$ label via the ATP pool in short-term incubations (8).

In a wide variety of cell types, PIs have been shown to constitute a source of an array of metabolites; some of these metabolites have important second messenger functions (9). Hydrolysis of PtdIns(4,5)P_2 by phosphoinositidase C (PIC) (Fig. 1) leads to the formation of the second messengers inositol(1,4,5)trisphosphate (Ins(1,4,5)P$_3$) and diacylglycerol (DAG), which participate, respectively, in Ca^{2+} modulation and activation of protein kinase C. The former can be sequentially dephosphorylated to inositol(1,4)bisphosphate, inositol 4-phosphate and inositol, or it can be phosphorylated to inositol(1,3,4,5)tetrakisphosphate (9). DAG, the other product of PtdIns(4,5)P_2 and PtdIns(4)P hydrolysis, could be phosphorylated by a DAG kinase to phosphatidate or it could be sequentially deacylated by DAG and monoacylglycerol lipases. PIs themselves can be substrates for the generation of other metabolites, the 3-phosphorylated inositol lipids (Fig. 1). The role of these meabolites is still unclear and constitutes the subject of active research (10,11).

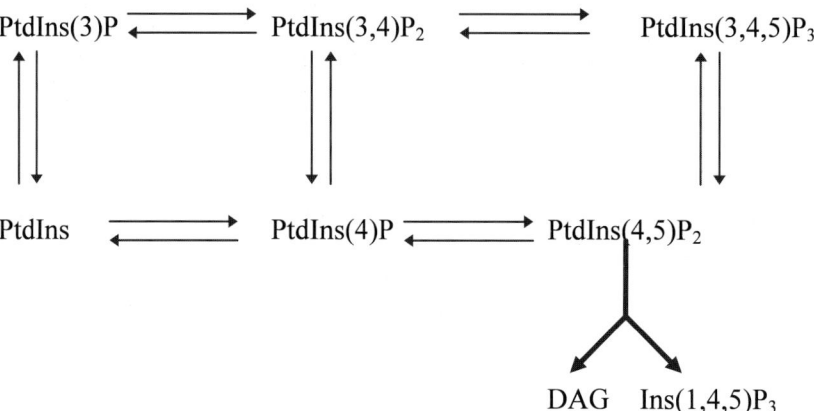

Figure 1. **Inositol lipid metabolism**. *The known inositol lipids are illustrated, together with interconversions that have been documented in vitro (not all of them have been demonstrated in vivo). In bold are reactions believed to be rate limiting or receptor controlled: the 3-phosphorylation of PtdIns, the 3-phosphorylation of PtdIns(4,5)P_2, and the hydrolysis of PtdIns(4,5)P_2 by PIC (modified from ref. (11)).*

Activation of PIC takes place in many cells as a result of receptor occupancy. Several PIC isozymes have been recognized: they vary in molecular weight, amino acid sequence and mode of regulation (12,13). In spermatozoa, PIC has been partially characterized (14-16), but the identity of the isozymes has not been reported.

Recent work has revealed that stimulation of capacitated spermatozoa with a variety of agonists leads to hydrolysis of PIs. Using the mouse as a model system, it has been found that stimulation with either ZP or progesterone results in hydrolsis of both PtdIns(4)P and PtdIns(4,5)P_2, and the concomitant generation of DAG (17) (Fig.2). In capacitated human spermatozoa, a follicular fluid fraction (whose activity relates to its progesterone content) is capable of inducing hydrolysis of both PtdIns(4)P and PtdIns(4,5)P_2 (18); however, there is no information as to whether ZP would cause similar hydrolysis in this species. It could be predicted that it would, essentially because (a) this seems to be a generalized phenomenon in spermatozoa of several species in response to natural agonists (including sea-urchin, (19)), and (b) it is likely that crucial events in the sequence leading to fusion are shared by a variety of taxa.

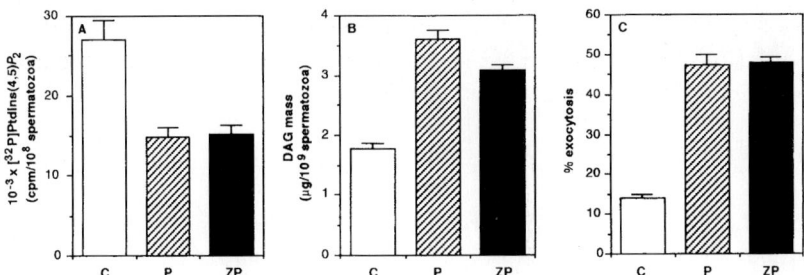

Figure 2. **Lipid changes and exocytosis in spermatozoa stimulated with progesterone or zona pellucida.** *A, levels of PtdIns(4,5)P$_2$ 5 min after stimulation with 15 µM progesterone (P), 1 zona pellucida (ZP)/µl, or in control (C) samples. B, changes in DAG 2.5 min after stimulation. C, exocytosis (as revealed by the presence of an 'AR' pattern after chlortetracycline staining), 15 min after stimulation (modified from ref. (17)).*

An important interaction between progesterone and ZP has also been unveiled (17), which sheds light on the relationship between different components of the egg's coats in the initiation of exocytosis. It has been found that progesterone is capable of priming the sperm cell for the subsequent action of ZP. This is seen not only in the number of cells that exhibit exocytosis (i.e. that complete membrane fusion), but it is also evident in the generation of the key messenger DAG and the hydrolysis of two of its sources, PtdIns(4)P and PtdIns(4,5)P_2 (Fig. 3). These findings suggest that the concentrations of agonists needed to initiate exocytosis may be lower than previously thought. They also indicate that a sequential exposure of the spermatozoon to these agonists (as it traverses the egg coats) would maximize activation of transduction mechanisms and generation of second messengers. This may be important for events taking place late in the sequence leading to membrane fusion as, for instance, they require high intracellular Ca^{2+} to be activated (8,20,21).

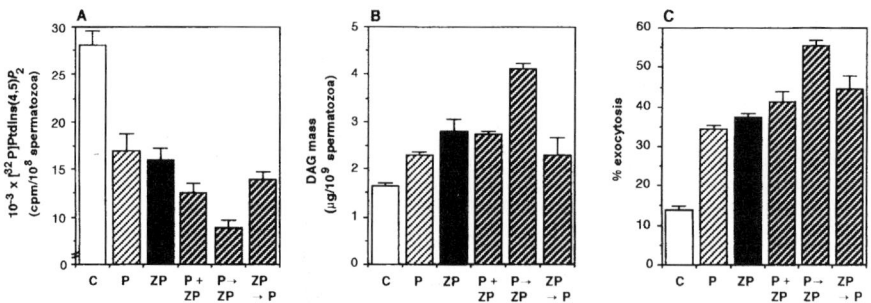

Figure 3. **The sequential exposure to progesterone and zona pellucida results in maximal hydrolysis of PtdIns(4,5)P$_2$, generation of DAG, and exocytosis in mouse spermatozoa**. *A, levels of PtdIns(4,5)P$_2$ 5 min after no stimulation (C), stimulation with 2.5 µM progesterone (P) and/or 0.5 zona pellucida (ZP)/µl, after stimulation for 3 min with P followed by ZP during 2 min, or the latter sequence in reverse order (i.e. 3 min ZP plus addition of P during the last 2 min). B, levels of DAG 5 min after spermatozoa were treated as described for the preceding panel. C, exocytosis (% of 'AR' pattern after staining with chlortetracycline) after spermatozoa were simulated with P, ZP or both for 15 min, or they were exposed first to P or ZP for 3 min and were then exposed to the other agonist for the rest of the incubation period (total 15 min) (modified from ref. (17)).*

Recent work has shown that another agonist, epidermal growth factor (EGF), is also capable of inducing PI hydrolysis and DAG formation (and exocytosis) in capacitated mouse spermatozoa (4) (Fig. 4). An EGF receptor has been identified in spermatozoa from various species including man (22, 23), and it has been shown that stimulation with EGF leads to receptor tyrosine phosphorylation (22). In addition, PI hydrolysis, DAG generation, and exocytosis elicited by EGF do not take place if cells are pre-exposed to protein tyrosine kinase (PTK) inhibitors (4).

These results strongly indicate that EGF has a role in the initiation of exocytosis; however, it is not clear what is the relationship between its action and that of ZP. It is evident that EGF is acting via its own receptor, rather than on a ZP receptor; this conclusion comes not only from the identification of an EGF receptor on spermatozoa, but also from experiments demonstrating that ZP could stimulate exocytosis above the levels seen when EGF was used at maximal concentrations (4). It appears that EGF would act as a co-factor during fertilization and, thus, its role in the initiation of exocytosis deserves futher attention.

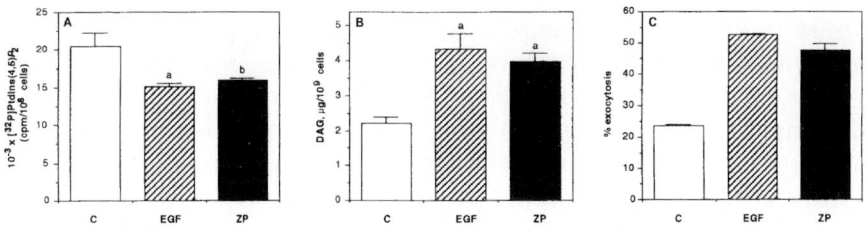

Figure 4. **Lipid changes and exocytosis in mouse spermatozoa stimulated with EGF.** A, levels of PtdIns(4,5)P$_2$ 5 min after stimulation with 100 ng EGF/ml, 1 zona pellucida (ZP)/μl, or in control (C) samples. B, changes in DAG 2.5 min after similar stimulations. C, exocytosis (% 'AR' pattern after chlortetracycline staining), 15 min after stimulation (modified from ref. (4)).

REGULATION OF PIC ACTIVATION AND PI HYDROLYSIS

Based on deduced amino acid sequences, PICs have been classified into 3 families (or types): PIC-b, PIC-g, and PIC-d (12). Each type contains more than one subtype (designated by adding Arabic numbers after the Greek letters; e.g. PIC-b1, PIC-b2). A classification based on enzyme purification and biochemical characterization has also been presented (13).

Regulation of PIC (and, hence, hydrolysis of PIs) is under the control of several transducing mechanisms. Importantly, different types of PIC isozymes are regulated by distinct mechanisms (9, 12, 3). One mechanism of PIC activation is phosphorylation by PTK, and the isozymes regulated in this way are the PIC-gs. Another mechanism is modulation by the a subunit of heterotrimeric GTP-binding proteins (G-proteins), with PIC-b being the target isozyme. This pathway is pertussis toxin-insensitive (24). There is, in addition, a pertussis toxin-sensitive pathway which employs G_i or G_o proteins and PIC enzymes other than b or g (24). The mechanism of PIC-d activation has not yet been identified. Another important regulator of PIC that has been recognized for a long time is Ca^{2+}, and yet there is little information regarding which isoforms are regulated by this cation (13). There is no clear evidence in somatic cells as to whether an elevation of intracellular Ca^{2+} is sufficient for activation of PIC. Nevertheless, hydrolysis of PIs occurs in some cells *after* influx of Ca^{2+} from the extracellular space, which suggests that elevation of intracellular Ca^{2+} is necessary for PIC activation in these cell systems (25).

There is still no account in the literature as to which PIC isozymes are involved in PI hydrolysis in spermatozoa. There is, however, some indirect information on possible early transducing pathways that could be involved in PIC activation and PI hydrolysis. This information relates to whether agonist-stimulated exocytosis is blocked by G-protein- or PTK-inhibitors, and whether these reagents are able to inhibit the relevant transducing processes, i.e. ADP-ribosylation of G_i proteins, or phosphorylation of putative PTK substrates (e.g. p95). Thus, it is possible to speculate on potential mechanisms activating this enzyme.

Hydrolysis of PIs by PIC-γ could take place after stimulation with ZP, progesterone, or EGF. This is supported by the observation that these agonists elicit activation of sperm PTK (22,26,27), and that exocytosis induced by these agonists is blocked by PTK inhibitors (4,28,29). On the other hand, ZP-induced exocytosis is inhibited by pertussis toxin (30,31) which may suggest the existent of a PIC other than b or g. However, it is also possible that pertussis toxin-sensitive G-proteins may modulate other aspects of sperm function such as Ca^{2+} influx (31,32) or even PTK activation (33). Neither progesterone-, nor EGF-stimulated exocytosis are inhibited by pertussis toxin (4,34), which would suggest either the presence of PIC-b or, simply, that these agonists only activate a PIC-g pathway. Further studies are needed to clarify these issues.

There is abundant information to suggest that Ca^{2+} may be a major regulator of PIC in spermatozoa. Whether the isozyme involved is PIC-d, or a novel type of Ca^{2+}-regulated PIC, is not known and would have to be resolved experimentally in future investigations. Evidence indicating the importance of Ca^{2+} in the regulation of PIC can be summarized as follows. Early studies on events underlying acrosomal exocytosis revealed that treatment with the divalent cation ionophore A23187 in the presence of Ca^{2+} caused a rapid and substantial hydrolysis of $PtdIns(4)P$ and $PtdIns(4,5)P_2$ (8). This phenomenon was identified in several mammalian species (including man) after stimulation with A23187/Ca^{2+} (Fig. 5) (8). Likewise, stimulation of sea-urchin sperm with the calcium ionophore ionomycin caused hydrolysis of both $PtdIns(4)P$ and $PtdIns(4,5)P_2$ (19). Hydrolysis of both PIs takes place in response to A23187 even if low Ca^{2+} is present in the extracellular milieu (~20 μM), but it does not occur if extracellular Ca^{2+} is chelated with EGTA (8). This led to the suggestion that Ca^{2+} influx was necessary for activation of PIC (35), a proposal that has now received considerable support.

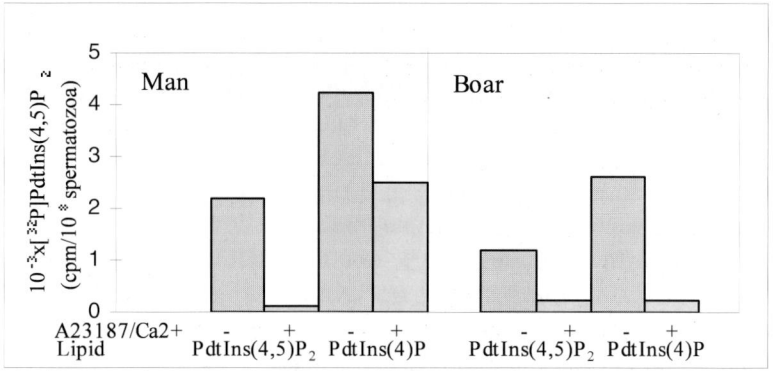

Figure 5. **Changes in PtdIns(4,5)P_2 and PtdIns(4)P in spermatozoa of different species stimulated with A23187 and Ca^{2+}.** *Spermatozoa from man, boar, mouse and ram were stimulated with 1 µM A23187 (10 µM for human sperm) and 3 mM Ca^{2+} for 5 min. Values given are means; standard deviations were never higher than 10-20% of the mean values (modified from ref. (8)).*

Using natural agonists of acrosomal exocytosis, it has been found that stimulation of spermatozoa under conditions that prevent Ca^{2+} entry does not result in PtdIns(4)P and PtdIns(4,5)P_2 breakdown. Thus, treatment with ZP in the absence of extracellular Ca^{2+} (i.e. no Ca^{2+} available for influx), or with extracellular Ca^{2+} available, but in the presence of a Ca^{2+} channel blocker, did not result in hydrolysis of PIs (17, 36). Similarly, treatment with progesterone, either with no extracellular Ca^{2+}, or in the presence of a Ca^{2+} channel blocker, did not lead to PI hydrolysis (18). Similar observations were made using sea-urchin spermatozoa, where it was found that PI hydrolysis stimulated by a fucose-sulphate glycoconjugate was prevented if the Ca^{2+} channel antagonist verapamil was included (19).

Although this appears to be solid evidence in favour of channel mediated Ca^{2+} entry, and an ensuing Ca^{2+}-regulated PIC activation, it could be argued that the elevation of intracellular Ca^{2+} could be modulated in another way. Since pertussis toxin and PTK inhibitors prevent ZP-induced Ca^{2+} influx (31, 32), it could be speculated that activation of PIC by G-proteins and/or tyrosine phosphorylation may be necessary for the generation of inositol phosphates, mobilization of Ca^{2+} from internal stores, and store-regulated ("capacitative") Ca^{2+} influx. This argument, however, cannot be reconciled with the observation that PI hydrolysis takes place only after Ca^{2+} entry. On the other hand, the observation that Ca^{2+} influx is prevented by G-protein and/or PTK inhibitors could be explained by arguing that there could be a link between these transducing mechanisms and mechanisms leading to Ca^{2+} channel opening. In this context, knowledge from other cell systems may help to recognize potential regulatory processes that may exist in spermatozoa. In particular, since both ZP and progesterone elicit PTK activity, a parallel with processes stimulated by growth factors (whose receptors have intrinsic PTK activity) could be illustrative. For instance, it has been found that EGF can provoke a rapid Ca^{2+} influx in human epidermoid carcinoma A431 cells (a widely used system because it expresses 10-100 times more EGF receptors on their surface than most other cells), and that this is prevented by Ca^{2+} channel blockers such as La^{3+} (37). This influx is independent from release of Ca^{2+} from intracellular stores (37). It has been postulated that the mechanism underlying EGF-stimulated Ca^{2+} entry is related to activation of pathways leading to leukotriene C_4 formation and Ca^{2+} channel opening (38). Thus, there seems to be a direct link between a receptor with PTK activity and Ca^{2+} entry via channels (interestingly, PTK activity may not necessarily be that of the EGF receptor (39)). Thus, it is possible that, in spermatozoa, activation of PTK may eventually result in Ca^{2+} channel opening before (or in the absence of) mobilization from stores. It is noteworthy that progesterone stimulation of PTK activity in human sperm takes place in the absence of extracellular Ca^{2+} (with EGTA included) (29), which would be in agreement with the proposal that PTK activation / channel opening precedes Ca^{2+} entry. Unfortunately, it has not been reported whether ZP-stimulated PTK activity would take place in the absence of Ca^{2+}; this would obviously help to clarify mechanisms of Ca^{2+} entry operating in the sperm cell.

    The situation with regards to G-protein involvement in Ca^{2+} entry is less clear. Although G-protein inhibitors would block Ca^{2+} influx elicited by ZP (31, 32), they do not prevent Ca^{2+} influx stimulated by progesterone (34). It is known that G-proteins may modulate events activated by tyrosine phosphorylation (33, 38), but how (or whether) this interaction takes place in spermatozoa is not known. Nevertheless, it seems that both G-proteins and PTK appear to be necessary for early events in acrosomal exocytosis, although neither may be sufficient to drive the cell to the final stage of membrane fusion. Obviously a great deal of work will be necessary to clarify these aspects of signal transduction in spermatozoa.

RELEVANCE OF PI HYDROLYSIS FOR EXOCYTOSIS

Hydrolysis of PIs has been implicated in a variety of cell functions, and it is considered to be an important source of messengers during exocytosis. It is therefore pertinent to consider whether PI hydrolysis plays a role in acrosomal exocytosis. Work carried out using a model system in which exocytosis is triggered with the ionophore A23187 has revealed that there is a tight link between occurrence of PI hydrolysis and exocytosis, i.e. conditions that lead to exocytosis also result in hydrolysis of PtdIns(4)P and PtdIns(4,5)P_2, whereas inhibition of PI breakdown is accompanied by lack of exocytosis (8). The best example corresponds to experiments in which it was found that neomycin, an aminoglycoside antibiotic that binds to the PIs, prevented A23187-induced hydrolysis of PtdIns(4)P and PtdIns(4,5)P_2 and, in parallel experiments, inhibited acrosomal exocytosis. The effect appeared to be specific because addition of neomycin once hydrolysis of PIs was completed (but before initiation of other downstream events) did not block exocytosis. Moreover, blockade by neomycin was reversed by addition of exogenous DAG, a product of PI breakdown, which indicated that the antibiotic was not affecting downstream events (40). Evidence using natural agonists is lacking and it would therefore be highly desirable to examine whether neomycin, or other reagents such as the PIC inhibitor U73122 would block ZP- or progesterone-induced hydrolysis of PIs and exocytosis.

ROLE OF PI BREAKDOWN IN THE SEQUENCE LEADING TO MEMBRANE FUSION

Generation and role of inositol phosphates

Hydrolysis of PI leads to the generation of inositol phosphates. In many cells, the latter have clear second messenger roles in the modulation of intracellular Ca^{2+} levels (9). Although stimulation of spermatozoa to undergo exocytosis results in generation of inositol phosphates, their role is less apparent because its formation takes place after an elevation of intracellular Ca^{2+} due to influx from the extracellular space. All the work carried out so far suggests that the inositol phosphates have no apparent role in events leading to acrosomal exocytosis.

In ram spermatozoa, stimulation with A23187 leads to Ins(1,4,5)P_3 generation which, obviously, takes place after Ca^{2+} entry (41). It could be argued that this is not a valid example, were it not for the fact that when sperm cells are stimulated with natural agonists, inositol phosphates are also generated after Ca^{2+} entry. Thus, in progesterone-stimulated human sperm,

La^{3+} (a Ca^{2+} channel blocker) prevents generation of Ins(1,4,5)P_3 (18). Similarly, in sea urchin sperm, the generation of Ins(1,4,5)P_3 seen after stimulation with a fucose-sulphate glycoconjugate is prevented if the Ca^{2+} channel blocker verapamil is also included (42). A similar situation can be inferred from experiments in which mouse sperm cells were stimulated with ZP; although Ins(1,4,5)P_3 was not quantified directly, measurements of DAG levels (the product of PI hydrolysis that is generated in parallel to Ins(1,4,5)P_3) revealed that inclusion of the Ca^{2+} channel blocker La^{3+} reduced the ability of ZP to induce DAG formation (and by inference Ins(1,4,5)P_3 formation) (17). One can therefore conclude that it is highly unlikely that inositol phosphates have a role in events leading to membrane fusion during exocytosis.

Generation of DAG

The other product of PI hydrolysis is DAG. Stimulation of spermatozoa with a variety of agonists led to a substantial formation of DAG: treatment with ZP, progesterone or EGF resulted in high levels of DAG in mouse spermatozoa (4, 17), whereas stimulation of human spermatozoa with progesterone also led to DAG formation (43). A considerable generation of DAG was also noted after A23187 in spermatozoa from man (43) and other species (mouse: (17); ram: (40); boar: (36)).

The mass of PIs in the sperm membranes is small and the amount of DAG generated after sperm stimulation is greater that the one potentially deriving from PI hydrolysis. It is thus important to note that DAG could be generated by mechanisms other than PI hydrolysis. DAG can also be generated by hydrolysis of phosphatidylcholine (PtdCho) via two pathways (Fig. 6): (a) activation of phospholipase C (PLC) or (b) the sequential action of phospholipase D (PLD) and phosphatidate phosphohydrolase (44).

This latter pathway appears to be the main mechanism for DAG generation in various somatic cells (44), and in sea urchin spermatozoa (45). However, several lines of evidence indicate that it is not important for DAG generation in mammalian spermatozoa. Work carried out using the ram sperm model revealed that there was no significant activation of PLD after Ca^{2+} entry and that there were no links between this little PLD activity and exocytosis (46). In mouse spermatozoa, treatment of capacitated cells with ZP or progesterone resulted in no activation of PLD (17). In addition, human sperm stimulated with either progesterone or A23187 revealed no PLD activation (43).

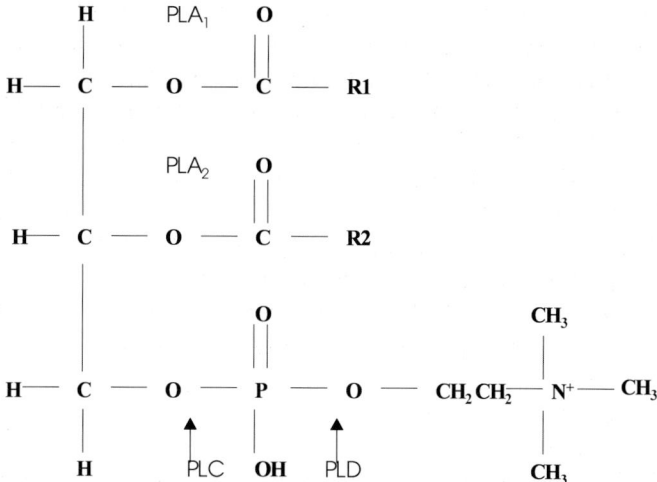

Figure 6. **Hydrolysis of phosphatidylcholine.** *Schematic structure of phosphatidylcholine with sites of cleavage by phospholipases C, D, A1 and A2. R1 and R2 are hydrocarbon chains of long chain fatty acids.*

On the other hand, evidence for PLC as a major mechanism for DAG formation has been obtained in studies using ram, mouse and human spermatozoa. Incubation with phospholipid precursors that resulted in no labelling of the PIs has revealed that stimulation with A23187 or natural agonists such as progesterone or ZP led to a considerable formation of DAG (and little phosphatidate) (17,47,48). PtdCho is the major substrate for PLC (47,48), and this enzyme can use both diacyl- and alkyl-acyl-PtdCho as a source of diglycerides (17,47,48). Activation of PLC seems to require low levels of Ca^{2+} (similar to what was observed with PIC) because stimulation of ram sperm with A23187 in the absence of added Ca^{2+} (~20 µM extracellular Ca^{2+}) resulted in levels of DAG similar to those seen with millimolar Ca^{2+}. However, the cation is clearly necessary for PLC activation, because inclusion of EGTA abolished the response (47). A preliminary characterization of bull and rabbit PLC has been presented (16).

The question that arises is whether the DAG generated by PI hydrolysis modulates other mechanisms of DAG formation and, furthermore, whethe there are other potential messenger roles for this metabolite.

Role(s) of DAG
In many cells the main role of DAG is to activate protein kinase C. In spermatozoa, there is abundant evidence to indicate that DAG exerts messenger roles independently of kinase C activation. So far, there is some circumstantial evidence to suggest that the DAG / protein kinase C pathway could be involved in events underlying exocytosis (49). However, direct

evidence of substrate phosphorylation as a result of activation of this pathway has yet to be presented.

Studies using the model in which ram spermatozoa are stimulated with A23187/Ca^{2+} have revealed that DAG participates in the modulation of two events after Ca^{2+} entry. One event modulated by this messenger is activation of PtdCho-PLC. This stems from the following observations: First, inhibition of PI breakdown by inclusion of neomycin (8) or Mg^{2+} (47) decreases the mass of DAG generated after stimulation (the latter reflects mainly PtdCho-PLC activity (47)). Second, pretreatment of spermatozoa with exogenous DAGs results in higher values of DAG upon stimulation with A23187/Ca^{2+}. This effect is clearly not mediated via protein kinase C because both the 1,2- and the 1,3-isomers of DAG were able to stimulate PtdCho-PLC activity (47) (only 1,2-DAG can stimulate kinase C).

Further studies with this model system revealed that DAG has another important messenger role as modulator of phospholipase A_2 (PLA_2), an enzyme with a key role in the generation of metabolites important for membrane fusion (20). It has been found that the activation of PLA_2 which takes place after Ca^{2+} entry (20) is stimulated if the endogenous levels of DAG are increased, either by inhibition of its catabolism, or by addition of exogenous permeable DAGs (50). Similarly to what was observed with PtdCho-PLC, both 1,2- and 1,3-DAG would stimulate PLA_2 activity, which indicates that DAG action is not mediated via protein kinase C (50).

Finally, it is possible that DAG has other messenger roles in spermatozoa, and work to be carried out in the future would certainly have to address this question.

OTHER ROLES FOR PIS DURING EXOCYTOSIS

Recent investigations in other systems have revealed that PIs may have other roles in cell function. Although no evidence exists, so far, to indicate that PIs have other roles in sperm function, it is important to summarize them briefly here.

One important aspect of PI metabolism which is being unveiled at present is the signalling system involving 3-phosphorylated inositol lipids (see Fig. 1). Although it is not known what the physiological functions of 3-phosphorylated lipids are, there has been considerable advance in the characterization of their metabolism (10,11). The principal route for PtdIns(3,4,5)P_3 synthesis is by 3-phosphorylation of PtdIns(4,5)P_2 by a PI3-kinase. This takes place in response to various agonists and involves regulation by either G-proteins or PTK and, perhaps, ras. In addition, 3-phosphorylation of PtdIns by a PtdIns-specific 3-kinase has been documented. It is thought that PtdIns(3,4,5)P_3 (and perhaps other related PIs) may act as a second messenger; PtdIns(3,4,5)P_3, in particular, has been implicated in membrane ruffling, superoxide generation in neutrophils and glucose transport control in adipocytes (11).

Another system in which PtdIns(4,5)P_2 appears to be involved is that related to the cytoskeleton, which is probably a separate issue entirely from that related to inositides in the plasma membrane. Tight binding of polyPIs and proteins has been known for some time, and it may involve a wide range of components of the cytoskeleton (51). The most studied interactions are those of PtdIns(4,5)P_2 with gelsolin and with profilin (11).

CONCLUSIONS

It is now clear that the PIs play a central role during exocytosis in mammalian spermatozoa. Stimulation of sperm cells with a variety of agonists leads to hydrolysis of both PtdIns(4)P and PtdIns(4,5)P_2. This PI breakdown is essential for subsequent exocytosis and serves mainly to generate messenger DAG. This metabolite has crucial roles in the activation of Ca^{2+}-dependent events which are instrumental in bringing about membrane fusion.

REFERENCES

1. Ward CR, Kopf GS. Molecular events mediating sperm activation. Dev Biol 1993; 158: 9-34.
2. Yanagimachi R. Mammalian fertilization. In: Knobil E, Neill JD, eds. The Physiology of Reproduction. New York: Raven Press, 1994: 189-317.
3. Meizel S, Pillai MC, Diaz-Perez E, Thomas P. Initiation of the human sperm acrosome reaction by components of human follicular fluid and cumulus secretions including steroids. In: Bavister BD, Cummins J, Roldan ERS, eds. Fertilization in Mammals. Norwell, MA: Serono Symposia, 1990: 205-22.
4. Murase T, Roldan ERS. Epidermal growth factor stimulates hydrolysis of phosphatidylinositol 4,5-bisphosphate, generation of diacylglycerol and exocytosis in mouse spermatozoa. FEBS Lett 1995; 360: 242-46.
5. Nikolopoulou M, Soucek DA, Vary JC. Changes in the lipid content of boar sperm plasma membranes during epididymal maturation. Biochim Biophys Acta 1985; 815: 486-98.

6. Parks JE, Arion JW, Foote RH. Lipids of plasma membrane and outer acrosomal membrane from bovine spermatozoa. Biol Reprod 1987; 37: 1249-58.
7. Berruti G, Franchi M. Calcium and polyphosphoinositides: their distribution in relation to the membrane changes occurring in the head of boar spermatozoa. Eur J Cell Biol 1986; 41: 238-45.
8. Roldan ERS, Harrison RAP. Polyphosphoinositide breakdown and subsequent exocytosis in the Ca^{2+}/ionophore-induced acrosome reaction of mammalian spermatozoa. Biochem J 1989; 259: 397-406.
9. Berridge MJ. Inositol trisphosphate and calcium signalling. Nature 1993; 361: 315-25.
10. Stephens LR, Jackson TR, Hawkins PT. Agonist-stimulated synthesis of phosphatidylinositol (3,4,5)-trisphosphate: a new intacelullar signaling system? Biochim Biophys Acta 1993; 1179: 27-75.
11. Divecha N, Irvine RF. Phospholipid signalling. Cell 1995; 80: 269-78.
12. Rhee SG, Choi KD. Multiple forms of phospholipase C isozymes and their activation mechanisms. Adv Second Messenger Phosphoprot Res 1992; 26: 35-61.
13. Cockcroft S, Thomas GMH. Inositol-lipid-specific phospholipase C isoenzymes and their differential regulation by receptors. Biochem J 1992; 288: 1-14.
14. Ribbes H, Plantavid M, Bennet PJ, Chap H, Douste-Blazy L. Phospholipase C from human sperm specific for phosphoinositides. Biochim Biophys Acta 1987; 919: 245-54.
15. Vanha-Perttula T, Kasurinen J. Purification and characterization of phosphatidylinositol-specific phospholipase C from bovine spermatozoa. Int J Biochem 1989; 21: 997-1007.
16. Hinkovska-Galchev V, Srivastava PN. Phosphatidylcholine and phosphatidylinositol-specific phospholipases C of bull and rabbit spermatozoa. Mol Reprod Dev 1992; 33: 281-86.
17. Roldan ER, Murase T, Shi QX. Exocytosis in spermatozoa in response to progesterone and zona pellucida. Science 1994; 266: 1578-81.
18. Thomas P, Meizel S. Phosphatidylinositol 4,5-bisphosphate hydrolysis in human sperm stimulated with follicular fluid or progesterone is dependent upon Ca^{2+} influx. Biochem J 1989; 264: 539-46.
19. Domino SE, Garbers DL. Stimulation of phospholipid turnover in isolated sea urchin sperm heads by the fucose-sulfate glycoconjugate that induces an acrosome reaction. Biol Reprod 1989; 40: 133-41.
20. Roldan ERS, Fragio C. Phospholipase A_2 activation and subsequent exocytosis in the Ca^{2+}/ionophore-induced acrosome reaction of ram spermatozoa. J Biol Chem 1993; 268: 13962-70.

21. Roldan ERS, Fragio C. Phospholipase A_2 activity and exocytosis of the ram sperm acrosome: regulation by bivalent cations. Biochim Biophys Acta 1993; 1168: 108-14.
22. Naz RK, Ahmad K. Presence of expression products of c-erbB-1 and c-erbB-2/HER2 genes on mammalian sperm cell, and effects of their regulation on fertilization. J Reprod Immunol 1992; 21: 223-39.
23. Lax Y, Rubinstein S, Breitbart H. Epidermal growth factor induces acrosomal exocytosis in bovine sperm. FEBS Lett 1994; 339: 234-38.
24. Martin TFJ. Receptor regulation of phosphoinositidase C. In: Taylor CW, ed. Intracellular Messengers. Oxford: Pergamon Press, 1993: 63-87.
25. Eberhard DA, Holz RW. Intracellular Ca^{2+} activates phospholipase C. Trends Neurosci 1989; 11: 517-20.
26. Leyton L, Saling PM. 95kD sperm proteins bind ZP3 and serve as tyrosine kinase substrates in response to zona binding. Cell 1989; 57: 1123-30.
27. Naz RK, Ahmad K, Kumar R. Role of membrane phosphotyrosine proteins in human spermatozoal function. J Cell Sci 1991; 99: 157-65.
28. Leyton L, LeGuen P, Bunch D, Saling PM. Regulation of mouse gamete interaction by a sperm tyrosine kinase. Proc Natl Acad Sci USA 1992; 89: 11692-95.
29. Tesarik J, Moos J, Mendoza C. Stimulation of protein tyrosine phosphorylation by a progesterone receptor on the cell surface of human sperm. Endocrinology 1993; 133: 328-35.
30. Endo Y, Lee MA, Kopf GS. Evidence for the role of a guanine nucleotide-binding regulatory protein in the zona pellucida-induced mouse sperm acrosome reaction. Dev Biol. 1987; 119: 210-16.
31. Florman HM, Tombes RM, First NL, Babcock DF. An adhesion-associated agonist from the zona pellucida activates G protein-promoted elevations of internal Ca^{2+} and pH that mediate mammalian sperm acrosomal exocytosis. Dev Biol 1989; 135: 133-46.
32. Bailey JL, Storey BT. Calcium influx into mouse spermatozoa activated by solubilized mouse zona pellucida, monitored with the calcium fluorescent indicator, Fluo-3. Inhibition of the influx by three inhibitors of the zona pellucida induced acrosome reaction: Tyrphostin A48, pertussis toxin, and 3-quinuclidinyl benzilate. Mol Reprod Dev 1994; 39: 297-308.
33. Yang L, Baffy G, Rhee SG, Manning D, Hansen CA, Williamson JR. Pertussis toxin-sensitive G_i involvement in epidermal growth factor-induced activation of phsopholipase C-γ in rat hepatocytes. J Biol Chem 1991; 266: 22451-58.

34. Tesarik J, Carreras A, Mendoza C. Differential sensitivity of progesterone- and zona pellucida-induced acosome reactions to pertussis toxin. Mol Reprod Dev 1993; 34: 183-89.
35. Roldan ERS, Harrison RAP. Molecular mechanisms leading to exocytosis during the sperm acrosome reaction. In: Bavister BD, Cummins J, Roldan ERS, eds. Fertilization in Mammals. Norwell, MA: Serono Symposia, 1990: 179-96.
36. Roldan ERS. unpublished results.
37. Moolenar WH, Defize LHK, de Laat SW. Calcium in the action of growth factors. CIBA Found Symp 1986; 122: 212-31.
38. Hudson PL, Pedersen WA, Saltsman WS, Liscovitch M, MacLaughlin DT, Donahoe PK, Blusztajn JK. Modulation by sphingolipids of calcium signals evoked by epidermal growth factor. J Biol Chem 1994; 269: 21885-90.
39. Filhol O, Chambaz EM, Gill GN, Cochet C. Epidermal growth factor stimulates a protein tyrosine kinase which is separable from the epidermal growth factor receptor. J Biol Chem 1993; 268: 26978-82.
40. Roldan ERS, Harrison RAP. The role of diacylglycerol in the exocytosis of the sperm acrosome. Biochem J 1992; 281: 767-73.
41. Harrison RAP, Roldan ERS, Lander DJ, Irvine RF. Ram spermatozoa produce inositol 1,4,5-trisphosphate but not inositol 1,3,4,5-tetrakisphosphate during the Ca^{2+}/ionophore-induced acrosome reaction. Cell Signalling 1990; 2: 277-84.
42. Domino SE, Garbers DL. The fucose-sulfate glycoconjugate that induces an acrosome reaction in spermatozoa stimulates inositol 1,4,5-trisphosphate accumulation. J Biol Chem 1988; 263: 690-95.
43. O'Toole CMB, Roldan ERS, Fraser LR. A role for diacylglycerol in human sperm acrosomal exocytosis. J Reprod Fert Abstr Ser 1994; 13: 8 (abstr 15).
44. Exton JH. Phosphatidylcholine breakdown and signal transduction. Biochim Biophys Acta 1994; 1212: 26-42.
45. Domino SE, Bocckino SB, Garbers DL. Activation of phospholipase D by the fucose-sulfate glycoconjugate that induces an acrosome reaction in spermatozoa. J Biol Chem 1989; 264: 9412-19.
46. Roldan ERS, Dawes EN. Phospholipase D and exocytosis of the ram sperm acrosome. Biochim Biophys Acta 1993; 1210: 48-54.
47. Roldan ERS, Murase T. Polyphosphoinositide-derived diacylglycerol stimulates the hydrolysis of phosphatidylcholine by phospholipase C during exocytosis of the ram sperm acrosome. J Biol Chem 1994; 269: 23583-89.
48. O'Toole CMB, Roldan ERS, Fraser LR. unpublished results.

49. Breitbart H, Lax J, Rotem R, Naor Z. Role of protein kinase C in the acrosome reaction of mammalian spermatozoa. Biochem J 1992; 281; 473-76.
50. Roldan ERS, Fragio C. Diradylglycerols stimulate phospholipase A_2 and subsequent exocytosis in ram spermatozoa. Biochem J 1994; 294: 225-32.
51. Jamney PA. Phosphoinositides and calcium as regulators of cellular actin assembly and disassembly. Ann Rev Physiol 1994; 56: 169-91.

Role of membrane tyrosine kinases in human sperm function

Rajesh K. Naz

Reproductive Immunology and Molecular Biology Laboratories, Department of Obstetrics and Gynecology, The Albert Einstein College of Medicine, New York 10461, USA

ABSTRACT

The role of membrane tyrosine phosphorylation and receptor tyrosine kinases was investigated in human sperm function especially during capacitation/acrosome reaction and sperm-zona pellucida binding. Sperm capacitation/acrosome reaction increases degree of tyrosine phosphorylation per sperm cell, the number of cells that were phosphorylated, and also induced subcellular site shift in phosphorylation pattern of sperm. During capacitation/acrosome reaction, 7-14 proteins belonging to four predominant molecular regions (190, 97, 43 and 29 kD) were phosphorylated/autophosphorylated. Two of these proteins of 95 and 51 kD were phosphorylated at tyrosine residues with enhanced phosphorylation after treatment with thymosin $\alpha 1$ (Tα1). Treatment with anti-FA-1 monoclonal antibody, that is specifically directed to a single sperm protein of 51 kD, reduced phosphorylation/autophosphorylation of all the relevant proteins including tyrosine phosphorylation of 95 kD as well as 51 kD protein. Many of the proteins that were phosphorylated/autophosphorylated during capacitation/acrosome reaction were also involved in human sperm-zona pellucida binding. Four sperm proteins of 95, 63, 51, and 14-18 kD that showed binding with the zona pellucida, three (95, 51 and 14-18 kD proteins) demonstrated the presence of phosphotyrosine residues, and one, the 51 kD protein, that was found out to be the well-characterized FA-1 antigen, also demonstrated autophosphorylating activity. These findings indicate that tyrosine *phosphorylation of sperm membrane proteins, especially of 95 kD and 51 kD (FA-1 antigen) proteins, has a definite role in human sperm capacitation/acrosome reaction and zona pellucida binding. The human sperm receptor(s) for zona pellucida, especially FA-1 antigen, also seems to fall in the category of receptor tyrosine kinase family. There may be a signal transduction pathway(s) operating during human sperm capacitation /acrosome reaction, and blocking phosphorylation of a single protein (e.g. FA-1 antigen of 51 kD) by a specific antibody or activation (e.g. unidentified Tα1 receptor) by Tα1 can affect phosphorylation/tyrosine phosphorylation of other relevant proteins by signal transduction pathway(s). These findings may find clinical applications in the specific diagnosis and treatment of male infertility and in immunocontraception.*

Le rôle fonctionnel des phosphorylations des tyrosines membranaires ainsi que celui des récepteurs de type tyrosine kinase des spermatozoïdes ont été étudiés au cours de la capacitation/ réaction acrosomique et l'interaction gamétique. La capacitation / réaction acrosomique du sperme augmente le degré de phosphorylation des tyrosines par spermatozoïde, le nombre de cellules qui ont été phosphorylées et également entraine des modifications qualitatives dans le profil des phosphorylations intra-cellulaires. Durant la capacitation/ réaction acrosomique, 7- 14 protéines appartenant à quatre régions moléculaires prédominantes (190, 97, 43 et 29 kD) sont phosphorylées/ autophosphorylées. Deux de ces protéines de 95 et 51 kD sont phosphorylées sur des résidus tyrosine avec une augmentation des phosphorylations aprés traitement à la tymosine α1 (Tα1). Un traitement avec l'anticorps monoclonal anti-FA1, qui reconnaît spécifiquement une protéine spermatique de 51 kD, réduit les phosphorylations/ autophosphorylations de toutes les protéines concernées incluant la phosphorylation des protéines de 95 et 51 kD. De nombreuses protéines ayant été phosphorylées/ autophosphorylées pendant la capacitation/ réaction acrosomique sont également impliquées dans la liaison spermatozoide/ zone pellucide. Quatre protéines spermatiques de 95, 63, 51 et 14-18 kD intervenant dans la liaison avec la zone pellucide, trois protéines spermatiques (95, 51 et 14-18 kD) ayant montré la présence de résidus phosphotyrosines et 1 protéine de 51kD caractérisée comme étant l'antigène FA1, ont toutes montré une activité d'autophosphorylation. Ces résultats indiquent que la phosphorylation des tyrosines des protéines spermatiques membranaires et spécialement des protéines de 95 et 51 (FA1) kD a un rôle précis dans la capacitation / réaction acrosomique et la liaison avec la zone pellucide. Le(s) récepteur(s) spermatique(s) de la zone pellucide et spécialement l'antigène FA1 semble(nt) également appartenir à la famille des récepteurs de type tyrosine kinase. Il pourrait y avoir une voie de transduction du signal activée au cours de la capacitation/ réaction acrosomique et le blocage de la phosphorylation d'une seule protéine (antigène FA1 de 51 kD) par un anticorps spécifique ou l'activation par Tα1 (récepteur Tα1 non identifié) pourrait affecter la phosphorylation/tyrosine phosphorylation des autres protéines importantes. Ces résultats pourraient trouver des applications cliniques dans le diagnostic et le traitement de l'infertilité masculine ainsi que dans la contraception vaccinale.

INTRODUCTION

Since the initial discovery of phosphorylase kinase catalyzing transfer of phosphate from ATP to glycogen phosphorylase by Fischer and Krebs (1), protein phosphorylation, especially at the tyrosine residues, has been shown to have a definite role in the regulation of function of various receptors (2). Protein phosphorylation is the most prevalent form of post-translational modification in metozoan cell and along with allosteric modulation, it is recognized as a universal mechanism for regulating function of proteins involved in many biological processes. The receptors for several growth factors are themselves tyrosine protein kinases that are activated by ligand binding (2). Protein tyrosine kinases regulate cell proliferation and differentiation, and the tyrosine phosphorylation may be the primary, or even the exclusive, indication of signal transduction. The receptor tyrosine kinases participate in transmembrane signaling, whereas the intracellular tyrosine kinases take part in signal transduction within the cell including signal to nucleus (3). All the receptor tyrosine kinases posses a large glycosylated extracellular ligand binding domain, a single hydrophobic transmembrane region, and a cytoplasmic domain that contains tyrosine kinase catalytic domain (2-4). The tyrosine kinase catalytic domain is the most conserved portion and among other highly conserved sequences of unknown function, it contains a consensus sequence, GlyXGlyXXGlyX (15-20) Lys, that functions as a part of the binding site for ATP.

Based upon the above studies carried out mostly in somatic/cancer cell lines, our laboratory investigated the role of tyrosine phosphorylation in sperm function. The aim of the present article is to review our findings on the role of membrane tyrosine phosphorylation and receptor tyrosine kinases in human sperm function especially in capacitation and/or acrosome reaction, and in binding with zona pellucida of the oocyte.

ROLE OF MEMBRANE TYROSINE PHOSPHORYLATION/YROSINE KINASES IN HUMAN SPERM CAPACITATION/ACROSOME REACTION

The molecules and mechanisms involved in signal transduction pathways leading to sperm capacitation and exocytosis are not clearly understood (5). In contrast to mouse sperm that presumably undergo acrosome reaction on the zona pellucida (ZP) surface, the sperm of other mammalian species including human can be induced to acrosome reach in response to various stimuli besides ZP proteins.

Thymosin α1 (Tα1) a synthetic 28 amino acid peptide (3.108 kD) of thymic origin increases (upto 2.6 fold) the human sperm capacitation and the acrosome reaction (6). Also, the monoclonal antibody (mab) to the well-characterized human sperm membrane glycoprotein of 51 kD, designated fertilization antigen-1 (FA-1), completely blocks the human sperm capacitation and the acrosome reaction (7-9). Our laboratory conducted a study to investigate the role of tyrosine phosphorylation/tyrosine kinases in human sperm capacitation/acrosome reaction and the modulation by these two molecules, namely Tα1 and anti-FA-1 monoclonal antibody (mab). This was examined using *in vitro* ^{32}P metabolic labeling experiment, *in vitro* kinase assay, Western blot procedure and immunofluoresence assay (10, 11). The tyrosine phosphorylation was determined using anti-phosphotyrosine monoclonal antibody (PTA) (PY20) that specifically reacts with phosphotyrosine containing proteins and does not react with phosphoserine and phorphothreoine residues. Results of metabolic labeling indicated ^{32}P incorporation into at least 7 proteins (200, 112, 104, 48, 42, 31 and 25 kD) predominantly belonging to four molecular regions (190, 97, 43 and 29 kD). The treatment with Tα1 enhanced phosphorylation of all these proteins in a concentration-dependent manner, besides specifically phosphorylating two additional proteins (77, 72 kD). In *in vitro* kinase assay, 14 proteins (122, 105, 95, 89, 73, 62, 48, 46 40, 33, 30, 28, 25 and 22 kD), belonging to similar four regions, were autophosphorylated and treatment with Tα1 enhanced phosphorylation in all these proteins in a concentration-dependent manner. Of the 7-14 proteins belonging to the four predominant molecular regions (190, 97, 43 and 29 kD) that were phosphorylated/autophosphorylated, two predominant proteins namely 95 and 51 kD belonging to two of these molecular regions (97 and 43 kD) were phosphorylated at tyrosine residues with enhanced tyrosine phosphorylation after Tα1 treatment.

Tα1 induced stimulation only in membrane protein extracts of non-capacitated sperm and not of already capacitated sperm. These findings indicate that autophosphorylation of membrane proteins depends upon the physiological stage of the sperm cell, and the capacitation induces changes/modifications of membrane proteins that define the subsequent autophosphorylation characteristics of these proteins. To exercise an effect, Tα1 has to be present during capacitation when those changes/modifications are taking place, and once those changes/modifications have occurred, Tα1 is unable to further enhance phosphorylation/autophosphorylation of the relevant proteins.

The results of phosphorylation/autophosphorylation experiments agree with the findings in the zona-free hamster ova-human sperm penetration assay (SPA). As observed in phosphorylation/autophosphorylation experiments, Tα1 increased the penetration index in SPA in a concentration-dependent manner (6). SPA seems to be a measure of `capacitation' of human sperm (12) and these findings indicate that phosphorylation/ autophosphorylation has a vital role in capacitation of human sperm. These correlations among various assays may indirectly suggest the use of ^{32}P metabolic labeling assay and/or in vitro kinase assay for measuring the fertilizing capacity of human sperm as a diagnostic technique for evaluating sperm function in male-factor infertility.

The exact signal transduction pathway(s) involved in stimulation of phosphorylation and hence capacitation is not clear at the present time, because receptor for Tα1 binding has not been delineated as yet on sperm or in any other somatic/immune or non-immune cell/cancer cell line. It is possible that sperm cell membrane has a specific receptor for Tα1 that after activation by ligand binding subsequently phosphorylates other relevant membrane proteins by signal transduction pathway. Some of the important components required for signal transduction pathway such as p21 ras protein (13), cyclin/cdc^2 protein kinase (14) guanine nucleotide binding proteins (15) and c-Myc protein (16) have been shown to be present in human sperm cell. It is also possible that with or without binding with the yet-unidentified receptor, Tα1 per se activates a specific/nonspecific protein kinase, directly or indirectly, that subsequently phosphorylates the relevant sperm membrane proteins. Various protein kinases including protein kinase C have been shown to be present in human sperm cell (17). This hypothesis could explain the enhancement of autophosphorylation in in vitro kinase assay, but for enhancement of phosphorylation in ^{32}P metabolic labeling experiments either Tα1 has to be internalized into sperm cell or the reactive protein kinase has to be present in sperm membrane that is accessible for Tα1 action.

Treatment of human sperm with anti-FA-1 mAb reduced/blocked phosphorylation/ autophosphorylation of the relevant proteins predominantly belonging to the four molecular regions in ^{32}P metabolic labeling experiments and in in vitro kinase assay, and also reduced/blocked tyrosine phosphorylation of 95 kD as well as 51 kD proteins (10,11). These findings are intriguing in view of the fact that anti-FA-1 mAb specifically binds only to a single protein band of 51 ± 2 kD (corresponding to dimeric form of FA-1 antigen) on immunoblot involving human sperm membrane-solubilized proteins, and completely blocks human sperm penetration without affecting percent sperm motility in SPA (10,11). It was interesting to find that besides reducing/ blocking phosphorylation/ autophosphorylation/ tyrosine phosphorylation of 51 ± 2 kD protein, it also reduced/blocked phosphorylation of other proteins including tyrosine phosphorylation of 95 kD protein. These findings suggest that there may be a signal transduction pathway(s) operating during human sperm capacitation\acrosome reaction, and blocking phosphorylation of a single protein (e.g. FA-1 antigen) by a specific antibody or activation by ligand binding (e.g. Tα1 binding to unidentified Tα1 receptor) can affect phosphorylation/tyrosine phosphorylation of other relevant proteins by signal transduction pathway(s).

The proteins belonging to 95 kD region have recently drawn special attention. We have isolated a 95 kD protein, designated FA-2 antigen, from human sperm using a sperm-specific mAb (18), a 95 kD protein(s) is involved in human sperm-zona binding (discussed below), and a similar protein of 95 kD has been delineated in human sperm that shows increased tyrosine phosphorylation after homologous ZP exposure (10), and after treatment with progesterone (19), platelet aggregation factor (20) and Tα1 (10, 11). Also, other studies carried out using the mouse sperm have reported a similar 95 kD protein in the sperm membrane that has tyrosine kinase activity and autophosphorylates in response to homologous ZP exposure and after capacitation/acrosome reaction (21, 22). These studies indicate that 95 kD sperm membrane protein may be evolutionarily conserved across species (mouse and human), and in humans, 95 kD protein can be activated/tyrosine phosphorylated by various exogenous stimuli (including Tα1, PAF and progesterone) besides ZP.

Immunofluorescence results on fixed human sperm revealed that the capacitation and zona exposure increased the degree of tyrosine phosphorylation per sperm cell, and the number of sperm cells that were tyrosine phosphorylated, expecially in the acrosomal regions of the sperm head (10). Interestingly, with these changes, there was also a shift in the site of phosphotyrosine-specific fluorescence from the tail regions of non-capacitated sperm to the acrosomal regions of capacitated/zona-exposed sperm cells. These changes were enhanced by Tα1 and reduced/blocked by anti-FA-1 mab. Using other systems, there are reports indicating a shift in subcellular localization of various proteins after tyrosine phosphorylation. In human epidermoid carcinoma A431 cells, it has been shown the the binding of epidermal growth factor (EGF) to its receptor rapidly triggers redistribution of phospholipase C-r$_1$ from a predominantly cytosolic localization to the membrane- bound activity, followed by phosphorylation at tyrosine residues (23). Since acrosomal region of the sperm cell is involved in sperm-zona interaction, the shift in phosphotyrosine-specific fluorescence site seems to have a physiological significance. Indeed, incubation of sperm cells with PTA showed a drastic inhibition of human sperm binding and penetration in SPA (10). A role of phosphorylation in the regulation of the function of various potassium and calcium channels has been proposed (24). Since Ca^{2+} is required for capacitation/acrosome reaction of human sperm cells, the phosphorylation of tyrosine residues may regulate the fertilizing capacity of sperm through the modulation of Ca^{2+} (and/or possibly other ions) influx. It is also possible that some of the sperm surface proteins that are tyrosine phosphorylated during capacitation/acrosome reaction are also involved in zona pellucida binding, and serve as substrates for tyrosine kinase activity.

ROLE OF MEMBRANE TYROSINE PHOSPHORYLATION/TYROSINE KINASES IN HUMAN SPERM-ZONA PELLUCIDA BINDING

Although the glycoprotein composition the zona pellucida (ZP) from several mammalian species has been relatively well elucidated (5) only paucity of information is available regarding the molecular identities and biochemical characteristics including tyrosine phosphorylation activity of the sperm surface molecules that are involved in zona binding especially in human (25, 26). A study was conducted in our laboratory to investigate: (1) the molecular identities of various sperm proteins and zona pellucida proteins that are involved in sperm-zona binding in humans, (2) whether these proteins that are involved in sperm-zona binding have phosphotyrosine residues and/or tyrosine kinase activity, and (3) to further elucidate the involvement of FA-1 antigen in sperm-zona binding in humans. The findings of this study are discussed below:

The sperm proteins that reacted with zona proteins belonged to four major molecular regions, namely 95 kD (double band), 63 kD (one band), 51 kD (one band) and 14-18 kD (three bands) regions; of all these 63 kD and 51 kD were most prominent (27). Also, there was another band of 34 kD seen in some (two out of five) experiments. The zona protein that reacted strongest with the sperm proteins belonged to molecular region of 55 kD (ZP3). Out of the four molecular regions of sperm proteins that interacted with the zona proteins (ZP3 of 55 kD), the three namely 95 kD, 51 kD and 14-18 kD proteins but not the 63 kD protein, demonstrated the presence of phosphotyrosine residues (27). One, out of these three proteins, the 51 kD protein, also showed the autophosphorylating activity in the *in vitro* kinase assay on the PTA-beads. There was variation in the autophosphorylating kinase activity when the assay was carried out on the beads versus carried out in solution. These type of variations in *in vitro* kinase assays have been reported in other systems (28). On the PTA-beads, two zona proteins of 55 kD (ZP3) and 220 kD (ZP1/ZP2) that bind to sperm proteins also demonstrated autophosphorylating activity.

The results of our investigation indicate that tyrosine phosphorylation of sperm and zona pellucida binding proteins may play a vital role in the sperm-zona interaction/binding. Treatment with solubilized human ZP increased the tyrosine phosphorylation of the 95 kD sperm protein (10). Also, treatment of human sperm with PTA that predominantly reacts with two sperm proteins namely 95 kD and 51 kD proteins on the Western blots, also inhibited (completely blocked) sperm binding to the zona pelucida in the hemizona assay (29). It is interesting to note that treatment of human sperm with PTA also inhibits sperm penetration in SPA (10), indicating an effect on sperm capacitation and/or acrosome reaction. Based upon these findings, one may speculate that binding between the sperm and zona pellucida proteins is of enzyme-substrate type, involving hydrophobic and ionic interactions through o-phospho-L-tyrosine residues of the interacting epitope(s) resulting in tyrosine phosphorylation of the binding proteins through the tyrosine kinase activity of the complementary molecule.

The purified human FA-1 antigen of 51 kD did not show the presence of phosphotyrosine residues nor any autophosphorylating activity in the *in vitro* kinase assay. Among the four molecular regions of sperm proteins that bind zona pellucida, there was a protein of 51 kD that showed phosphotyrosine residues and autophosphorylating activity, and the binding of this protein with zona pellucida protein was inhibited by the o-phospho-L-tyrosine. To examine that whether the 51 kD was the FA-1 antigen or not, we performed two sets of experiments. The 51 kD among the four zona pellucida binding sperm proteins showed specific binding with the anti-FA-1 mab in the Western blot procedure, and the purified unlabeled FA-1 antigen competed with the ^{125}I-labeled 51 kD protein for binding with the zona pellucida protein in a concentration-dependent manner. These data confirm that the 51 kD protein, that is a tyrosine kinase receptor involved in sperm capacitation/acrosome reaction and zona pelucida binding, is indeed the FA-1 antigen. Anti-FA-1 antibodies (both monoclonal and polyclonal) have been shown to inhibit sperm-zona binding in a variety of species including humans (8, 9, 26, 29, 30).

The differences between 51 kD sperm protein and the purified FA-1 antigen for reaction with PTA and autophosphorylating activity may be due to the purification procedure involving immunoaffinity chromatography that causes a loss of phosphorylating activity of FA-1 antigen. Various procedures and detergents can differently affect the glycosylation and phosphorylation patterns of purified proteins. It is also possible that the FA-1 antigen requires the presence of other zona-binding sperm protein(s) for phosphorylation/autophosphorylating activity, thus suggesting the presence of signal transduction pathway in the human sperm cell. The immunoaffinity purification that results in elimination of these additional proteins causes a loss of tyrosine phosphorylation/autophosphorylating activity of the purified FA-1 antigen.

CONCLUSION

These findings indicate that the sperm proteins that bind to zona pellucida protein, ZP3 of 55 kD, have molecular identities of 95 kD, 63 kD, 51 kD and 14-18 kD, respectively. Three of these four proteins, namely the 95 kD, 51 kD and 14-18 kD, have phosphotyrosine residues and seem to involve the o-phospho-L-tyrosine epitope in sperm-zona pellucida interaction, and one of these three, 51 kD protein (FA-1 antigen), also has autophosphorylating activity. Interestingly, the complementary zona pellucia protein, ZP3 of 55 kD, also demonstrated autophosphorylating activity. Many of these sperm proteins that participate in sperm-zona pellucida binding are also involved in sperm capacitation/acrosome reaction. These culumlative findings indicate a vital role of protein tyrosine phosphorylation and tyrosine receptor kinases in sperm capacitation/acrosome and sperm-zona pellucida binding in humans.

Acknowledgements
We thank Ms. Margaret O'Connell for excellent typing assistance. This work was supported by a grant from NIH, HD 2445 to R.K.N.

REFERENCES

1. Fischer EH, Krebs EG. The conversion of phosphorylase b to phosphorylase a. J Biol Chem 1955; 216:121-132.
2. Ullrich A, Shlessinger J. Signal transduction by receptors with tyrosine kinase activity. Cell 1990; 61:203-212.
3. Pawson T. Protein modules and signalling network. Nature 1995; 373:573-580.

4. Smith JA, Francis SH, Corbin JD. Autophosphorylation: a salient feature of protein kinases. Mol Cell Biol 1993; 127/128:51-70.
5. Yanagimachi R. Mammalian fertilization. In: Knobil E, Neill JD, eds. The Physiology of Reproduction New York: Raven Press, 1994; 189-318.
6. Naz RK, Kaplan P, Goldstein AL. Thymosin alpha-1 enhances the fertilizing capacity of human sperm cell: implication in diagnosis and treatment of male infertility. Biol Reprod 1992; 47:1064-1072.
7. Naz RK, Alexander NJ, Isahakia M, Hamilton, MD. Monoclonal antibody to a human sperm membrane glycoprotein that inhibits fertilization. Science 1984; 225:342-344.
8. Naz RK, Phillips TM, Rosenblum BB. Characterization of the fertilization antigen-1 for the development of a contraceptive vaccine. Proc Natl Acad Sci USA 1986; 83:5713-5717.
9. Kaplan P, Naz RK. The fertilization antigen-1 does not have any proteolytic/acrosin activity, but its monoclonal antibody inhibits sperm capacitation and acrosome reaction. Fertil Steril 1992; 58:396-402.
10. Naz RK, Ahmad K, Kumar R. Role of membrane phosphotyrosine proteins in human spermatozoal function. J Cell Sci 1991; 99:157-165.
11. Ahmad K, Naz RK. Thymosin alpha-1 and FA-1 monoclonal antibody affect fertilizing capacity of human sperm by modulating protein phosphorylation pattern. J Reprod Immunol, in press.
12. Gould JE, Overstreet JW, Yanagimachi H, Yanagimachi R, Katz DF, Hanson FW. What functions of sperm cell are measured by in vitro fertilization of zona-free hamster eggs? Fertil Steril 1983; 40:344-352.
13. Naz RK, Ahmad K, Kaplan P. Expression and function of ras-proto-oncogene proteins in human sperm cells. J Cell Sci 1992; 102:487-494.
14. Naz RK, Ahmad K, Kaplan P. Involvement of cyclins and cdc^2 serine/threonine protein kinase in human sperm cell function. Biol Reprod 1993; 48:720-728.
15. Kopf G. Mechanisms of signal transduction in mouse sperm. Ann NY Acad Sci 1989; 564:289-302.
16. Naz RK, Ahmad K, Kumar G. Presence and role of c-myc proto-oncogene product in mammalian sperm cell function. Biol Reprod 1991; 44:842-850.
17. Roten R, Paz GF, Hamonnai ZT, Kalina M, Naor Z. Protein kinase C is present in human sperm: possible role of flagellar motility. Proc Natl Acad Sci USA 1990; 87:7305-7308.
18. Naz RK, Morte C, Garcia-Framis V, Kaplan P, Martinez P. Characterization of a sperm-specific monoclonal antibody and isolation of a 95-kilodalton fertilization antigen-2 from human sperm. Biol Reprod 1993; 49:1236-1244.

19. Tesarik J, Moos J, Mendoza C. Stimulation of protein tyrosine phosphorylation by a progesterone receptor on the cell surface of human sperm. Endocrinology 1993; 133:328-335.
20. Baldi E, Falsetti C, Gervasi G, Carloni V, Casano R, Forti G. Stimulation of platelet aggregation factor synthesis by progesterone and A23187 in human spermatozoa. Biochem J 1992; 292:209-216.
21. Leyton L, Saling PM. 95 kD sperm protein binds ZP3 and serves as tyrosine kinase substrate in response to zona binding. Cell 1989; 57:1123-1130.
22. Leyton L, LeGuen P, Bunch D, Saling PM. Regulation of mouse gamete interaction by sperm tyrosine kinase. Proc Natl Acad Sci USA 1992; 89:11692-11695.
23. Todderud G, Wahl MI, Rhee SG, Carpenter G. Stimulation of phospholipase C-r_1 membrance association by epidermal growth factor. Science 1990; 249:296-298.
24. Huganir RL, Delcour AH, Greengard P, Hess GP. Phosphorylation of the nicotine acetylcholine receptor regulates its rate of densensitization. Nature 1986; 321:774-776.
25. Naz RK, Chaturvedi MM, Aggarwal BB. Role of cytokines and proto-oncogenes in sperm cell function: relevance to immunologic infertility. Am J Reprod Immuno 1994; 32:26-27.
26. Naz RK, Sacco A, Singh O, Pal R, Talwar GP. Development of contraceptive vaccines for humans using antigens derived from gametes (spermatozoa and zona pellucida) and hormones (human chorionic gonadotrophin): current status. Hum Reprod Update 1995; 1:1-18.
27. Naz RK, Ahmad K. Molecular identities of human sperm proteins that bind human zona pellucida: nature of sperm-zona interaction, tyrosine kinase activity and involvement of FA-1. Mol Reprod Develop 1994; 39:397-408.
28. Kumar R, Shepard HM, Mendelsohn J. Regulation of phosphorylation of the c-erbB-2/HER2 gene production by a monoclonal antiboby and sperm growth factor(s) in human mammary carcinoma cells. Mol Cell Biol 1991; 11:979-986.
29. Kadam AL, Fateh M, Naz RK. Fertilization antigen (FA-1) completely blocks human sperm binding to human zona pellucida: FA-1 antigen may be sperm receptor for zona pellucida in humans. J Reprod Immunol, in press.
30. Naz RK, Brazil C, Overstreet JW. Effects of antibodies to sperm surface fertilization antigen-1 on human sperm-human zona interaction. Fertil Steril 1992; 57:1304-1310.

Human sperm acrosome reaction. Eds P. Fénichel, J. Parinaud.
Colloque INSERM/John Libbey Eurotext Ltd © 1995. Vol. 236, pp. 257-276.

Role of cAMP pathways: cross-talk mechanisms for the acrosome reaction

Christopher De Jonge

Department of Obstetrics and Gynaecology, University of Nebraska Medical Center, Omaha, Nebraska, USA

Abstract

The acrosome reaction (AR) can be induced in vitro by a variety of naturally occurring and synthetic compounds, e.g., follicular fluid and calcium ionophore A23187, respectively. The events that culminate in the AR of human spermatozoa have been shown to involve at least two second messenger pathways (e.g., Zaneveld, et al., 1991). One signal transduction pathway demonstrated to have a role in the human sperm AR involves the generation of the second messenger adenosine 3':5'-cyclic monophosphate (cAMP) by the amplifying enzyme adenylate cyclase, ultimately leading to the activation of cAMP-dependent kinase (PKA) (De Jonge et al., 1991a). The PKA pathway stimulators forskolin and dibutyryl cyclic AMP (dbcAMP) induced an ARmax at 1.0µM and 1.0mM, respectively, in capacitated spermatozoa. The ED_{50} and $\Delta ARmax$ values were: 0.01 µM and 17% for forskolin and 0.069mM and 13% for dbcAMP. To more firmly establish a role for the PKA pathway in the AR, inhibitors of PKA were added at the end of the capacitation period and prior to stimulation by inducers. For example, when the PKA inhibitor KT5720 was used, a dose-dependent reduction of the forskolin and dbcAMP-induced AR was detected. Collectively, these results provide evidence for the role of the PKA pathway in the AR. Additional substantive support for the involvement of the PKA pathway in the AR comes from experiments to determine the effect of human natural cycle periovulatory follicular fluid (hFF) and solubilized human zona pellucida (sZP). When hFF was added (10%, 20% and 30% v:v) to capacitated spermatozoa, a signifcant (p<0.05) stimulation of the AR was detected. The PKA inhibitor, KT5720 (50 nM, 100 nM), prevented hFF (20%) stimulation of the AR when added at the end of the capacitation period and 5 min prior to the addition of hFF. These data demonstrate that hFF stimulates the human sperm AR and, in part, through the PKA pathway. Capacitated spermatozoa incubated with 2, 4 and 6 sZP showed a dose-dependent increase in the AR. Pretreatment of spermatozoa with KT5720 significantly lowered the AR induced by 4 sZP, but not completely, suggesting the involvement of additional signal transduction pathways. To investigate pathway "crosstalk", the following experiments were conducted: l) stimulators of the PKA and PKC pathway were combined and tested at the ARmax and ED_{50} concentrations for each; and 2) spermatozoa were pretreated with a PKA inhibitor and then stimulated using a PKC pathway stimulator; were tested. The results for (1) indicate an additive AR response for ED_{50} concentrations. The results for (2) demonstrate that a PKA inhibitor prevents induction of the AR by a PKC stimulator, and vice versa. Collectively, the results suggest a convergent mechanism of crosstalk between the PKA and PKC pathways leading to the human sperm acrosome reaction.

La réaction acrosomique (RA) peut être induite par de nombreux composants naturels ou synthétiques tels que, respectivement, le liquide folliculaire ou le calcium ionophore A 23187. Il a été démontré que les événements qui aboutissent à la réaction acrosomique du spermatozoïde humain semblent impliquer au moins deux voies de transmission du signal (Zaneveld et al, 1991). Une des voies de transmission du signal mise en évidence dans la RA du sperme humain implique la génération comme second messager de l'adénosine monophosphate 3',5' cyclique (cAMP) par l'intermédiaire de l'adénylate cyclase, conduisant en fin de compte à l'activation d'une kinase AMPc dépendante (PKA) (De Jonge et al 1991). Les stimulateurs de la PKA, la forskoline et le dibutiryl cAMP (dbc AMP), induisent une RA maximale sur des spermatozoïdes capacités a 1µM et 0.1mM respectivement. Les valeurs de ED_{50} et du ΔRA max sont: $0.01\mu M$ et 17 % pour la forskoline et 0.069 mM et 13% pour le dbc AMP. Afin d'établir de façon plus ferme le rôle de la voie de la PKA dans la réaction acrosomique, des inhibiteurs de la PKA ont été ajoutés en fin de temps de capacitation avant la stimulation par des inducteurs. Ainsi, par exemple, lors de l'utilisation du KT5720, inhibiteur de la PKA, on observe une diminution de l'induction de la RA par la forskoline et le dbcAMP. L'ensemble de ces résultats permet de prouver le rôle de la voie de la PKA dans la réaction acrosomique. Des expériences sur l'effet du liquide folliculaire humain (hLF) et de zones pellucides solubilisées (sZP) viennent soutenir l'implication de la voie de la PKA dans la réaction acrosomique. On observe une augmentation significative (p<0.05) de la *stimulation de la RA lorsque du hLF (10%, 20%, 30% v/v) est ajouté à des spermatozoïdes capacités. L'inhibiteur de la PKA (KT5720) (50 nM, 100 nM) empêche la stimulation de la RA par le hLF(20%), lorsqu'il est ajouté 5 minutes avant le hLF en fin de capacitation. Ces résultats démontrent que le hLF stimule la RA en partie par l'intermédiaire de la voie de la PKA. L'incubation de spermatozoïdes capacités en présence de 2, 4, 6 sZP montre une augmentation dose dépendante de la RA. Le pré-traitement des spermatozoïdes par du KT5720 diminue de façon significative mais non totale l'induction de la RA par 4sZP, ce qui suggère l'implication d'autres voies de transmission du signal. Afin d'étudier l'intrication des voies de transmission les expériences suivantes ont été réalisées: 1) Combinaison des stimulateurs de la PKA et de la PKC aux concentrations RA_{max} et ED_{50} pour chacun d'entre eux. 2) traitement des spermatozoïdes avec un inhibiteur de la PKA et stimulation par un activateur de la PKC. Les résultats obtenus en 1) montrent une réponse RA additive pour les concentrations correspondant aux ED_{50}. Les résultats obtenus en 2) démontrent qu'un inhibiteur de la PKA empêche la stimulation de la RA par la PKC et vice versa. L'ensemble de ces résultats suggère un mécanisme convergent d'interactions entre PKA et PKC conduisant à la réaction acrosomique du spermatozoïde humain.*

INTRODUCTION

The acrosome reaction (AR) of human spermatozoa is an exocytotic process necessary for fertilization. In order for the AR to occur in vivo and under most in vitro conditions the spermatozoa must first undergo capacitation. Capacitation involves the reorganization and/or removal of sperm membrane proteins and lipids, after which the sperm membranes become competent for fusion in response to AR inducing agents. During the AR the contents of the acrosomal vesicle become exposed, allowing for dissolution of the aerosomal matrix and dispersion of its enzymatic components. The activation and release of acrosin facilitates the enzyme-dependent penetration of the zona pellucida by the spermatozoon (e.g., 1,2,3).

During transit through the female reproductive tract, and at the point of gamete interaction, the human spermatozoon encounters many potential modulators of the AR, e.g., oviductal and follicular fluid, cumulus oophorus and zona pellucida. The influence of some of these biological materials on the human sperm AR has recently been described. Literature data demonstrate that human follicular fluid has a stimulatory effect on the AR (see e.g., 4, 5, 6, 7). Cumulus oophorus also has been shown to stimulate the AR (see e.g., 4, 6).

Additionally, the last and principle barrier for species-specific fertilization, i.e., the zona pellucida, stimulates the AR (see e.g., 8, 9). Until now the mechanism(s) by which these biological materials stimulate the acrosome reaction have remained largely obscure.

In somatic cells, exocytosis can be stimulated by a variety of signaling pathways. For example, the binding of an extracellular signal to a membrane receptor can lead to changes in a guanine nucleotide binding protein (G protein) which can influence the activity of a number of potential targets, e.g., an amplifying enzyme. The amplifying enzyme converts a precursor molecule into a second messenger that can activate, among other targets, a protein kinase and lead to the phosphorylation of a protein integral in the exocytotic process (see e.g., 10).

The events that culminate in the AR of human spermatozoa have been shown to involve at least two second messenger pathways (3). Evidence for the involvement ofthe two pathways in the AR eomes as a result oftesting ehemical modulators that mimic pivotal stimulatory eomponents in eaeh pathway, e.g., cAMP analogues and synthetic diacylglycerols. In addition, inhibitors that act at the target of these stimulatory molecules, e.g., cAMP-dependent kinase and Ca^{2+}, phospholipid dependent kinase, prevented induction of the reaction. The first signal transduction pathway demonstrated to have a role in the human sperm AR involves the generation of the second messenger adenosine 3':5'-cyclic monophosphate (cAMP) by the amplifying enzyme adenylate cyclase, ultimately leading to the activation of cAMP-dependent kinase (PKA) (11). The second signaling pathway demonstrated to play a role in the AR involves the amplifying enzyme phospholipase C that converts phosphatidylinositol 4,5-bisphosphate into the second messengers inositol 1,4,5-trisphosphate (InsP3) and diacylglycerol (DAG). DAG, in a Ca^{2+} and phospholipid dependent process, activates protein kinase C (12) .

The existence of several AR stimulatory pathways has lead to the question of whether the pathways function independently from one another or whether interaction, i.e., "crosstalk", occurs between them (13). For example, different patterns of crosstalk have been demonstrated in a variety of somatic cells types ,e.g., hepatocytes for the glucagonreceptor,reticulocytes, S49 mouse Iymphoma cells and epidermal cells for the ‚l3-adrenoceptor (e.g., 14). Crosstalk between signaling paths is thought to provide for sensitive control mechanisms for regulating cellular response(s) to varying stimuli. Thus, if crosstalk occurs between signal transduction pathways in spermatozoa, then it could potentially provide these cells with the unique ability to sense and respond to the multiple and varied signals encountered during transit through the female reproductive tract.

This review will present data demonstrating a role for the cAMP-dependent kinase (PKA) pathway in the human sperm AR and second messenger pathway crosstalk in AR stimulation.

MATERIALS AND METHODS

Chemicals
Calcium ionophore A23187, dibutyryl cyclic AMP (dbcAMP), 8-bromo cAMP, isobutylmethylxanthine, papaverine, Walsh cAMP-dependent protein kinase inhibitor (kinase A inhibitor, crude from rabbit muscle), adenosine, 2'-0-methyladenosine, 2',3'-dideoxyadenosine, forskolin, 4a-phorbol 12,13-didecanoate, 4,B-phorbol 12,13-didecanoate, 1,2-dioleoyl-snglycerol, 1,2-dioctanoyl-sn-glycerol, Ficoll (Type 400), human serum albumin (HSA, fraction V), Bismark brown Y, Rose bengal, dimethyl sulfoxide (DMSO), HEPES and all salts (cell culture tested) were obtained from Sigma Chemical Company (St. Louis, MO). Calphostin C and KT5720 were obtained from Kamiya Biomedical Company (Thousand Oaks, CA). 1-Ethyl4 (isopropylidenehydrazino) 1-H-pyrazalo-[3,4-6] pyridine-5-carboxylic acid (SQ 20009) was a gift from Dr. Gregory Kopf. N-[2-(methylamino)ethyl]-5-isoquinolinesulfonamide dihydrochloride (H-8) was obtained from Seikagaku America, Inc. (St. Petersburg, FL). All modulatorswere dissolved in dimethyl sulfoxide (<1% final concentration of dimethyl sulfoxide in capacitation medium which has previously been shown to have no effect on sperm motility or acrosomal status, see e.g., 15), except dbcAMP, Walsh inhibitor, adenosine, H-8, SQ 20009, 2'-0-methyladenosine, 2',3'-dideoxyadenosine which were dissolved in distilled water.

Capacitation medium
Modified-Biggers, Whitten and Whittingham medium (BWW, pH 7.4), which lacked glucose, sodium pyruvate and sodium lactate and contained 35 mg/ml of HSA, was used as capacitation medium for the spermatozoa (15). The medium containing this HSA concentration has previously been shown to maintain sperm motility during incubation to induce capacitation and after modulator treatment (11, 12, 15).

Sperm preparation
Semen was obtained from apparently healthy volunteers by masturbation. Initial semen quality was determined using standard parameters after complete liquefaction (16). Only samples with 70% or greater motility, quantitated using a hemacytometer and cell counter and distinguishing between immotile and motile cells, were used for experimentation. Semen was layered over 11% Ficoll in 0.12 M sodium chloride and 0.025 M

HEPES, at pH 7.4, and centrifuged at 500 x g for 30 minutes. The supernatant was removed and the sperm pellet resuspended in 1 ml of capacitation medium and centrifuged at 200 x g for 2 minutes. The supernatant was discarded and the sperm pellet resuspended in capacitation medium to give a final sperm concentration of 5.0 x 106 sperm cells/ml. Sperm motility was reassessed and if there was greater than a 15% reduction in motility or less than 68% overall motility the specimen was rejected (15).

Stimulator and inhibitor testing
The procedure for stimulator and inhibitor testing was the synchronous acrosome reaction assay (15). Briefly, 0.5 ml aliquots of washed spermatozoa in capacitation medium were pipetted into plastic centrifuge tubes and incubated at 37°C in a 5% CO_2 atmosphere incubator for O and 3 hours. An acrosome reaction stimulator was added at each time point to one of two tubes, the same concentration of vehicle was added to the other tube and served as a control, and the incubation continued for an additional 15 minutes. An aliquot of capacitation medium containing spermatozoa was removed from each tube and placed on a hemacytometer for assessment of the percentage of motile cells ("motility"), distinguishing between immotile and motile cells and quantitating the populations using a cell counter, before stopping the reaction using 0.5ml of 3% glutaraldehyde. No significant ($p>0.05$) difference in motility or the percentage acrosome reaction was detected between the 0 hour control and 0 hour treatments or 3 hour control (data not shown).

Inhibitors of the acrosome reaction were added at the end of the incubation period, i.e., after spermatozoa had become capacitated, 5 minutes prior to the addition of activator and the assay continued as described above. Calphostin C, an inhibitor of PKC, has been shown to have a dependence on light for its inhibitory properties to be most effective (17). Therefore, following the addition of Calphostin C and during the time-course of incubation for testing this compound, an incandescent light was directed at all test tubes.

The first phase of this investigation was to determine if a dose-dependent AR response could be detected after treatment of spermatozoa with various acrosome reaction stimulators at varying concentrations. Initial test concentrations were based upon previous unpublished observations and the literature data (11, 12). Stimulator concentrations tested varied from the maximal AR stimulatory dose to a concentration where no significant ($p>0.05$) difference in the percentage AR was detected between spermatozoa treated with stimulator and the nontreatment control. The ED_{50} dose for each stimulator was calculated from the dose response curve for each (see Statistical Analysis).

Cross-talk (13)
Further characterization of each pathway was provided by pretreating capacitated spermatozoa with either a PKA or PKC inhibitor followed by treatment with an stimulator for the same pathway at the ARmax dose. The difference between the ARmax and the %AR in the non treatment control at 3 hours was calculated and is termed the ΔARmax. Subsequent to this series, the following experiments were conducted. PKA and PKC inhibitor concentrations were varied from a dose where no significant (p>0.05) difference in the %AR could be detected after challenge with the appropriate pathway stimulator to a dose where a significantly (P<0.05) greater %AR was detectable in comparison to the control.

The purpose of the second phase of this investigation was to determine if crosstalk occurs between the PKA and PKC pathways and if so, to try to characterize the mechanism by which the pathways are related and how this relationship might affect the net cellular response, i.e., the AR. To test for interactions between the pathways, stimulators and inhibitors of each pathway were tested in various combinations. Specifically, stimulators for each pathway were tested in combination at their ED_{50} concentration (ED_{50} + ED_{50}). Next, a kinase inhibitor for one pathway was tested to determine the effect on the AR when spermatozoa were treated with a stimulator for the alternative pathway, e.g., PKC inhibitor + PKA stimulator (ED_{50} dose) and PKA inhibitor + PKC stimulator (ED_{50} dose). The final series of experiments to investigate pathway crosstalk involved testing a PKA or PKC inhibitor followed by the combination of PKA stimulator (ED_{50} dose) and PKC stimulator (ED_{50} dose).

Sperm acrosome evaluation
Acrosomal status was evaluated using a double stain technique (15). This method for determining acrosomal status has been validated by transmission electron microscopy (18). Briefly, spermatozoa were fixed for 30 minutes in 3% glutaraldehyde in 0.1 M sodium cacodylate. Subsequently, the samples were washed twice by centrifugation (1000 x g for 3 min) using distilled water. The final sperm pellet was resuspended in ~50µl of distilled water, the sample transferred onto microscope slides and smears prepared. After air drying, the slides were incubated in 0.8% Bismark brown Y (pH 1.8) at 37°C for 10 minutes, followed by two 10-dip washings in distilled water. The slides were then incubated in 0.8% rose bengal (pH 5.3) at room temperature for 20-23 minutes, followed by two 10-dip washings in distilled water. The slides were then passed through an alcohol dehydration series (50%, 95% and 100%) with 20 dips in each. Finally, the slides were immersed in Histo-Clear (National Diagnostics, Manville, NJ) for 10 minutes and then allowed to air dry. The acrosomal status of the spermatozoa was assessed (200 cells

per treatment) microscopically under oil immersion (1000X). Slides were read blind by a single observer and were occasionally checked by another observer.

Statistical analysis

The mean, standard deviation and 90% confidence intervals were calculated. Each data set represents at least three experiments using at least two different donors. Frequency data were statistically compared using Bartlett's test for homogeneity and Dunnet's multiple comparison test. Following generation of the dose-response curves the data were analyzed using Table-Curve (Jandel Scientific) and the ED_{50} for each activator was calculated. An alternative method used for calculating these values was by transformation ofthe data and determination ofthe optimal linear correlation coefficient. Percentage inhibition was calculated by subtracting the percentage AR for control (baseline or background AR) from each treatment, then the stimulator-only treatment was normalized to 100% and the percent inhibition was calculated forthe inhibitor-treated groups.

RESULTS

Chemical Characterization of PKA Pathway Involvement in the AR (11, 12, 13)

Amplifying enzyme

An adenylate cyclase activator, forskolin, stimulated a dose-dependent AR using concentrations from 0.005 µM to 10 µM (see Table 1). The maximum %AR (ARmax) was elicited by a concentration of 1.0 µM. The ED_{50} calculated from the dose-response curve was 0.01 µM. The ΔARmax, derived from the difference between the ARmax and the %AR in the non-treatment control at 3 hours, was calculated as 17%.

It was important to confirm forskolin's specificity of action by testing the effect of adenylate cyclase inhibitors on the forskolin-induced AR. Adenosine, 2'-0-methyladenosine and 2',3'dideoxyadenosine (the latter two compounds are agonists of the inhibitory "P-site" on adenylate cyclase) prevented the forskolin-induced AR when added (1 and 5 mM, final conc. for each compound) to spermatozoa at either the onset or completion of capacitation and prior to forskolin stimulation (10 µM, final conc.) (Table 2). Adenylate cyclase inhibition by adenosine could be bypassed by the addition of dbcAMP (1 mM, final conc.), resulting in stimulation ofthe AR.

Forskolin [M]	% Motility [2]	% AR
0	81 ± 7	8 ± 2 (7-9)
10μM	77 ± 7	24 ± 1* (23-25)
1μM	80 ± 6	25 ± 5 * (21-29)
0.1μM	75 ± 5	20 ± 3* (18-22)
0.01μM	79 ± 5	17 ± 2* (15-19)
0.005μM	83 ± 5	12 ± 2 (10-14)

Table 1: **Stimulatory effect of forskolin on the acrosome reaction of capacitated human spermatozoa.**[1]

[1] *See text for experimental detail; n=3. The values represent the mean ± SD with 90 % confidence intervals. Reprinted with permission.*
[2] *Motility did not change significantly ($p>0.05$) in any of the test samples as compared to untreated controls*
* *Significantly ($p<0.05$) different from the 3 hour non treatment control*

Forskolin [M]	Inhibitor [M]	% Motility[2]	% AR
0	0	78 ± 7	12 ± 4 (10-14)
10μM	0	80 ± 8	39 ± 6*(36-42)
10μM	adenosine (1mM)	79 ± 8	17 ± 6 (9-25)
10μM	adenosine (5mM)	78 ± 7	14 ± 6 (6-22)
10μM	2'-O-methyl(1mM)	78 ± 5	12 ± 4 (5-19)
10μM	2'-O-methyl(5mM)	82 ± 6	12 ± 4 (5-19)
10μM	2',3'-dideoxy(1mM)	79 ± 1	14 ± 3 (9-19)
10μM	2',3'-dideoxy(5mM)	72 ± 6	15 ± 2 (12-18)

Table 2: **The effect of adenosine and two adenosine analogues on the forskolin-induced acrosome reaction of capacitated spermatozoa**[1]

[1] *see text for experimental detail; n=4 for adenosine and n=3 for analogues of adenosine. The value represent the mean ± SD with 90 % confidence intervals.*
[2] *Motility did not change significantly ($p>0.05$) in any of the tests samples as compared to untreated controls.*
* *Significantly ($p<0.05$) different from the 3 hours non treatment control*

Second messenger

A membrane-permeable analogue of the intracellular second messenger cAMP, dibutyryl cAMP (dbcAMP), stimulated a dose-dependent AR using concentrations ranging from 0.05 mM to 1.0 mM (see Table 3). The ARmax concentration for dbcAMP was 1.0 mM. From the doseresponse curve, the

ED$_{50}$ was calculated to be 0.069 mM. The ΔARmax was calculated to be 13%.

To identify when calcium influx might occur in relationship to the action of cAMP, spermatozoa were incubated in capacitating medium without CaCl$_2$ (Ca^{2+} chelating agents were not used) and then stimulated to undergo the AR using either calcium ionophore A23 187 (10 µM, final conc.) or dbcAMP (1 mM). A23 187 had no significant (p>0 .05) stimulatory effect on the AR (7 ± 2% AR) in comparison to non-treated controls (10 ± 1% AR). In contrast, dbcAMP caused a significant (p < 0.01) stimulation of the AR (33 ± 4% AR). These results indicate that the action of cAMP likely occurs after calcium.

DBC AMP [M]	% MOTILITY[2]	% AR
0	79 ± 6	9 ± 2 (7-11)
1mM	72 ± 11	22 ± 3*(20-24)
0.5mM	66 ± 11	21 ± 4* (17-25)
0.1mM	68 ± 13	19 ± 4* (15-23)
0.05mM	80 ± 7	12± 3 (9-15)

Table 3: **Stimulatory effect of dbcAMP on the acrosome reaction of capacitated human spermatozoa** [1]

[1] *see text for experimental detail; n=3. The values represent the mean ± SD with 90 % confidence intervals. Reprinted with permission.*
[2] *Motility did not change significantly (p>0.05) in any of the tests samples as compared to untreated controls.*
* *Significantly (p<0.05) different from the 3 hours non treatment control*

Cyclic nucleotide phosphodiesterase

A phosphodiesterase is responsible for the hydrolysis of cAMP to AMP. Xanthine and nonxanthine phosphodiesterase inhibitors prevent cAMP to AMP conversion, and thus they were tested to determine the effect on the AR When isobutylmethylxanthine (IBMX) was added (1 mM, final conc.) to capacitated spermatozoa, a significant (p<0.05) stimulation of the AR occurred in comparison with the control (Table 4). Likewise, the non-xanthine inhibitors papaverine (10 and 100 µM final conc.) and SQ 20009 (1 µM, final conc.) stimulated an AR that was significantly (p<0.01) greater than the non-treatment control.

Inducer	[M]	% Motility²	% AR
0		75 ± 3	10 ± 3 (4-18)
dbc AMP	1mM	76 ± 4	30 ± 6*(20-40)
IBMX	1mM	76 ± 4	29 ± 3* (24-34)
SQ20009	1µM	74 ± 2	23 ± 1*(22-24)

Table 4: **The effect of phosphodiesterase inhibitors on the dbcAMP-induced acrosome reaction of capacitated human spermatozoa**

[1] *see text for experimental detail; n=3. The values represent the mean ± SD with 90 % confidence intervals.*
[2] *Motility did not change significantly (p>0.05) in any of the tests samples as compared to untreated controls.*
* *Significantly (p<0.05) different from the 3 hours non treatment control*

INDUCER	INHIBITOR [M]	% MOTILITY²	% AR
0	0	85 ± 6	10 ± 3 (9-11)
dbcAMP (1mM)	0	83 ± 4	22 ± 6*(19-25)
Forskolin (1µM)	0	84 ± 5	22 ± 2*(21-23)
Forskolin (1µM)	KT5720 (100nM)	80 ± 7	9 ± 2(8-10)
Forskolin (1µM)	KT5720 (50nM)	79 ± 7	15 ± 3*(13-17)
Forskolin (1µM)	KT5720 (25nM)	81 ± 7	15 ± 4*(13-17)
dbcAMP (1mM)	KT5720 (100nM)	79 ± 8	10 ± 1 (9-11)
dbcAMP (1mM)	KT5720 (50nM)	84 ± 5	14 ± 1*(13-15)
dbc AMP (1mM)	KT5720 (25nM)	82 ± 5	16 ± 1*(15-17)

Table 5: **The effects of protein kinase A activators and a proteine kinase A inhibitor on the acrosome reaction of capacitated human spermatozoa** [1]

[1] *see text for experimental detail; n=3. The values represent the mean ± SD with 90 % confidence intervals.Reprinted with permission.*
[2] *Motility did not change significantly (p>0.05) in any of the tests samples as compared to;untreated controls.*
* *Significantly (p<0.05) different from the 3 hours non treatment control*

Protein kinase

The effect of PKA inhibitors, Walsh protein kinase A inhibitor (10 and 100 µM), H-8 (1 and 10 µM) and KT5720 (25, 50 and 100 nM), on the dbcAMP-induced AR was tested. The maximal stimulatory dose of dbcAMP (1 mM) was used in all cases. All the inhibitors prevented the dbcAMP-induced AR depending on the type and dose of inhibitor. For example, the maximum concentration (100 nM) of KT5720 prevented the forskolin and dbcAMP-induced AR (see Table 5).

However, at the lower inhibitor concentrations complete inhibition was not detected. KT5720 at 25 nM and 50 nM caused a 58% inhibition of the forskolin-induced AR and a 50% and 67% inhibition of the dbcAMP-induced AR, respectively. A similar inhibitory dose-dependence was observed with H-8.

Biological Characterization of PKA Pathway Involvement in the AR (7,9)
Human follicular fluid

The effect of periovulatory natural cycle follicular fluid on the human sperm acrosome reaction was tested (Table 6). When hFF was added (n=3; 30% final conc.) to non-capacitated spermatozoa, no significant (p>0.05) stimulation of the AR was detected in comparison to the untreated control. The addition of varying hFF doses (n=3) to capacitated spermatozoa resulted in a significant (p<0.03) stimulation of the AR at each dose in comparison to the untreated capacitated control.

INDUCER	KT5720	%AR[b]
0	0	8 ± 2 (6-11)[d]
20%hFF	0	30 ± 3 (26-33)[e]
20%hFF	50nM	9 ± 2 (7-11)[d]
0sZP*	0	16 ± 2 (13-20)[$]
4sZP	0	48 ± 1 (46-50)[@]
4sZP	50nM	34 ± 1 (33-36)[o]

Table 6: **The effect of cAMP-dependant kinase inhibitor on the human follicular fluid and solubilised human zona pellucida induced acrosome reaction** [a]

[a] *See De Jonge et al., 1994 and Biefeld et al., 1994 for experimental detail. N=3; mean ± SD (95% confidence limits)*
[b] *% AR values with dissimilar superscripts are significantly (p<0.01) different relative to their respective control*

In addition, stimulation of the AR under these conditions was significantly correlated (r=0.960, p<0.04) with hFF concentration. No significant (p>0.05) difference in sperm motility was detected between the 3 hr control (82%) and sperm treated with hFF (e.g., 30% hFF = 77%).

A PKA inhibitor, KT5720, was tested to determine if hFF stimulates the AR via the PKA pathway, (Table 6). When KT5720 (50 nM and 100 nM, final conc.) was added to capacitated spermatozoa, 5 min prior to the addition of hFF (20% final conc.), no significant (p>0.05) stimulation of the AR by hFF was detected at either concentration of KT5720 in comparison to the untreated capacitated control. The percent AR for hFF-treated spermatozoa was significantly (p< 0.0001) greater than control or inhibitor-treated spermatozoa. No significant (p>0.05) difference in sperm motility was detected between the control (85%) and either the hFF (85%) or hFF + inhibitor treated (82%) spermatozoa.

Zona pellucida

The effect of solubilized human ZP on the AR of capacitated spermatozoa was evaluated (Table 6). Also, the AR-inducing ability of six solubilized zona-free oocytes (representing the greatest number of zonae studied) was tested. A significant (P<0.02) stimulation of the AR was detected for all concentrations of zonae. In addition, the AR response was dose-dependent. In contrast, solubilized zona-free oocytes failed to cause a significant (P>0.05) stimulation of the AR.

KT 5720 was tested to determine the effect on the AR when spermatozoa were stimulated with 4 solubilized ZP (Table 6). KT5720 significantly (P<0.01) reduced the solubilized ZP-induced AR in comparison to spermatozoa treated with solubilized ZP alone. However, complete inhibition was not detected as compared to the untreated control.

A combination of inhibitors (PKA/PKC/PKG) was also studied (data not shown). The combination of inhibitors caused a significantly (P<0.02) greater inhibition of the solubilized ZP-induced AR than individual inhibitors.

Second messenger pathway crosstalk characteristics (13)

To determine if the %AR could be enhanced by using a combination of stimulatory compounds of the PKA and protein kinase C (PKC) pathways, the ARmax dose for forskolin and dbcAMP and ARmax doses of activators of the PKC pathway were tested (Table 7). No increase in the %AR was detected beyond that obtained using an activator individually at its ARmax dose when activators from each pathway were added in combination at their ARmax dose. Furthermore, although not presented, the ΔAR values for each combination of stimulators did not exceed the ΔAR for the individual compound.

To determine if the PKA and PKC pathways interact synergistically to stimulate the AR, activators from the PKA and PKC pathways were tested in combination at their ED_{50} concentrations (Table 8). A mathematically additive stimulation of the AR was detected when the PKA and PKC stimulators ($ED_{50} + ED_{50}$) were added in combination in comparison to single activator treatment. No combination of stimulators tested caused a greater than additive response. However, when the ΔAR for each condition was calculated it was found that the ΔAR for the stimulator combinations either equalled or exceeded the sum of the ΔAR's for the single compound that comprised the stimulator combination, e.g., dbcAMP (ΔAR=6%) + 1,2-dioctanoyl (ΔAR= 13%) < dbcAMP + 1,2-dioctanoyl (ΔAR=24%).

INDUCER [M]	INDUCER² [M]	%MOTILITY³	% AR
0	0	81 ± 4	9 ± 2 (8-10)
Forskolin(0.01μM)	0	83 ± 6	15 ± 2*(14-16)
dbcAMP(0.069mM)	0	82 ± 3	15 ± 1*(14-16)
0	1,2-dioctanoyl(35μM)	79 ± 9	22 ± 3*(20-24)
0	1,2-dioleoyl (33μM)	80 ± 3	21 ± 3*(19-24)
0	4α (21nM)	84 ± 5	16 ± 3*(14-18)
Forskolin (0.01μM)	1,2-dioctanoyl (35μM)	83 ± 5	28 ± 3*(27-29)
Forskolin (0.01μM)	1,2-dioleoyl (33μM)	82 ± 3	28 ± 3*(26-30)
Forskolin (0.01μM)	4α (21nM)	84 ± 1	23 ± 5*(19-27)
dbc AMP (0.069mM)	1,2-dioctanoyl (35μM)	78 ± 9	33 ± 5*(19-37)
dbc AMP (0.069mM)	1,2-dioleoyl (33μM)	81 ± 12	31 ± 5*(27-35)
dbc AMP (0.069mM)	4α (21nM)	84 ± 3	25 ± 6*(20-30)

Table 7: **The effect of proteine kinase A activators with proteine kinase C at ED$_{50}$ concentrations on the acrosome reaction of capacitated human spermatozoa**

[1] See text for experimental detail, n=3. The values represent the mean ± SD with 90% confidence intervals. Reprinted with permission.

[2] 1,2-dioctanoyl represents 1,2-dioctanoyl-sn-glycerol, 1,2-dioleoyl represents 1,2-dioleoyl-sn-glycerol. 4α represents 4α-phorbol-12,13-didecanoate.

[3] No significant (p>0.05) change in sperm motility occured after incubation to induce capacitation or after treatment with modulators.

* Values are significantly (p<0.05) different from 3 hr non treatment control.

Inducer [M]	Inducer[2] [M]	%Motility[3]	% AR
0	0	80 ± 4	7 ± 1 (6-8)
Forskolin(10μM)	0	79 ± 6	22 ± 2*(20-24)
dbcAMP(1.0mM)	0	75 ± 2	23 ± 2*(14-16)
0	1,2-dioctanoyl(50μM)	78 ± 5	28 ± 2*(26-30)
0	1,2-dioleoyl (50μM)	78 ± 2	28 ± 2*(27-29)
0	4α (0.1μM)	80 ± 3	30 ± 3*(27-33)
Forskolin (1.0μM)	1,2-dioctanoyl (50μM)	82 ± 3	29 ± 3*(26-32)
Forskolin (1.0μM)	1,2-dioleoyl (50μM)	79 ± 1	27 ± 3*(25-29)
Forskolin (1.0μM)	4α (0.1μM)	80 ± 2	30 ± 3*(27-33)
dbc AMP (1.0mM)	1,2-dioctanoyl (50μM)	80 ± 4	28 ± 3*(26-30)
dbc AMP (1.0mM)	1,2-dioleoyl (50μM)	77 ± 5	28 ± 2*(26-30)
dbc AMP (1.0mM)	4α (0.1μM)	81 ± 2	29 ± 2*(27-31)

Table 8: **The effect of proteine kinase A activators with protein kinase C activators at maximal activating concentrations on the acrosome reaction of capacitated human spermatozoa** [1.]
See table 7 legend for description of symbols. Reprinted with permission.

Inducer[2]	Inhibitor	% Motiltity[3]	% AR
0	0	86 ± 4	9 ± 2 (8-10)
1,2-dioctanoyl(35μM)	0	83 ± 2	18 ± 3*(16-20)
1,2-dioleoyl (33μM)	0	79 ± 6	17 ± 3*(15-19)
4α (21nM)	0	82 ± 6	15 ± 1*(14-16)
1,2-dioctanoyl (35μM)	KT5720 (50nM)	82 ± 3	9 ± 2 (8-10)
1,2-dioleoyl (33μM)	KT5720 (50nM)	84 ± 5	9 ± 2 (8-10)
4α (21nM)	KT5720 (50nM)	85 ± 4	10 ± 2 (9-11)

Table 9: **The effect of PKC activator and a PKA inhibitor on the acrosome reaction of capacitated human sperm.** [1]
[1] *See text for experimental detail, n=3. The values represent the mean ± SD with 90%confidence intervals. Reprinted with permission.*
[2] *See table 7*
[3] *Motility did not change significantly (p>0.05) in any of the test samples as compared to untreated controls*
* *Values are significantly (p<0.05) different from 3 hr non treatment control.*

To determine whether an inhibitor for one pathway could prevent induction of the AR by a stimulator of the alternative pathway, capacitated spermatozoa were pretreated (5 min.) with KT5720 (50 nM) and then stimulated to AR using the ED_{50} dose of either 1,2-dioctanoyl, 1,2dioleoyl-sn-glycerol or 4β-phorbol 12,1 3-didecanoate. None of the PKC stimulators were able to bypass the KT5720-mediated inhibition of PKA and induce the AR (Table 9). Capacitated spermatozoa were pretreated (5 min.) with Calphostin C (25 nM and 50 nM) and then stimulated with either forskolin or dbcAMP at their ED_{50} dose to induce the AR. Calphostin C, at both concentrations, prevented induction of the AR by each of the PKA stimulators in comparison with non-treatment controls(Table 10).

INDUCER	INHIBITOR	% MOTILTITY [2]	% AR
0	0	83 ± 2	8 ± 1 (7-9)
dbcAMP (0.069mM)	0	86 ± 4	16 ± 1*(15-17)
Forskolin (0.01μM)	0	85 ± 4	14 ± 1*(13-14)
dbcAMP (0.069mM)	Calphostin C(50nM)	85 ± 2	9 ± 1 (8-10)
dbcAMP (0.069mM)	Calphostin C(25nM)	83 ± 6	9 ± 1 (8-10)
Forskolin (0.01μM)	Calphostin C(50nM)	85 ± 2	8 ± 1 (7-9)
Forskolin (0.01μM)	Calphostin C(25nM)	83 ± 3	9 ± 1 (8-10)

Table 10: **The effect of PKA activators (ED_{50}) and a PKC inhibitor on the acrosome reaction of capacitated human spermatozoa[1]**
[1] *See text for experimental detail, n=3. The values represent the mean ± SD with 90%confidence intervals. Reprinted with permission.*
[2] *Motility did not change significantly (p>0.05) in any of the test samples as compared to untreated controls.*
* *Significantly (p<0.05) different from 3 hours non treatment control.*

Finally, combinations of PKA and PKC stimulators at EDso doses were added to capacitated spermatozoa pretreated (5 min.) with an inhibitor of either PKA or PKC. When capacitated spermatozoa were pretreated with KT5720 (50 nM) and then stimulated with the combination of either dbcAMP and PKC stimulators or forskolin and PKC stimulators, no induction of the AR was detected in comparison to non-treatment controls (data not shown, see ref. 13). When capacitated spermatozoa were pretreated with Calphostin C (50 nM) and then treated using a combination of PKC and PKA stimulators at EDso doses, no induction of the AR was detected in comparison to the non-treatment control (data not shown, see ref. 13).

DISCUSSION

The mechanism(s) by which human spermatozoa undergo acrosomal exocytosis has long been questioned. Hypotheses concerning various aspects of the reaction have been tested, e.g., pH, membrane factors, and supported by experimental evidence. However, no clear integration of these events has been convincingly detailed. While on the surface the acrosome reaction may appear to be a relatively simple process, recent reports have revealed it's complexity. It is becoming increasingly evident that the acrosome reaction can be elicited by the activation of one or more signal transduction pathways.

This report presents convincing evidence for the role of the cAMP-dependent pathway in the human sperm acrosome reaction. Factors that target specific loci in the cAMP-dependent kinase pathway were used to determine if support for involvement of the entire pathway could be amassed. Starting with the amplifying enzyme, adenylate cyclase (AC), it was shown that AR stimulation could be achieved if an agonist for AC was used. Further, it was shown that antagonists of the enzyme prevented AR stimulation. Lastly, AC inhibition could be bypassed, e.g., by influencing a downstream component, to effect the AR by using an analogue (dbcAMP) of the product (cAMP) of AC activity.

Also include herein are data that provide evidence for interplay or "crosstalk" between signalling pathways, in particular between the PKA and PKC pathways. Several types of pathway crosstalk can be characterized, and they are: 1) independent; 2) antagonistic; 3) sequential; and 4) convergent. To determine if crosstalk might occur in the sequence of events leading to the AR exocytosis and in what manner, experiments were performed using stimulators for each pathway in various combinations at ARmax and ED_{50} concentrations. The use of stimulator combinations at their ED_{50} doses was to elucidate whether the pathways function independently or convergently. In these types of sytems, stimulator treatment combinations at less than maximal concentrations would be anticipated to yield an additive or nearly additive response. The results demonstrate that the combination of stimulators induced an AR that was equivalent to the addition of a single stimulator at its ARmax dose. These results, i.e., an additive response, fit a pattern that would be consistent with both of these crosstalk models, i.e., independence or convergence. If the data are evaluated relative to the ΔAR (data not shown), then evidently the combination of stimulators at their ED_{50} doses causes an additive to greater than additive, i.e., synergistic, response. This response would not be characteristic of an independent system but would accommodate a model for convergence

Stimulators of each pathway were used at their ARmax dose to try to further elaborate whether independent or convergent crosstalk occurs in the AR process. Stimulator combinations at ARmax doses caused no increase in the percentage AR beyond that obtained when a stimulator was added alone. It would be expected that if the pathways acted independently then the combined stimulator treatment at ARmax doses would cause an additive response, but this didn't occur. Alternatively, if the pathways functioned convergently a less than additive AR response would be anticipated when using the ARmax doses, and this was detected. Finally, if the PKA and PKC pathways were acting antagonistically, then the combination of stimulators of the two pathways, regardless of concentration, would have resulted in minimal to no stimulation of the AR. The AR response that was detected argues against this model of crosstalk. When the data are taken collectively the following conclusion can be made: the acrosome reaction that occurs as a result of PKA and PKC stimulation does not likely occur as a result of antagonistic or independent mechanisms of crosstalk, but rather the AR may occur through sequential or convergent interactions.

To determine if the pathways function sequentially, and to further rule out the possibility of independence, a stimulator for one pathway and an inhibitor for the other were tested. The rationale being that if the pathways were operating sequentially, then depending on the modulator combination being tested, e.g., PKA stimulator with PKC inhibitor, the stimulator of one pathway could bypass the kinase inhibitor-mediated inhibition of the other pathway. If the pathways were independent then no inhibition would occur regardless of modulator combination. The data demonstrate that kinase inhibitors of each pathway prevented induction of the AR by a stimulator of the alternative pathway. It can be reasoned from these data that the PKA and PKC pathways do not operate independent of one another and it appears unlikely that they operate sequentially.

CONCLUSION

In conclusion, based upon the data presented herein it can be reasoned that a convergent pattern of crosstalk is the most likely manner in which the PKA and PKC pathways interact in the sequence of events that culminate in human sperm acrosomal exocytosis. It may be that for spermatozoa a convergent pattern of crosstalk exists to provide for built in redundancy to ensure that the greatest potential for successful AR stimulation is in place. Additionally, it may provide a mechanism to "salvage" the reaction from not occurring should one pathway be defective. While these data are by no means conclusive they emphasize the need for continued research in this area.

Acknowledgements
The data and conclusions presented resulted from the efforts of many individuals with whom I have had the distinct honor and pleasure of working with over the last several years and without their contributions the many

projects that are synopsized herein would not have been possible. Appreciation is extended to the Editors of the Journal of Andrology for their permission to use previously published material.

REFERENCES

1. Wasserman PM. Early events in mammalian fertilization. Ann Rev Cell Biol 1987:3109-42.
2. Yanagimachi R. Mammalian fertilization. In: Knobil E, Neill J, eds. The Physiology of Reproduction. New York: Raven Press, Ltd., 1988:135-85.
3. Zaneveld LJD, De Jonge CJ, Anderson RA, Mack SR. Human sperm capacitation and the acrosome reaction. Human Reprod 1991;6:1265-74.
4. Tesarik J. Comparison of acrosome reaction-inducing activities of human cumulus oophorus, follicular fluid and ionophore A23 187 in human sperm populations of proven fertilizing ability in vitro. J Reprod Fertil 1985; 74: 383-8.
5. Suarez SS, Wolf DP, Meizel S. Induction of the acrosome reaction in human spermatozoa by a fraction of human follicular fluid. Gamete Res 1986; 14: 107-21.
6. Meizel S. Pillai MC, Diaz-Perez E, Thomas P. Initiation of the human sperm acrosome reaction by components of human follicular fluid and cumulus secretions including steroids. In: Bavister BD, Cummins J, Roldan ERS eds. Fertilization in Mammals. Norwell, Massachusetts: Serono Symposia, USA, 1991: 205-22.
7. De Jonge CJ, Barratt CLR, Radwanska E, Cooke ID. The acrosome reaction inducing effect of human follicular and oviductal fluid. J Androl 1993; 14:359-65.
8. Cross NL, Morales P, Overstreet JW, Hanson FW. Induction of acrosome reactions by the human zona pellucida. Biol Reprod 1988;38:235-44.
9. Bielfeld P, Zaneveld LJD, De Jonge CJ. The zona pellucida-induced acrosome reaction of human spermatozoa is mediated by protein kinases. Fertil Steril 1994; 61: 536-41.
10. Berridge MJ. The molecular basis of communication within the cell. Sci Amer 1985;253: 142-52.
11. De Jonge CJ, Han H-L, Lawrie H, Mack SR, Zaneveld LJD. Modulation of the human sperm acrosome reaction by effectors of the adenylate cyclase /cyclic AMP second-messenger pathway. J Exp Zool 1991a; 258:113-25.

12. De Jonge CJ, Han H-L, Mack SR, Zaneveld LJD. Effect of phorbol diesters, synthetic diacyl glycerols, and a protein kinase C inhibitor on the human sperm acrosome reaction. JAndrol 1991b;12:62-70.
13. Doherty CM, Tarchala SM, Radwanska E, De Jonge CJ (1995). Characterization of two second messenger pathways and their interactions in eliciting the human sperm acrosome reaction. JAndrol 1995; 16:36-46.
14. Houslay MD. "Crosstalk": a pivotal role for protein kinase C in modulating relationships between signal transduction pathway.Eur J Biochem 1991; 195:9-27.
15. De Jonge CJ, Mack SR, Zaneveld LJD. Synchronous assay for human sperm capacitation and the acrosome reaction.J Androl 1989;10:232.
16. Zaneveld LJD, Jeyendran RS . Modern assessment of semen for diagnostic purposes . Sem Reprod Endocrinol 1988:6:323-37.
17. Bruns RF, Miller FD, Merrimen RL, Howbert JJ, Heath WF, Kobayashi E, Takahashi I, Tamaoki T, Nakano H. Inhibition of protein kinase C by Calphostin C is light-dependent. Biochem Biophys Res Commun 1991; 176: 288-93.
18. Mack SR, De Jonge CJ, Bielfeld P, Zaneveld LJD. Acrosome reaction of human spermatozoa: Comparative evaluation by triple stain and electron microscopy. Mol Androl 1990; 2; 265-79

Chapter IV
Chapitre IV

Clinical applications
Applications cliniques

Methods for evaluating the acrosomal status of human sperm

Nicholas L. Cross

Department of Physiological Sciences, Oklahoma State University, Stillwater, Oklahoma 74078-035, USA

ABSTRACT

Many assays are now available for assessing the acrosomal status of human sperm. Sperm may be evaluated by brightfield microscopy, fluorescence microscopy, or flow cytometry using simple, accurate assays. Some aspects of the assays still remain to be improved, to provide better methods for brightfield microscopy and to facilitate assaying large numbers of samples

A l'heure actuelle de nombreux tests d'évaluation du statut acrosomique sont disponibles. Le sperme peut être analysé en microscopie à fond clair, à fluorescence ou encore en cytométrie de flux en utilisant des tests simples et précis. Cependant quelques aspects de ces tests restent encore à améliorer afin de proposer de meilleures méthodes adaptables en microscopie à fond clair d'une part et d'autre part permettant de faciliter l'analyse d' un plus grand nombre d'échantillons.

INTRODUCTION

Acrosomal exocytosis is a critical event in the fertilization process, and the ability to discern whether or not sperm acrosome-react is an essential tool in the study of sperm function. The human acrosome has so far defied attempts to visualize it with phase contrast or differential contrast optics due to its small size and optical properties, and for many years research was limited by the need to use electron microscopy to determine if sperm were acrosome-reacted. In the past decade, however, many simpler techniques have been developed, and now the major problem is deciding which assay to use. In this paper I describe the most common techniques and I suggest some desirable features that might be incorporated into new assays.

TECHNIQUES FOR BRIGHTFIELD MICROSCOPY	TECHNIQUES FOR FLUORESCENCE MICROSCOPY
	Peanut Agglutinin (3)
	Pisum Sativum Agglutinin (4,5)
Triple stain (1)	Ricinus communis agglutinin (6)
Coomassie blue (2)	Anti-Acrosin antiserum (5)
	Monoclonal HS21 (7,8)
	Monoclonal HS63 (9)
	Monoclonal GB24 (10)
	Monoclonal C11H (3)

Table I. **Assays that have been directly compared to transmission electron microscopy.** *Some of these assays do not agree exactly with electron microscopy. Consult the original references for details.*

VALIDATING AN ASSAY.

How does one know that an assay gives correct results? Transmission electron microscopy is usually considered the best standard of comparison (Table I), even though under some conditions, a few sperm may be hard to categorize (1, 4, 10). An alternative to using electron microscopy is to compare the new assay against a well established light microscope assay. But when a discrepancy is found, electron microscopy should be used to help resolve the issue. It is also important that electron microscopy is used to check the results when new inhibitors or inducers of the acrosome reaction are employed.

Most methods for detecting acrosome-reacted sperm work because they reveal either the loss of acrosomal material (acrosomal contents or outer acrosomal membrane) or exposure to the extracellular space of acrosomal components (the inner acrosomal membrane or the not-yet-dispersed acrosomal contents).

ASSAYS THAT REVEAL THE LOSS OF ACROSOMAL MATERIAL.

Assays that detect the presence or absence of acrosomal material require the sperm to be permeable to the probe. When sperm are treated with stains for brightfield microscopy, the harsh conditions of the fixative and staining solutions disrupt the sperm membrane. When a lectin or an antibody is to be used, the sperm are usually permeabilized with ethanol or methanol and then exposed to the probe. All of these assays show acrosome-intact sperm as labeled over the entire anterior head. Acrosome-reacted sperm lose much or all of the component that produces the labeling pattern, so they have no label over the anterior head. With most probes an equatorial band of label persists in reacted sperm, but a few probes do not react with the equatorial segment so the head of a reacted sperm is unlabeled.

Talbot and Chacon (6, 11) developed the first light microscope methods for assessing human acrosomal status. Their triple-stain procedure, in which trypan blue serves as a viability stain, and Bismark brown Y and Rose Bengal reveal acrosomal status, is often criticized for producing too-subtle distinctions between intact and reacted sperm. It is still in use, however, sometimes varied by omitting the trypan blue (12).

There are other stains that can be observed by brightfield microscopy. Coomassie blue (2) and silver staining (13, 14) have been directly or indirectly compared to transmission electron microscopy, with satisfactory results. Binding of a monoclonal antibody to an intraacrosomal antigen has been visualized using alkaline phosphatase-antialkaline phosphatase (15) but the labeling is of low intensity.

Fluorescence assays are better than brightfield assays because the labeling has higher contrast, and the difference between reacted and intact patterns is much more obvious. Lectin-based assays are very fast, requiring as little as five minutes to label the sperm. Pisum sativum agglutinin (16) binds to acrosomal contents; peanut agglutinin (17) binds to the outer acrosomal membrane. Ricinus communis agglutinin produces a labeling pattern similar to the other two lectins, although its site of binding has not been identified (6). Many modified versions of these assays have been described (18-21).

Polyclonal and monoclonal antibodies have been produced that bind to exocytosis-labile components. Labeling with antibodies is slower than with lectins, in part because exposure to a second, fluoresceinated antibody is required. Examples include polyclonal anti-sperm antibody, anti-acrosin antiserum, and anti-outer acrosomal membrane antiserum as well as monoclonal antibody HS21(16, 5, 22, 7).

ASSAYS THAT REVEAL EXTERNALIZED ACROSOMAL MATERIAL.

The acrosome reaction exposes to the extracellular space a new set of sperm components, including the inner acrosomal membrane and the acrosomal contents. Some assays are designed to detect the emergence of these components. In these assays the sperm are not permeabilized so the probe will only have access to the target if the sperm is acrosome-reacted.

The heads of acrosome-intact sperm are essentially unlabeled; the acrosomal region of reacted sperm are labeled. The probes include Con A, soybean trypsin inhibitor and monoclonal antibodies GB24 and MH61 (10, 23-25). They are visualized by fluorescence microscopy.

In a different approach, Ohashi et al. (26) devised a semi-quantitative assay that employs beads coated with a monoclonal antibody that binds to the anterior head of acrosome-reacted sperm. The formation of mixed aggregates of beads and sperm is a function of the number of acrosome-reacted sperm.

These assays have some advantages over assays in which the sperm must be permeabilized. It may be possible to carry out the assay on living sperm, so the acrosomal status of motile sperm can be determined. Alternatively, the first step of the assay can be fixation with formaldehyde (23), so that the experimenter has precise control of the time at which sperm are assayed - a useful feature if the population is changing rapidly. (Sperm can be formaldehyde-fixed before permeabilizing them to label with a probe for an intracellular marker, but the fixation conditions may have to be carefully controlled (18)).

CHLORTETRACYCLINE.

Chlortetracycline produces patterns that reveal acrosomal status, although the mechanism by which it works is unknown. Treating human sperm with chlortetracycline produces three or four patterns of head fluorescence (4, 27). The relative abundance of these patterns changes with the length of incubation in vitro and following treatment with agents that induce acrosome reactions. A pattern representing acrosome-reacted sperm has been identified, as well as one believed to be characteristic of capacitated sperm.

CELL VIABILITY.

Some dying sperm acrosome-react, so it is sometimes necessary to determine if an experimental treatment is altering the number of reacted sperm by affecting sperm viability. If experimental and control groups are being compared and the experimental treatment does not change the number of motile sperm, then one can safely conclude that acrosome reactions induced by the experimental treatment were not secondary to cell death. On the other hand, if the experimental treatment changes the number of motile sperm, or if the total number of reacted sperm is being measured rather than the increment caused by an experimental treatment, then it is wise to detect dead sperm and exclude them from the analysis. Dead sperm can be revealed by supravital staining (11, 16, 28) or by their failure to swell in hypotonic solutions (22). Both of these procedures are believed to detect sperm that have disrupted plasma membranes.

It is well to be aware of the limitations of this approach. A sperm can probably be dead and still have a continuous membrane and therefore not be excluded from the count. On the other hand, some of the excluded dead sperm may have died after having a normal acrosome reaction. Although these uncertainties are potential sources of error, the error will be negligible if the number of reacted, living sperm is much greater than the number of dead sperm, as is usually the case. If there are many dead sperm, then an assay that can be applied to living sperm can be used so the motility of each sperm can be assessed (10).

PROBLEMS OF ANALYSIS.

The best assays produce clear differences between acrosome-intact and -reacted sperm (and between viable and nonviable, if a test for viability is included). Nevertheless, all assays will produce some patterns that are not easy to assign to a group. When this occurs, it is best to tabulate the questionable sperm separately rather than trying to force sperm into a bimodal distribution. The size of the ambiguous group must be small compared to the other categories for the assay to be meaningful. In my experience with the Pisum sativum assay, this category rarely exceeds 2% of the sperm.

Some researchers identify an intermediate pattern in which the probe binds in a diffuse or patchy distribution and consider this to be a early stage of the acrosome reaction (for example, references 4 and 21). To prove that this interpretation is correct, transmission electron microscopy should be used to show that the number of sperm in an early stage of the acrosome reaction is the same as the number of sperm with the intermediate labeling pattern, and the intermediate pattern should display a precursor-product relationship with the fully reacted pattern. That is, after treating sperm with an inducer of the acrosome reaction, the intermediate pattern should appear before the fully reacted pattern and then the intermediate pattern should decline as the fully reacted pattern increases. To my knowledge, these two easily-obtained pieces of evidence are not available in any case that a intermediate pattern has been identified.

The follicular fluid-stimulated acrosome reaction is virtually complete in three minutes (29). If the acrosome reaction is this fast under all circumstances, then the number of incompletely reacted sperm will be very small except when there are many capacitated sperm and they are assayed within three minutes of exposure to an inducer. There are suggestions that acrosome reactions induced by A23187 may proceed more slowly, however. Following A23187 treatment, the number of sperm scored as reacted using soybean trypsin inhibitor increases with a half-time of about five minutes, but the number scored as reacted using Pisum sativum increases with a half-time of about 20 minutes (data from Figure 4A of reference 24). Soybean trypsin inhibitor is applied to living cells, and is believed to react with externalized acrosomal contents. Pisum sativum agglutinin also reacts with acrosomal contents, but it is applied to permeabilized cells, so it scores a sperm as reacted only when the acrosomal contents are fully dispersed. The differing results from these two probes can be reconciled if A23187 causes the acrosomal contents to be externalized rapidly and then the contents disperse slowly. Unfortunately the sperm were not inspected with electron microscopy, so we can not be sure that this explanation is correct.

FLOW CYTOMETRY.

Flow cytometry provides an objective measure of cell fluorescence and it can provide data on a large number of cells, improving the sensitivity of the assay. It is also considerably less fatiguing for the operator than microscope-based assays. Flow cytometry has been applied to sperm labeled with monoclonal antibodies (10, 25, 30), peanut agglutinin (31), and Pisum sativum agglutinin (28). The monoclonals that recognize antigens that are externalized by the acrosome reaction are particularly useful for flow cytometry because they avoid the need to permeabilize the cells, a treatment which often causes the sperm to aggregate. Supravital dyes have been incorporated into some of these procedures (28, 30).

FUTURE PROSPECTS.

Can the present procedures be improved? First, we need better techniques for dealing with large numbers of samples. Our present protocol permits us to process (wash, fix, and label) about 100 samples simultaneously (32), but inspecting 200 sperm in each of those samples would take about five hours at the microscope. Few people care to spend more than two uninterrupted hours scoring sperm. If the clinical interest in assessing acrosomal function continues to grow, we can expect to see microscope-based assays become automated and flow cytometry-based assays become more common. Second, the techniques for brightfield microscopy should be made less ambiguous. Wider use of probes bound to beads or particles may be helpful in this regard. Finally, it would be useful to have an assay that clearly reveals the earliest stage of the acrosome reaction in living sperm. In the ideal assay, living sperm would be loaded with a nontoxic, soluble, fluorescent probe that would be sequestered in the acrosome. As soon as membrane fusion occurred the probe would be released from the acrosome. One could simply inspect motile sperm and observe whether they have a fluorescent acrosome to determine their acrosomal status.

REFERENCES

1. Mack SR, De Jonge C, Bielfeld P, Zaneveld LJD. Acrosome reaction of human spermatozoa: comparative evaluation by triple stain and electron microscopy. Mol Androl 1990; 2:265-279.
2. Aarons D, Boettger-Tong H, Biegler B, George G, Poirier GR. The acrosomal status of human sperm evaluated by Coomassie Blue staining and electron microscopy. Mol Androl 1993; 5: 31-37.
3. Kallajoki M, Virtanen I, Suominen J. The fate of acrosomal staining during the acrosome reaction of human spermatozoa as revealed by a monoclonal antibody and PNA lectin. Int J Androl 1986; 9: 181-194.
4. DasGupta S, Mills CL, Fraser LR. Ca^{2+}-related changes in the capacitation state of human spermatozoa assessed by a chlortetracycline fluorescence assay. J Reprod Fertil 1993; 99:135-143.
5. Tesarik J, Drahorad J, Testart J, Mendoza C. Acrosin activation follows its surface exposure and precedes membrane fusion in human sperm acrosome reaction. Development 1990; 110: 391-400.
6. Talbot P, Chacon RS. A new procedure for rapidly scoring acrosome reactions of human sperm. Gamete Res 1980; 3:211-216.
7. Wolf DP, Boldt J, Byrd W, Bechtol DB. Acrosomal status evaluation in human ejaculated sperm with monoclonal antibodies. Biol Reprod 1985; 32:1157-1162.
8. Suarez SS, Wolf DP, Meizel S. Induction of the acrosome reaction in human spermatozoa by a fraction of human follicular fluid. Gamete Res 1986; 14: 107-121.

9. Chao HT, Ng HT, Leng CH, Lee CY, Wei YH. Electron microscopic immunolocalization of a conserved sperm acrosomal antigen recognized by HS63 monoclonal antibody. Andrologia 1993; 25: 203-210.
10. Fenichel P, Hsi BL, Farahifar D, Donzeau M, Barrier-Delpech D, Yehy CJ. Evaluation of the human sperm acrosome reaction using a monoclonal antibody, GB24, and fluorescence activated cell sorter. J Reprod Fertil 1989; 87: 699-706.
11. Talbot P, Chacon RS. A triple-stain technique for evaluating normal acrosome reactions of human sperm. J Exp Zool 1981; 215:201-208.
12. De Jonge CJ, Mack SR, Zaneveld LJD. Synchronous assay for human sperm capacitation and the acrosome reaction. JAndrol 1989;10: 232-239.
13. Gosalvez J, Lopez-Fernandez C, De La Torre J, Suja JA, Rufas JS. A method for visualizing the acrosome by light microscopy. Stain Technol 1986; 61: 227-230.
14. Anderson RA, Feathergill KA, De Jonge CJ, Mack SR, Zaneveld JD. Facilitative effect of pulsed addition of dibutyryl cAMP on the acrosome reaction of noncapacitated human sperm. J Androl 1992;13:398-408.
15. Braun J, Hirsch T, Krause W, Ziegler A. Evaluation of the acrosome reaction using monoclonal antibodies against different acrosomal antigens - comparison with the triple stain technique. Int J Androl 1991;14: 431-436.
16. Cross NL, Morales P, Overstreet JW, Hanson FW. Two simple methods for detecting acrosome-reacted human sperm. Gamete Res 1986,15:213-226.
17. Mortimer D, Curtis EF, Miller RG. Specific labelling by peanut agglutinin of the outer acrosomal membrane of the human spermatozoon. J Reprod Fertil 1987; 81: 127-135.
18. Morales P, Cross NL. A new procedure for determining acrosomal status of very small numbers of human sperm. J Histochem Cytochem 1989; 37: 1291-1292.
19. Mendoza C, Carreras A, Moos J, Tesarik J. Distinction between true acrosome reaction and degenerative acrosome loss by a one-step staining method using Pisum satiuum agglutinin. J Reprod Fertil 1992; 95: 755-763.
20. Tesarik J, Mendoza C, Carreras A. 1993. Fast acrosome reaction measure: a highly sensitive method for evaluating stimulus-induced acrosome reaction. Fertil Steril 1993; 59:424-430.
21. Aitken RJ, Brindle JP. Analysis of the ability of three probes targeting the outer acrosomal membrane or acrosomal contents to detect the acrosome reaction in human spermatozoa. Hum Reprod 1993; 8: 1663-1669.

22. Sanchez R, Toepfer-Petersen E, Aitken RJ, Schill WB. A new method for evaluation of the acrosome reaction in viable human spermatozoa. Andrologia 1991; 23: 197-203.
23. Holden CA, Hyne RV, Sathananthan AH, Trounson AO. Assessment of the human sperm acrosome reaction using concanavalin A lectin. Mol Reprod Dev 1990; 25: 247-257.
24. Arts EG, Kuiken J, Jager S. A new method to detect acrosome reacted spermatozoa using biotinylated soybean trypsin inhibitor. Fertil Steril 1994; 62: 1044-1055.
25. Okabe M, Nagira M, Kawai Y, Matzno S, Mimura T, Mayumi T. A human sperm antigen possibly involved in binding and/or fusion with zona free hamster eggs. Fertil Steril 1990; 54:1121-1126.
26. Ohashi K, Saji F, Dato M, Okabe M, Mimura T, Tanizawa 0. Evaluation of acrosomal status using MH61-beads test and its clinical application. 1992; Fertil Steril 58:803-808.
27. Lee MA, Trucco GS, Bechtol KB, Wummer N, Kopf GS, Blasco L, Storey BT. Capacitation and acrosome reactions in human spermatozoa monitored by a chlortetracycline fluorescence assay. Fertil Steril 1987; 48: 649-658.
28. Henley N, Baron C, Roberts KD. Flow cytometric evaluation of the acrosome reaction of human spermatozoa: a new method using a photoactivated supravital stain. Int J Androl 1994;17: 78-84.
29. Yudin AI, Gottlieb W, Meizel S. Ultrastructural studies of the early events of the human sperm acrosome reaction as initiated by human follicular fluid. Gamete Res 1988; 20:11-24.
30. Tao J, Du JY, Critser ES, Critser JK. Assessment of the acrosomal status and viability of human spermatozoa simultaneously using flow cytometry. Hum Reprod 1993; 8: 1879-1885.
31. Purvis K, Rui H, Scholberg A, Hesla S, Clausen OP. Application of flow cytometry to studies on the human acrosome. JAndrol 1990; 11: 361-366.
32. Cross NL. Multiple effects of seminal plasma on the acrosome reaction of human sperm. Mol Reprod Dev 1993; 35: 316-323.

Culture media, capacitation and acrosome reaction

Yves J.R. Ménézo

Laboratoire Marcel Mérieux et Institut National des Sciences Appliquées, Biologie 406, 69621 Villeurbanne Cedex, France

ABSTRACT

The concept of capacitation was proposed originally independently by Austin and Chang in 1951. Since that time, scientific litterature has not clearly sorted the various concepts involved in the major events preparing the male gamete for fertilization: capacitation and acrosome reaction. These events represent the switch from a stable state required for a prolonged storage in the male genital tract to a modified one necessary for the penetration of the oocytes.

Le concept de capcacitation a été proposé intialement par Austin et Chang indépendamment en 1951. Depuis, la littérature scientifique n'a pu clairement sélectionner les nombreux concepts impliqués dans les événements majeurs préparant le gamète mâle à la fécondation: la capacitation et la réaction acrosomique. Ces phénomènes représentent le passage d'un état stable nécessaire à un stockage prolongé dans le tractus génital mâle à un état modifié indispensable à la pénétration de l'oeuf.

INTRODUCTION

Capacitation process occurs normally in the female genital tract during sperm ascent. The use of monolayers of epithelial cells of female genital tract origin has allowed to realize this process in semi in-vitro conditions. It can be successfully performed nowadays in more or less defined media: this has enhanced our knowledge in the biochemical aspects of these events. At the time when the most important option followed to improve fertilization is the mechanical way through micro-injection, whatever the concerns and the absence of basic research to back the ART, in this review, we will analyze the possibility of action to increase the sperm fertilizing ability. Components of the culture media may act in several ways according to the target of the capacitation process : these different aspects will be reviewed here.

LIPIDS

The ratio cholesterol/phospholipids seems one of the key elements in the regulation of capacitation and AR. The most reliable model was proposed by Davis et al. (1) and involved a modification of the cholesterol/ phospholipid ratio in sperm membranes. All the compouns that could act on this ratio are potential target to prepare for fertilization. Albumin which is an universal ligand carrier can mediate these cholesterol efflux. However it is clear, to explain variations observed between experiments or laboratory, that the type of preparation of albumin can influence strongly the results. We have used and recommended (also for safety reasons) the use of ethanol precipitated, crystallized albumin. This process can partly remove a part of the lipids bound to the core of albumin thereby increasing the exchanges with the sperm membrane lipid content. Albumin prepared with thermal shock only, precipitates with its lipids and may be so less powerful to induce capacitation and AR. Serum addition as well as follicular fluid addition can play a role in this game through HDL and LDL; serum addition may be rather inhibitory due to the contribution of free and esterified cholesterol.

Lipids composition is related to membrane fluidity through variations of cholesterol content and the interaction with the proteins.Variations in the cholesterol content have direct effect on the acrosome status and mannose ligand binding sites (2). Destabilization of the membrane will increase the permeability to Ca^{2+}. The result being fusion of the membranes (Ca can chelate phospholipid molecules).

Membrane bound enzymes such as phospholipase A2 may change in configuration in relation to the loss of cholesterol from the sperm membranes: hydrolysis of phospholipids in the presence of Ca then releases lysophospholipids highly active in promoting AR. In the other hand, phospholipid methylation seems to be involved in sperm capacitation. Methylation needs the presence of S-Adenosyl methionine as cofactor. Bovine and human sperm do have a SAM synthetase activity (3). Phospholipid methylation must be of some relevance as an increase of a de novo synthesis of phospholipids in observed during capacitation in the bull and the pig. Moreover, inhibitors of phospholipid methylation inhibits AR in hamster spermatozoa. Methylation of IP3 is supposed to open membrane Ca^{2+} channels (4). Aracidonic acid may have a direct positive effect on A.R. in the Hamster (5).

METABOLIC SUBSTRATES, IONS AND CAPACITATION

The relation Ca^{2+}/ ATPase is also a key point. Ca^{2+} ATPase is an energy dependent enzyme that help to maintain a low Ca level in the cell. Capacitation requires high Ca levels in the cells. Sr^{++} ions can substitute fully to for Ca^{++} in human, but not Mg^{2+} or Zn^{2+}. This later cation can even be inhibitory for golden hamster sperm capacitation and AR. Potassium inhibits hyperactivation of sperm (see content of the oviduct and especially the ampulla). High K^+/Na^+ ratio seems favorable for survival and maintenance of fertilizing ability in rat, bovine and human sperm. Some cation at the level of trace elements can be deleterious : Fe^{2+} can react with ascorbic acid and form free radicals which are deleterious for sperm survival and fertilizing ability, especially through the formation of lipid peroxiides.

All the substrates that could increase the ATP and cAMP content are important for the capacitation process. So presence of glucose which increases the ATP and then cAMP content is important. In the contrary, for Rogers and Yanagimachi (6), glucose delays AR in the guinea pig. Analogs of glucose (deoxy glucose) can inhibit the AR may be by depleting the ATP content. For Sakkas et al. (7) glucose is necessary for in vitro fertilization in mouse. Glucose is an important metabolite: it allows the formation of NADPH through the pentose phoshate pathway; NADPH is necessary to prevent the peroxide formation either directly by himself or via regeneration of GS-SG. Fructose cannot replace glucose, moreover it seems to alter the acrosomal membrane during storage of bovine sperm.(8).

Cyclic AMP is used for phosphoryllation of membrane proteins and other proteins involved in motility. Adenylate cyclase activity increases and phosphodiesterase decrease both maintaining a high content of cAMP, during in vitro incubation. It has been well documented that bicarbonate induces a rapid stimulation of adenyl cyclase and cAMP content (9).There are some good indications that bicarbonate have a role in early capacitation rather than in acrosome reaction (10). Ca^{++} and cAMP contents in capacitating hamster spermatozoa suggest that cAMP is a key factor inducing hyperactivation. Ca^{2+} might be also required for acrosin activity, the later being involved in the vesiculization of the acrosomal membrane.

AMINO ACIDS AND CAPACITATION

The sulfonated aminoacids hypotaurine (HT) and taurine (T) are known to be essential for sustaining sperm motility. It is important to know which one is the most useful and important as HT is also a reducing agent preventing the formation of free radicals (these compounds being important for AR) and

T is rather an osmoregulator. Both compounds are present at the time of fertilization in the milieus surrounding the gametes. Mrsny and Meizel (11) showed that they could act through an inhibition of the Na/K ATPase : the result being the maintenance of a high level of ATP available for cAMP synthesis and all the related events. Anyway these compounds are known to be essential for sustaining sperm motility during capacitation and A.R. However, according to de Lamirande and Gagnon (17) and Aitken (3), reactive oxygen species could play a role in capacitation and AR: hypotaurine is permanently present in the surrounding milieu at the time of fertilization i.e. follicular fluid and tubal secretion, whatever the specy (tubal épithelial cells have a CSD, cysteine sulfinate decarboxilase). Hypotaurine is even present in sperm cells and seminal plasma; there is a striking difference between bovine (250nMoles/109 spermatozoa) and human sperm (60nMoles/109 cells). it is probable that this obvious difference is the image of differences in quality of sperm. It is important to consider that the by-product of hypotaurine after scavenging of free radicals is taurine. In the other hand, Taurine may act as a inhibitor of methylation processs.

If we consider the phospholipid methylation, this process requires methionine: this coumpound is important in vitro for the synthesis of SAM. The SAM synthesis is more important in human sperm than in bovine sperm, and its synthesis is strongly inhibited by seminal plasma.This pathway is also used for the synthesis of polyamines which is considered as being low in ejacullated spermatozoa. Moreover methionine is also involved in the synthesis of hypotaurine and taurine (14).

PHARMACOLOGY OF SPERM

Action through the culture medium may include pharmacological stimulation. Sperm is a specialized cell with receptors: alfa and beta, A2. We have demonstrated that stimulation with NECA, a stable analog of adenosine can increase cAMP content and induce phosphoryllation of sperm proteins.

One must not forget that cathecholamines are present in the female genital tract. One surprising point is that these compounds can bind easily to albumin. They can be easily detected in significant amount in commercial preparations of albumin, even after ethanolic preparations (15). Cathecholamines do not seem to induce AR but rather to stimulate capacitation (16).

At the time of mechanical approach to fertilization it is rather encouraging that some way are open to improve sperm fertilizing ability.

ANTIBODIES AND CAPACITATION

The use of serum addition, at the time of fertilization, is always a possible risk (especially in case of idiopathic infertility) as the immunological history of the patients is always partially unknown. Moreover the presence of serum rather hinders capacitation (17).

Sperm antibodies can interfere with the fertilization process, but the ones that bind to the head are more deleterious that the tail binding ones. In addition, it depends mainly upon the epitopes against which they have been produced. First of all the lipid exchanges with albumin may be reduced by a heavy covering of proteins (Ab) on acrosomal membrane. Negative interactions may occur also especially when antibodies can have access to new epitopes appearing during membrane remodeling : this is the case for M Ab HS 11 which reacts only with capacitated, acrosome intact spermatozoa (18).

Washing sperm to reduce or to remove antisperm antibody are poorly efficient due to the high affinity of the binding. To strong treatments usually result in damaging sperm. In our experience we have chosen 2 ways: the induction of capacitation by pharmacological agents (NECA) and the use of complement. NECA induces a rapid increase in cAMP content and phosphoryllation of human sperm membrane proteins. Complement induces a lysis of some of the spermatozoa, but C3 molecules are now well known as ligand between sperm and oocytes. C3 has given interesting results, in IUI or IVF for patients with high antibody titers. Complement in some case they only way to isolate motile sperm from antibody related sperm clumps (19). Complement may bind to SP 40, a protein present in the seminal plasma as well as in serum. (20).

CONCLUSIONS

The possibilities to modulate capacitation and AR, through the culture media are important. The problem is that we still do not understand exactly were compounds of the culture medium act exactly. Albumin, Calcium and bicarbonate ions have direct effects; some compounds such as glucose, taurine have more indirect effects. Obviously the future is more in a better knowledge of spem pharmacology.

REFERENCES

1. Davis B.K., Byrne R., Hungund B. Studies on the mehanism of capacitation. II Evidence for lipid transfer between plasma membrane of rat sperm and Serumalbumin during capacitation in vitro. Biochim. Bipophys. Acta 1979, 558: 257-266
2. Benoff S., Hurley J., Cooper G.W., Mandel F.S., Rosenfeld D.L., Hershlag A. Head-specific mannose ligand receptor expression in human spermatozoa is dependent on capacitation associated membrane cholesterol loss. Human Reprod. 1993, 8: 2141-2154
3. Guerin P., Gharrib A., Ménézo Y. Synthesis of S-Adenosyl-Methionine/S-Adenosyl-Homocysteine in human and bovine ejaculated spermatozoa. Mol. Androl. 1991, 3: 9-17
4. Florman H.M., Corron M.E., Kim T.D.H., Babcock D.F. Activation of voltage-dependent calcium channels of mammalian sperm is required for zona pellucida-induced acrosome exocytosis. Dev. Biol. 1992, 152: 304-314
5. Meizel S., Turner K.O. The effects of products and inhibitors of arachidonic metabolism on the Hamster sperm acrosome reaction. J. Exp. Zool. 1984, 231: 283-288
6. Rogers J.A., Yanagimachi R. Glucose effect on respiration : possible mechanisms for capacitation in guinea pig spermatozoa. Jexp. Zool. 1975, 207: 107-111
7. Sakkas D., Urner F., Ménézo Y., Leppens G. Effcet of glucose and fructose on fertilization, cleavage and viability of mouse embryos in vitro. Biol. Reprod. 1993, 49: 1288-1292
8. Aalseth E.P., Saacke R.G Alteration of the anterior acrosome of motile bovine spermatozoa by fructose and hydrogen ion concentration. J. Reprod. Fertil. 1987, 81: 625-634
9. Garbers D.L., Tubb D.J., Hyne R.V. A requirement of bicarbonate for Ca^{++} induced elevation of cyclic AMP in guinea pig spermatozoa. J. Biol. Chem. 1982, 257: 8980-8994
10. Shi D.X., Roldan E.R.S.. Bicarbonate/CO2 is not required for zona pellucida or progesterone-induced acrosomal exocytosis of mouse spermatozoa but is essential for capacitation. Biol. Reprod. 1995, 55: 540-546
11. Mrsny R.J., Meizel S. Inhibition of hamster na+/k+- ATPase activity by taurine and hypotaurine. Life Sci. 1985, 36: 271-275
12. De Lamirande E., Gagnon G. Human sperm hyperactivation and capacitation as part of an oxidative process Free rad. Biol. Med. 1993, 14: 157-166

13. Aitken J., Fisher H. Reactive oxygen speciesgeneration and human spermatozoa: the balance of benefit and risk. BioEssays 1994, 16: 259-267
14. Guérin P. Le metabolisme de la methionine dans le spermatozoïde et les cellules epitheliales tubaires. Transmethylations et biosynthese de l'hypotaurine Ph.D. thesis, 1994, No 94 ISAL
15. Khatchadourian Ch., Ménézo Y., Gérard M., Thibault Ch. Chatecholamines within the rabbit oviduct at fertilization time. Human Reprod. 1987, 2: 1-5
16. Meizel S., Working P.K. Further evidence suggesting the hormonal stimulation of hamster sperm acrosome reaction by catecholamines in vitro Biol. Reprod. 1980, 22: 211-216
17. Calvo L., Dennison Lagos L., Banks S.M., Fugger E.F., Sherins R.J. Chemical composition and protein source in the capacitation medium significantly affect the ability of human spermatozoa to undergo follicular fluid induced acrosome reaction. Human Reprod. 1993, 8: 575-580
18. Fann C.H., Lee C.Y.G.. Monoclonal antibodies affecting sperm-zona binding and/or zona induced acrosome reaction. J. Reprod Immunol. 1992, 21: 175-187
19. Ménézo Y., Fénichel P.. The use of complement in case of severe sperm agglutination. 49th American Fertility Society meeting, Montreal Canada, 1993, Abstr.
20. Kirsbaum L., Sharpe J.A., Murphy B., d'Apice A.J.F., Classon B., Hudson P., Walker I.D. Molecular cloning and characterization of the novel human complement associated protein, SP-40, 40 : a link between the complement and reproductive systems. EMBO J. 1993, 8: 711-718

Human sperm acrosome reaction. Eds P. Fénichel, J. Parinaud.
Colloque INSERM/John Libbey Eurotext Ltd © 1995. Vol. 236, pp. 295-313.

In vitro induction of the human sperm acrosome reaction

David Mortimer

SIVF, 4 O'Connell Street, Sydney NSW 2000, Australia

ABSTRACT

Our work on in-vitro induction of the human sperm acrosome reaction (AR) is summarized and, taken in conjunction with an overview of recent literature, used to establish a foundation for diagnostic and therapeutic applications of AR induction. It is concluded that assessment of spontaneous ARs is physiologically meaningless and that diagnostic tests must use an appropriate biochemical inducer of the AR. Ideally this would be the zona pellucida glycoprotein ZP3, but the scant supply of human zonae precludes this approach. Recombinant human ZP3 (rhZP3) does induce the AR, but is not yet commercially available - although it does represent the probable future for such diagnostic tests. Meanwhile, because follicular fluid cannot be standardized for quality control purposes, it is less ideal as an AR agonist. Progesterone and the calcium ionophore A23187 are the only viable alternatives, and it is recommended that one of these two agonists (most probably the latter) be employed until rhZP3 is available. Mild A23187 treatment must be used to minimize its toxic effect on the spermatozoa. In light of the need for the fertilizing spermatozoon to undergo its AR actually on the zona pellucida, the clinical application of AR induction remains confused, and probably has no value. However, capacitation promotion (e.g. pentoxifylline), so that spermatozoa which bind to the zona are optimally capable of undergoing an AR, may have clinical benefit.

Nos travaux sur l'induction in vitro de la réaction acrosomique (AR) sont résumés ici et, conjointement avec une revue de la littérature récente, servent de base pour des applications diagnostiques et thérapeutiques d'induction de la réaction acrosomique. La conclusion est que l'évaluation de la réaction acrosomique spontanée est physiologiquement dénuée de sens et que les tests diagnostiques doivent utiliser un inducteur biochimique de la RA approprié. Idéalement ce serait ZP3, une glycoprotéine de la zone pellucide, mais la faible quantité de zona humaines disponibles exclut une telle approche. La ZP3 humaine recombinante (rhZP3) induit la réaction acrosomique mais n'est pas encore commercialisée alors qu'elle représente l'avenir probable de ce type de tests de diagnostic. Le liquide folliculaire ne pouvant être standardisé, ce qui gêne le contrôle qualité, il est considéré comme un candidat peu fiable. La progestérone et le ionophore calcique A 23187 sont alors les seules alternatives plausibles et il est recommandé que l'un de ces deux agonistes (plus probablement le dernier) soit utilisé jusqu'à ce que le rhZP3 soit disponible. Des traitements doux au calcium ionophore doivent être utilisés afin de minimiser ses effets toxiques sur le spermatozoïde. Par contre face à l'évidence du besoin impératif pour le spermatozoïde fécondant d'accomplir sa RA au contact de la zone pellucide, l'application clinique de l'induction de la RA reste confuse et n'a probablement aucune valeur. Cependant favoriser la capacitation (par de la pentoxyfilline par exemple), afin que les spermatozoïdes se liant à la zone pellucide soient capables d'accomplir leur réaction acrosomique de façon optimale, pourrait avoir un effet clinique bénéfique.

INTRODUCTION

The acrosome reaction (AR) is a calcium-dependent process essential for fertilization in all eutherian mammals (review: 1). The ability to undergo the AR is developed over a period of several hours, usually within the female reproductive tract, by an incompletely-understood process known as capacitation. However, capacitation does involve a series of subcellular changes that result in intracellular alkalinization and an increased intracellular Ca^{2+} ion concentration ($[Ca^{2+}]_i$). Structurally, the AR consists of a cascade of events resulting in the formation of localized membrane fusions between the outer acrosomal membrane and the plasma membrane, creating fenestrations between the acrosome and the exterior. The appearance of these fenestrations is the typical morphological appearance of the AR and allows release of the acrosome contents, including the hydrolytic enzymes hyaluronidase and acrosin, which are traditionally believed to facilitate penetration of the fertilizing spermatozoon through the egg vestments.

Capacitated spermatozoa are, by definition, in a state ready to undergo the AR either spontaneously or in response to some biological trigger. While it was dogma that the AR occurred prior to the fertilizing spermatozoon's penetration of the oocyte-cumulus complex, perhaps induced by some component of the products of ovulation, the modern view is that the AR actually occurs on the zona pellucida (ZP), induced by ZP3 after binding to the zona's sperm receptor, not prior to or during penetration of the cumulus.

Although several authors have proposed studies of AR dynamics as an additional test of sperm fertilizing ability, consideration of the physiological regulation of the AR clearly indicates that spontaneous acrosome loss is non-physiological, even disadvantageous (1,2). Indeed, the reliance of early protocols for the zona-free hamster egg penetration test (HEPT) upon spontaneous capacitation and ARs is very probably the major reason that studies using such protocols are now known to have poor clinical relevance, with ionophore-optimized protocols having far greater sensitivity and specificity (e.g. 3).

Various workers have studied the induction of the human sperm AR by either human follicular fluid (hFF), the cumulus cell mass, or the ZP. A role for hFF as a specific physiological trigger of the AR is disputed, but high levels of ARs can be induced by ZP3, obtained by solubilizing zonae. Unfortunately, human zonae are too scarce for this to be useful in the routine diagnostic situation, although the advent of recombinant human ZP3 (rhZP3 (4)) should lead to the development of a new generation of diagnostic tests. For now, calcium ionophores, particularly the antibiotic A23187, have been used widely to induce ARs artificially in more-or-less capacitated human sperm populations, although early protocols which employed very high levels of ionophore often caused substantial concomitant loss of motility and/or vitality.

This paper summarizes the author's work on the in-vitro induction of the human sperm AR and uses it, in conjunction with a overview of other relevant literature, as a foundation for the rational diagnostic application of AR testing and the use of clinical AR induction.

EXPERIMENTS

Spontaneous acrosome reactions
Selected motile sperm populations were prepared from three ejaculates from each of ten donors using two-layer discontinuous Percoll gradients. They were incubated under the most physiological in-vitro conditions possible by using a complex "synthetic tubal fluid" culture medium (STF) based upon the composition of human oviduct fluid (5) with high albumin content (30 mg/ml, comparable to periovulatory oviduct fluid) at 37°C under 5% CO_2. ARs were assessed using FITC-conjugated peanut agglutinin (PNA) lectin labeling (6);

spermatozoa were considered reacted only if the equatorial segment alone showed PNA labeling.

Although only a minority of spermatozoa underwent a spontaneous AR, the incidence of acrosome loss after 36 h of incubation did approach the maximum level inducible using ionophore (Figure 1). Overall, spontaneous AR levels were higher than those reported in many other in-vitro incubation studies, a finding that was attributed to the more physiological nature of STF culture medium - perhaps due to its high albumin content or the inclusion of progesterone (7).

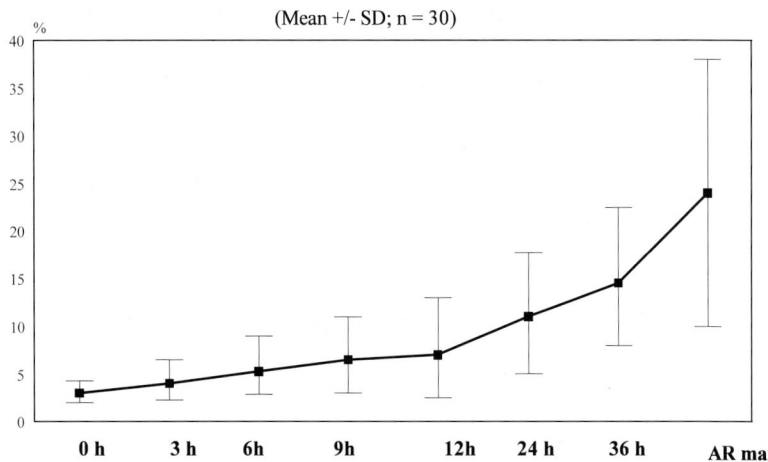

Figure 1: **Occurrence of spontaneous acrosome reactions by human spermatozoa** *in vitro* **during incubation for up to 36 hours (7).**

AR induction by follicular fluid

While many authors have shown that hFF induces the human sperm AR, such a role appears physiologically unfounded if the fertilizing spermatozoon undergoes its AR after binding to the ZP. This is further supported by the finding that prior exposure to human oviduct fluid decreases the AR responsiveness of human spermatozoa to hFF (8), as well as a report that failure of spermatozoa bound to the ZP to then undergo the AR is a cause of infertility (9). Certainly the incubation of human spermatozoa in hFF-supplemented culture media does promote the occurrence of acrosome loss, but it would seem to be more an expression of the high lability of capacitated human spermatozoa responding to a non-specific agonist of the AR. Furthermore, many such studies used low albumin concentrations so that hFF-supplementation will have resulted in substantially increased albumin concentration, perhaps thereby promoting capacitation by virtue of albumin's role as a sterol acceptor.

Selected populations of motile human spermatozoa were prepared from three ejaculates from each of five donors, again using discontinuous Percoll gradients, and incubated under physiologically-optimized conditions in STF medium for 6 h to induce capacitation. After exposure to hFF (5 to 100%) for 2h acrosomal status was assessed using FITC-PNA. All incubations were at 37°C under 5% CO_2 in air. The hFF was a pool prepared from large follicles whose mature oocytes had successfully fertilized *in vitro* and cleaved to at least 2-cell embryos; only uncontaminated follicular aspirates were used and the hFF was heat-inactivated to destroy complement which might cause artefactual loss of vitality. A23187 treatment was used as a positive control ("ARmax").

Exposure to hFF caused only relatively small proportions of spermatozoa to undergo ARs (Figure 2). These sub-populations were smaller than that capable of responding to a Ca^{2+}-influx generated by A23187. Our interpretation of these observations was that while hFF may act to stimulate or promote the human sperm AR it did not appear to be a specific inducer of it (10). Consequently, a role for hFF in the physiological regulation of human fertilization, at the relatively low concentrations that would be expected to be present in the tubal ampulla, is most unlikely.

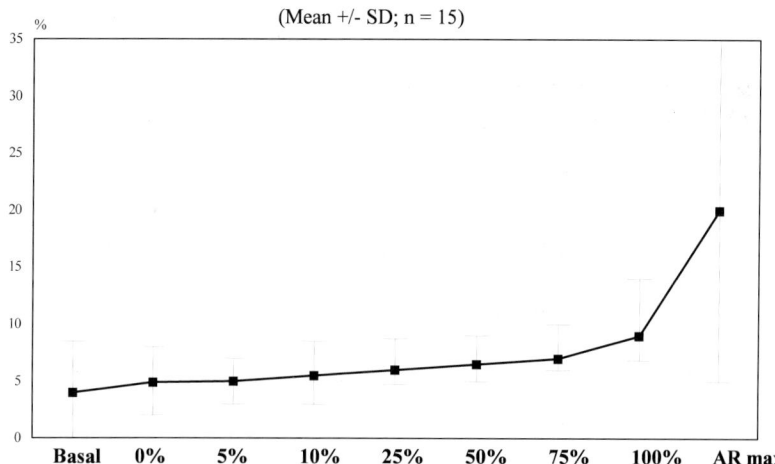

Figure 2: **Induction of acrosome reactions in capacitated human spermatozoa** *in vitro* **by 0 to 100% (v/v) follicular fluid (10).**

AR induction by cumulus

Early studies reported that capacitated human spermatozoa were induced to undergo the AR in the presence of the cumulus mass (11, 12). In a series of experiments to re-assess and expand upon this, populations of motile donor spermatozoa prepared by direct swim-up migration from liquefied semen into STF medium were preincubated for 5 h to induce capacitation. Aliquots were then coincubated for 2 h with pieces of cumulus mass, obtained either from superovulated hamsters or cut from mature human oocytes obtained for clinical IVF. Spontaneous and A23187-treated (10 µM for 20 min. followed by 2 h further incubation) controls were run in parallel with AR assessments in three sperm populations: "Around" = spermatozoa left in the sperm suspension after removal of the cumulus; "On" = spermatozoa loosely adherent to the cumulus surface, recovered from the washing medium; and "Within" = those spermatozoa recovered from the cumulus after hyaluronidase dispersion. All incubations were at 37°C under 5% CO_2, and acrosomal status was assessed using FITC-PNA lectin-labeling combined with Hoechst 33258 vital staining (6).

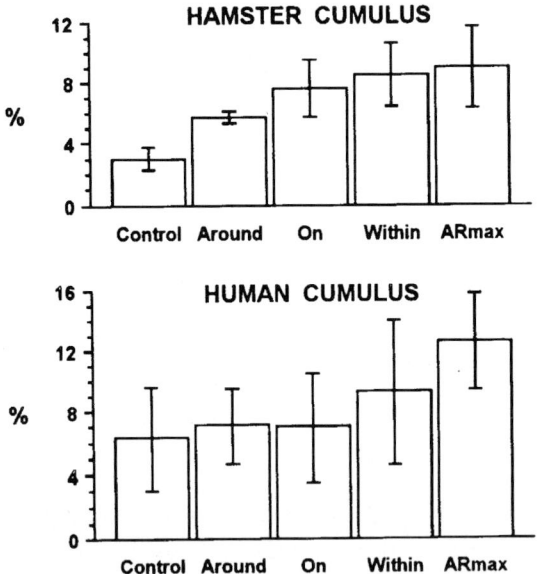

Figure 3: **Induction of acrosome reactions in live, capacitated human spermatozoa during coincubation with either hamster or human cumulus (values are mean ± SEM).**

Some component of both hamster and human cumulus masses induced an AR in some capacitated human spermatozoa (Figure 3). However, not only were the absolute levels of induced ARs very much a minority of spermatozoa, responses to cumulus were also not maximal, being only 74 and 63% of A23187-induced ARmax values for hamster and human cumulus respectively (13).

AR induction by A23187

Comparative data on the maximal induction of ARs using calcium ionophore obtained over several early studies are shown in Figure 4.

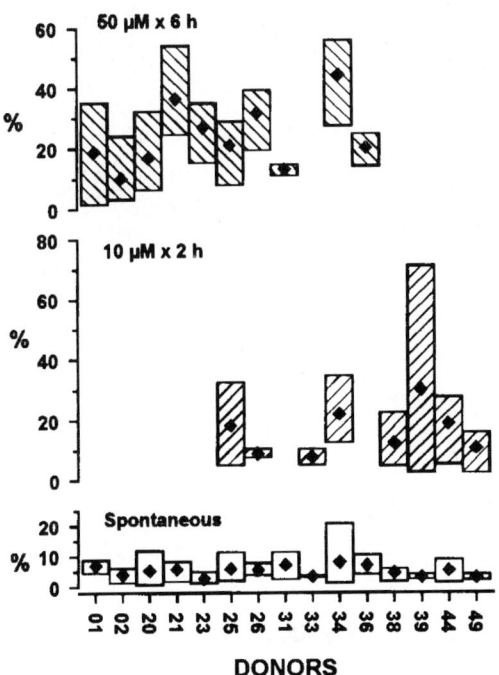

Figure 4: **Inter-ejaculate variability for control donors of either spontaneous acrosome reactions during a 6 h incubation *in vitro*, or acrosome reactions induced by severe or mild treatment with the calcium ionophore A23187.** Bars denote range ($n \geq 3$ samples, diamonds indicate medians).

The same donors were used several times each over a period of two years, during which time our protocol for inducing ARmax changed from a 6 h exposure to 50 µM to A23187 (7) to a 20 min. exposure to 10 µM A23187 after a 6 h preincubation followed by a further 2 h incubation (10). Regardless of the absolute levels of induced ARs, which were lower using the milder A23817 treatment, the variability in ARmax was very different between donors: some showed highly consistent values while others showed great intra-individual variation (14). These findings cause concern for the reliability of single assessments of AR inducibility using A23187 in some men (e.g. the acrosome reaction after ionophore challenge or "ARIC" test (15)), although cannot deny the clinical value of such tests (see below).

In a prospective clinical study of 36 patients and 5 control donors, we found that tests of AR dynamics permitted a good (78.6%) prediction of sperm fertilizing ability, defined as either in-vivo conception or fertilization in-vitro during a 5-year follow-up (Table I, Analysis A). No physiologically relevant correlations were found between any AR measure and other aspects of sperm function as tested by the HEPT (using a calcium deprivation protocol (6)) or a sperm-zona binding test (ZBT) using salt-stored human zonae pellucidae, indicating that although the HEPT is dependent upon the AR, different aspects of sperm function are measured by AR assessments and the HEPT (16).

STEP PREDICTOR VARIABLES	IN/OUT	R^2	ΔR^2
ANALYSIS A: SPERM FUNCTION TEST DATA ONLY			
1. HEPT % penetration	in	0.156	0.156
2. AR positive live sperm @24h	in	0.296	0.140
3. AR negative live sperm @24h	in	0.327	0.031
4. AR negative live sperm @ 6h	in	0.364	0.037

Prediction: Infertile = 83.3% (10 / 12)
Fertile = 76.7% (23 / 30)
Overall = 78.6% (33 / 42: 37 patients + 5 donors)

Table I: **Discriminant function analysis results for sperm fertilizing ability using acrosome reaction dynamics, zona-free hamster egg penetration test and sperm-zona binding test data either alone (Analysis A), or in conjunction with semen analysis and sperm preparation results (Analysis B).** See text for further explanation.

A similar finding has since been reported by others (17). Interestingly, in our study the ZBT had no predictive value, while inclusion of the sperm preparation yield, normal sperm morphology and ejaculate volume in the analysis improved the correct prediction of sperm function to 87.8%, with a 91.7% specificity (Table I, Analysis B). However, only 50% of the variance was accounted for, indicating that the predictor variables remained incomplete, and perhaps also prone to inherent error.

STEP PREDICTOR VARIABLES	IN/OUT	R^2	ΔR^2
ANALYSIS B: ALL AVAILABLE TEST DATA			
1. HEPT % penetration	in	0.164	0.164
2. AR positive live sperm @24h	in	0.338	0.174
3 AR negative live sperm @24h	in	0.367	0.029
4. AR negative live sperm @ 6h	in	0.412	0.045
5 Sperm penetration yield	in	0.434	0.022
6. HEPT penetration capacity	in	0.466	0.032
7. HEPT % penetration	out	0.452	-0.014
8. Normal sperm morphology in semen	in	0.474	0.022
9. Ejaculate volume	in	0.498	0.024

Prediction: Infertile = 91.7% (11 / 12)
Fertile = 86.2% (25 / 29)
Overall = 87.8% (36 / 41: 36 patients + 5 donors)

Table I: Discriminant function analysis results for sperm fertilizing ability using acrosome reaction dynamics, zona-free hamster egg penetration test and sperm-zona binding test data either alone (Analysis A), or in conjunction with semen analysis and sperm preparation results (Analysis B). See text for further explanation.

Influence of extracellular pH on the human sperm AR

Although the roles of ion transport and hydrolytic enzymes in the eutherian AR remain uncertain and perhaps subject to species differences it seems that an influx of K^+ ions, probably generated by the activity of a plasma membrane Na^+, K^+-ATPase, is an important initial step. This is accompanied by an H^+ ion efflux resulting in an increased intra-acrosomal pH (pH_i) preceding the morphological events of the AR. This alkalinization may allow activation and/or maximal activity of acrosomal enzymes and is accompanied by an influx of Ca^{2+} ions probably due to the activity of Ca^{2+}-translocating enzymes in the plasma membrane. Consequently, the effect of altering extracellular pH (pH_o) on the human sperm AR was investigated.

Motile sperm populations were prepared from three donors by direct swim-up migration from liquefied semen into STF medium and preincubated at pH 7.5 to 7.6 for 6 h to induce capacitation. Aliquots were then washed into modified Tyrode's medium (normal pH = 7.6). For the alkaline series (pH 8.0 and 8.4) the pH was adjusted using NaOH while for the acidic range (pH 6.8 and 7.2) adjustments were made using either HCl or H_2SO_4 as separate series. Mild A23187 treatment (see above) was used to determine the ARmax. All incubations were at 37°C under 5% CO_2 in air, and acrosomal status was assessed using the combined FITC-PNA + H33258 technique.

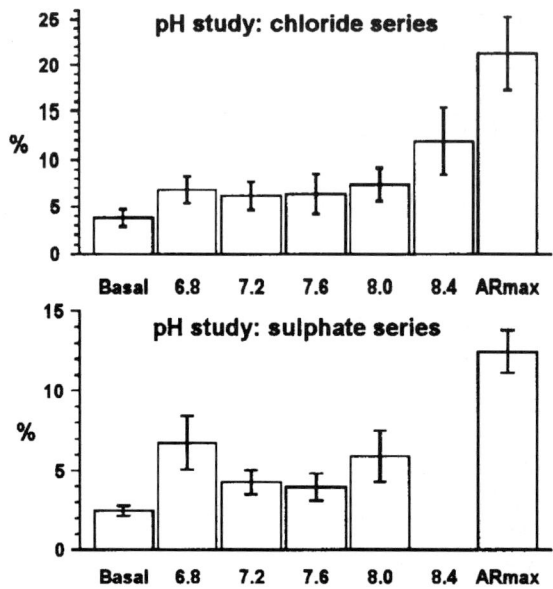

Figure 5: **Effect of changing extracellular pH on the occurrence of acrosome reactions in live, capacitated human spermatozoa *in vitro*** (values are mean ± SEM).

Increasing pH_o to 8.4 induced higher levels of ARs compared to the physiological range of pH 7.2 to 7.6, to about 40% of the maximum inducible using A23187 (Figure 5). Decreased pH_o (6.8) induced higher levels of ARs compared to the physiological range when sulphate, but not chloride ions were used (also to about 40% of ARmax). Consequently, shifting pH_o outside the physiological range does promote acrosome loss, although at acidic pH the effect may be due more to the presence of SO_4^- ions (18).

Induction of the human sperm AR by glycosaminoglycans

The ability of follicular fluid to induce ARs in capacitated spermatozoa is well documented in several species and, while this may be attributable to its progesterone content (e.g. 19, 20), some workers believe it contains a specific AR-inducing factor. There is also substantial evidence that glycosaminoglycans (GAGs), including heparin, can induce ARs in capacitated spermatozoa of other eutheria. Because many GAGs are heavily sulphated, and we had found that SO_4^- ions might induce the AR, we also investigated the ability of a range of GAGs to induce ARs in capacitated human spermatozoa (21).

Motile sperm populations were prepared from three donors by direct swim-up migration from liquefied semen into STF medium and preincubated for 6 h. Separate aliquots were then treated with 1, 10 and 100 µg/ml of either heparin sulphate (HEP), chondroitin sulphate A, B or C (CSA, CSB and CSC), hyaluronic acid (HYA), fucoidan (FUC) or ascophyllan (ASC) for 2 hours (all from Sigma); A23187 (10 µM x 20 min.) acted as the ARmax positive control. The pH of all treatments was maintained at 7.2 to 7.6 and incubations were at 37°C under 5% CO_2; acrosomal status was determined using FITC-PNA + H33258.

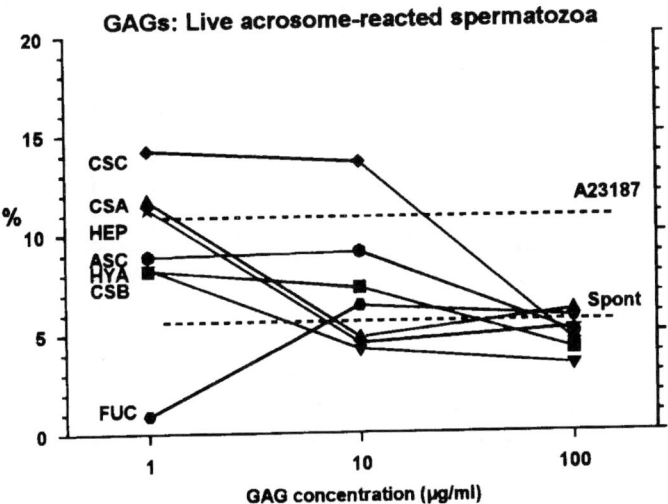

Figure 6: **Induction of acrosome reactions in live, capacitated human spermatozoa by a 2 h treatment with various glycosaminoglycans at 1, 10 and 100 mg/ml** *(CSA, CSB, CSC = chondroitin sulphates A, B and C; HEP = heparin sulphate; ASC = ascophyllan; FUC = fucoidan; HYA = hyaluronic acid). A23187 = ionophore positive control; Spont = spontaneous incidence of acrosome reactions or negative control.*

Most GAGs induced significant levels of ARs above the spontaneous control level (Figure 6), but the effect was maximal at 1 µg/ml frequently due to substantial decreases in sperm vitality at higher GAG concentrations. CSB, ASC and FUC were comparably effective, while CSC, CSA and HEP were as effective as A23187. Since hFF contains substantial quantities of a wide range of GAGs, these substances may also be at least partially responsible for the AR inducing ability of hFF - although the effect may be rather non-specific due to their heavy sulphation. While integration of these observations into a physiological model for the in-vivo regulation of fertilization is certainly difficult, the stimulatory effect of GAGs as AR inducers *in vitro* did have some potential application (see below).

Combined effect of GAGs and pH on the human sperm AR
In an attempt to avoid the often deleterious impact of A23187 on sperm vitality (and also upon oocytes) the combined effect of elevated pH_o and heparin sulphate was investigated. In a further series of three experiments, HEP was tested at 0, 1, 10 and 100 µg/ml at both pH 7.5 and pH 8.4. These results (Figure 7) confirmed both the stimulatory effect of elevated pH_o and of heparin (18).

Optimized clinical AR induction in human spermatozoa

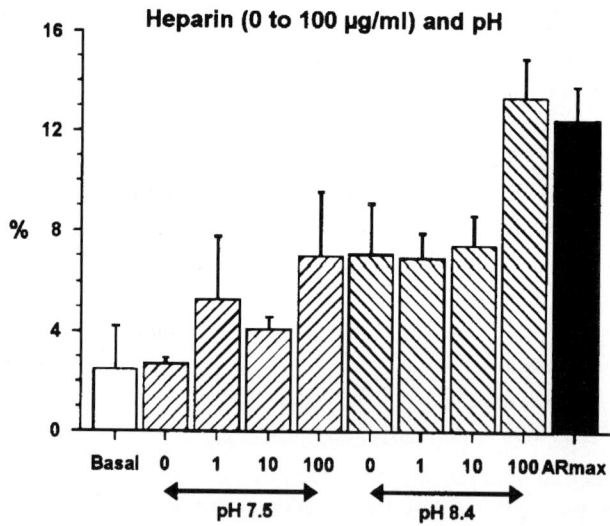

Figure 7: **Induction of acrosome reactions in live, capacitated human spermatozoa by treatment with heparin sulphate at either pH 7.5 or pH 8.4** (values are mean ± SEM).

At the time of sperm-oocyte fusion the fertilizing spermatozoon has completed its AR but retains an intact equatorial segment. Before intracytoplasmic sperm injection (ICSI), several units used sub-zonal insertion (SUZI) as a clinical sperm microinjection procedure. However, SUZI was dependent upon injecting a live, acrosome-reacted spermatozoon - with intact equatorial segment - into the perivitelline space. There was therefore great interest in developing techniques to induce physiological ARs without killing the spermatozoa (e.g. 22) and preferably avoiding ionophores.

Ejaculates from nine infertility patients were diluted with Hepes-buffered HTF (10 mg HSA/ml) containing 5 mM pentoxifylline to promote capacitation (23). After a 15 minute incubation, motile sperm populations were separated using discontinuous Percoll gradients and suspended in bicarbonate-buffered HTF medium. The following treatments were then undertaken to establish the optimum AR induction method for each man. All incubations were at 37°C under 5% CO_2 in air, and acrosomal status was assessed using the combined FITC-PNA + H33258 technique (24).

A   HTF medium (control)
B   HTF medium + 50% hFF x 6 h
C,D,E HTF medium + dbcGMP at 1, 5 or 10 µM x 6 h
F   HTF medium + 50% hFF x 24 h
G,H,I HTF medium + 50% hFF + dbcGMP at 1, 5 or 10 µM x 24 h
J   HTF at pH 8.4 + 1 mg/ml heparin + 1 mg/ml progesterone
K   10 µM dbcGMP then HTF at pH 8.4 + 1 mg/ml heparin + 1 mg/ml progesterone
L   A23187 at 2.5 µM in DMSO

Average results for the nine men are shown in Figure 8. However, maximum levels of live acrosome-reacted spermatozoa for each man ranged from 27.0 to 88.3% with the optimum treatment being variable between men: treatment A, E and F in one case each (max AR values 65.1, 49.9 and 76.0% respectively), treatment I in two cases (max AR values 72.8 and 84.8%), and treatment G in four cases (max AR values 27.0, 42.0, 51.9 and 88.3%). In no case was A23187 the most effective AR agonist, and in one case it caused a 97.8% loss of vitality.

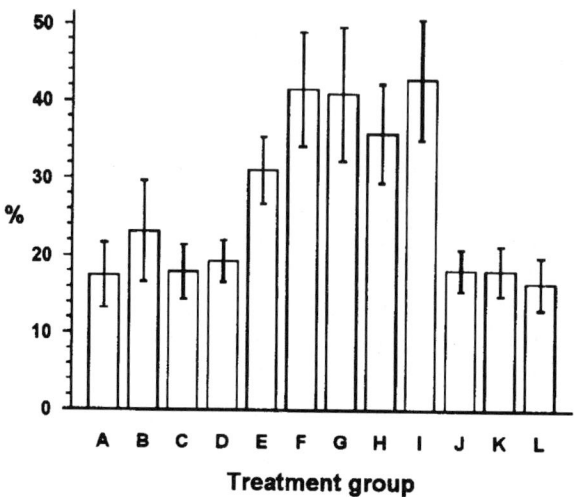

Figure 8: Optimized induction of acrosome reactions in live, capacitated spermatozoa from nine infertility patients using a range of treatments: *A = HTF medium control; B = HTF + 50% hFF x 6 h; C,D,E = HTF + dbcGMP at 1, 5 or 10 mM x 6 h; F = HTF + 50% hFF x 24 h; G,H,I = HTF + 50% hFF + dbcGMP at 1, 5 or 10 mM x 24 h; J = HTF at pH 8.4 + 1 mg/ml heparin + 1 mg/ml progesterone; K = 10 mM dbcGMP then HTF at pH 8.4 + 1 mg/ml heparin + 1 mg/ml progesterone; L = A23187 at 2.5 mM in DMSO. Values are mean ± SEM.*

OVERVIEW

Diagnostic value of AR testing

Although high levels of spontaneous AR loss have been associated with unexplained IVF fertilization failure (25), it has generally been concluded that assessment of spontaneous ARs is physiologically meaningless, and hence that the most informative diagnostic tests must use an appropriate biochemical inducer of the AR. The ideal inducer is the zona glycoprotein ZP3 but, until recombinant human ZP3 becomes commercially available, biological or biochemical agonists must be employed.

The hFF-induced AR assay is significantly associated with semen characteristics, and the frequency distribution of results differ markedly between fertile men and infertility patients (26). Such hFF-stimulated ARs have much greater prognostic value for IVF success than traditional semen characteristics (including Tygerberg morphology assessment) (27). Because hFF remains a biologically-derived material, only available with substantial intrinsic variability, it cannot be standardized, therefore rendering the achievement of technical quality control extremely difficult. Consequently, hFF as the AR agonist cannot be recommended for a standardized assay.

Progesterone (P) has been shown to induce significant increases in ARs in normospermic patients, but with no effect on spermatozoa from oligozoospermic men (28). Significantly lower AR rates after P challenge have been reported for patients showing IVF fertilization rates below 50%, with a significant correlation existing between fertilization rate and P-stimulated AR rate (29).

Unlike the HEPT, the AR response to A23187 shows only limited correlation with sperm kinematics (17). Consequently, AR induction assays cannot be used interchangeably with tests of sperm-oocyte fusion. A lack of response to A23187 has been associated with unexplained IVF fertilization failure by several groups (e.g. 15, 25, 30, 31), although some have found A23187 response to have poor practical value (32). This probably serves to emphasize the need for robust assay protocols with comprehensive quality control, such as has been established for the ARIC test.

Infertility patients with a high incidence of abnormal forms show a low spontaneous AR rate and a diminished P-stimulated AR response, although the "non-specific" response to A23187 is apparently conserved (33). However, whether this situation is due to dysfunction of the sperm P receptor and/or other membrane transduction systems remains unknown. Clinical significance also remains to be established these mechanisms have not yet been proven to cause defective fertilization. This illustrates the need to distinguish studies trying to elucidate cellular mechanisms from clinical studies where a relevant endpoint must be employed; it also provides further justification for using the real biological trigger of the AR rather than a, hopefully, unphysiological agonist.

Studies investigating a multitude of second messenger systems in attempts to elucidate specific aetiological lesions are also extremely premature. Not only does substantial crosstalk appear to exist between these systems, but we remain ignorant as to which are actually involved in the physiological AR. Although P does induce a transient rise in $[Ca^{2+}]_i$, a physiological role for P in inducing the AR remains unproved. However, we know that rises in both $[Ca^{2+}]_i$ and pH_i occur early in the AR process and, since both can be induced by A23187, ionophore treatment would seem to be the appropriate approach - although A23187 must be employed in a mild treatment protocol to minimize any direct toxic effect on the spermatozoa.

Pentoxifylline and the human sperm AR
Although pentoxifylline (POF) did not increase spontaneous AR rates, the response to A23187 may be significantly enhanced by pre-treatment with POF in control patients (34). This may also have been contributory to the very high AR levels seen in our own study described above.

Therapeutic induction of the human sperm AR
The clinical application of AR induction remains confused, especially if the fertilizing spermatozoon must undergo its AR on the ZP, after binding to the sperm receptor, ZP3. Artificial AR induction therefore seems to have no value, although capacitation promotion, so that spermatozoa which bind to the zona are optimally capable of undergoing an AR, may have clinical benefit. In this regard, the report that the fertilization rate of men with low ARIC results can be improved significantly by POF treatment demonstrates a rational application for POF treatment of spermatozoa in clinical IVF, provided that it is used carefully (23). Furthermore, because the greatest benefit has been reported for men whose ARIC results were improved by POF treatment (31), prior diagnostic investigation has a definite role.

Influence of sperm preparation methods
Finally, it is essential that spermatozoa either for diagnostic assessment or any clinical application must be prepared from semen in a non-traumatic way that avoids possible iatrogenic damage (e.g. free radical-induced membrane lipid peroxidation) that might impair their function (e.g. 35).

CONCLUSION

A clinical test employing a mild A23187-optimized AR assessment protocol seems to have excellent diagnostic value for identifying men at risk for sperm dysfunction, such as may be expressed either as prolonged idiopathic infertility or IVF fertilization failure. Furthermore, testing in conjunction with a controlled assessment of POF sperm pre-treatment will help identify those men whose AR dysfunction is amenable to simple pharmacological treatment at IVF. Standardized sperm preparation methods to avoid iatrogenic damage and optimize capacitation dynamics will help minimize the assay's variability due to intrinsic biological differences between men.

Acknowledgments
The author's unpublished work was supported by grant MA-9817 the Medical Research Council of Canada (13, 14, 16, 18, 21), and research funds from Sydney IVF (24).

REFERENCES

1. Yanagimachi R. Mammalian fertilization. In: Knobil E, Neill JD, eds. The Physiology of Reproduction. 2nd Ed. New York: Raven Press Ltd, 1994: 189-317.
2. Hunter RHF. Human fertilization in vivo, with special reference to progression, storage and release of competent spermatozoa. Hum Reprod 1987; 2: 329-332.
3. Aitken RJ, Buckingham DW, Fang HG. Analysis of the responses of human spermatozoa to A23187 employing a novel technique for assessing the acrosome reaction. J Androl 1993; 14: 132-141.
4. Van Duin M, Polman JEM, De Breet ITM, Van Ginneken K, Bunschoten H, Grootenhuis A, Brindle J, Aitken RJ. Recombinant human zona pellucida protein ZP3 produced by Chinese hamster ovary cells induces the human sperm acrosome reaction and promotes sperm-egg fusion. Biol Reprod 1994; 51: 607-617.
5. Mortimer D. Elaboration of a new culture medium for physiological studies on human sperm motility and capacitation. Hum Reprod 1986; 1: 247-250.
6. Mortimer D. Practical Laboratory Andrology. New York: Oxford University Press, 1994.
7. Mortimer D, Curtis EF, Camenzind AR, Tanaka S. The spontaneous acrosome reaction of human spermatozoa incubated in vitro. Hum Reprod 1989; 4: 57-62.
8. Zhu J, Barratt CLR, Lippes J, Pacey AA, Cooke ID. The sequential effects of human cervical mucus, oviductal fluid, and follicular fluid on sperm function. Fertil Steril 1994; 61: 1129-1135.
9. Liu DY, Baker HWG. Disordered acrosome reaction of spermatozoa bound to the zona pellucida: A newly discovered sperm defect causing infertility with reduced sperm-zona pellucida penetration and reduced fertilization in vitro. Hum Reprod 1994; 9: 1694-1700.
10. Mortimer D, Camenzind AR. The role of follicular fluid in inducing the acrosome reaction of human spermatozoa incubated in vitro. Hum Reprod 1989; 4: 169-174.
11. Tesarik J. Comparison of acrosome reaction-inducing activities of human cumulus oophorus, follicular fluid and ionophore A23187 in human sperm populations of proven fertilizing ability in vitro. J Reprod Fertil 1985; 74: 383-388.
12. Stock CE, Bates R, Lindsay KS, Edmonds DK, Fraser LR. Human oocyte-cumulus complexes stimulate the human acrosome reaction. J Reprod Fertil 1989; 86: 723-730.

13. Mortimer D, Camenzind AR. Human sperm-hamster cumulus coincubation and induction of the acrosome reaction. Ann Mtg Can Fertil Androl Soc, 1990.
14. Camenzind AR, Mortimer D. Intra-individual variability of human sperm acrosome reaction dynamics. Ann Mtg Can Fertil Androl Soc, 1990.
15. Cummins JM, Pember SM, Jequier AM, Yovich JL, Hartmann PE. A test of the human sperm acrosome reaction following ionophore challenge: Relationship to fertility and other seminal parameters. J Androl 1991; 12: 98-103.
16. Mortimer D. Évaluation de la réaction acrosomiale comme test de fécondance des spermatozoïdes humains. Contraception-Fertilité-Sexualité, 18: 552-553.
17. Aitken J, Buckingham D, Harkiss D. Analysis of the extent to which sperm movement can predict the results of ionophore-enhanced functional assays of the acrosome reaction and sperm-oocyte fusion. Hum Reprod 1994; 9: 1867-1874.
18. Mortimer D, Camenzind AR. Influence of extracellular pH upon the human sperm acrosome reaction. J Androl 1990; 11 (Suppl. 1): P-27.
19. Morales P, Llanos M, Gutierrez G, Kohen P, Vigil P, Vantman D. The acrosome reaction-inducing activity of individual human follicular fluid samples is highly variable and is related to the steroid content. Hum Reprod 1992; 7: 646-651.
20. Saaranen MJ, Calvo L, Dennison L, Banks S, Bustillo M, Dorfmann AD, Goldstein M, Thorsell L, Schulman JD, Sherins RJ. Acrosome reaction inducing activity in follicular fluid correlates with progesterone concentration but not with oocyte maturity or fertilizability. Hum Reprod 1993; 8: 1448-1454.
21. Mortimer D, Camenzind AR. The role of follicular fluid and glycosaminoglycans in the induction of the human sperm acrosome reaction in vitro. Serono Symposium "Gamete Biology", Newport Beach (USA), 1988.
22. Parinaud J, Vieitez G, Labal B, Richoilley G. Effect of sperm pre-treatments on the results of sub-zonal insemination (SUZI). Hum Reprod 1994; 9: 110-112.
23. Yovich JL. Pentoxifylline: Actions and applications in assisted reproduction. Hum Reprod 1993; 8: 1786-1791.
24. Mortimer D, Jones V. Optimized acrosome reaction induction in human spermatozoa. XI Ann Sci Mtg Fertil Soc Australia, 1992. Abstract 119FC.
25. Fénichel P, Basteris B, Donzeau M, Ayraud N, Farahifar D, Hsi BL. Dynamics of human sperm acrosome reaction: Relation with in vitro fertilization. Fertil Steril 1991; 55: 994-999.

26. Calvo L, Dennison-Lagos L, Banks SM, Sherins RJ. Characterization and frequency distribution of sperm acrosome reaction among normal and infertile men. Hum Reprod 1994; 9: 1875-1879.
27. Calvo L, Dennison-Lagos L, Banks SM, Dorfmann A, Thorsell LP, Bustillo M, Schulman JD, Sherins RJ. Acrosome reaction inducibility predicts fertilization success at in-vitro fertilization. Hum Reprod 1994; 9: 1880-1886.
28. Falsetti C, Baldi E, Krausz C, Casano R, Failli P, Forti G. Decreased responsiveness to progesterone of spermatozoa in oligozoospermic patients. J Androl 1993; 14: 17-22.
29. Krausz C, Bonaccorsi L, Luconi M, Fuzzi B, Criscuoli L, Pellegrini S, Forti G, Baldi E. Intracellular calcium increase and acrosome reaction in response to progesterone in human spermatozoa are correlated with in-vitro fertilization. Hum Reprod 1995; 10: 120-124.
30. Pampiglione JS, Tan SL, Campbell S. The use of the stimulated acrosome reaction test as a test of fertilizing ability in human spermatozoa. Fertil Steril 1993; 59: 1280-1284.
31. Yovich JM, Edirisinghe WR, Yovich JL. Use of the acrosome reaction to ionophore challenge test in managing patients in an assisted reproduction program: A prospective, double-blind, randomized controlled study. Fertil Steril 1994; 61: 902-910.
32. Parinaud J, Vieitez G, Moutaffian H, Richoilley G, Labal B. Relevance of acrosome function in the evaluation of semen in vitro fertilizing ability. Fertil Steril 1995; 63: 598-603.
33. Oehninger S, Blackmore P, Morshedi M, Sueldo C, Acosta AA, Alexander N. Defective calcium influx and acrosome reaction (spontaneous and progesterone-induced) in spermatozoa of infertile men with severe teratozoospermia. 1989). Fertil Steril 1994; 61: 349-354.
34. Tasdemir M, Tasdemir I, Kodama H, Tanaka T. Pentoxifylline-enhanced acrosome reaction correlates with fertilization in vitro. Hum Reprod 1993; 8: 2102-2107.
35. Mortimer D. Sperm preparation techniques and iatrogenic failures of invitro fertilization. Hum Reprod 1991; 6: 173-176.

Human sperm acrosome reaction. Eds P. Fénichel, J. Parinaud.
Colloque INSERM/John Libbey Eurotext Ltd © 1995. Vol. 236, pp. 315-325.

Acrosomal function and sperm fertilizing ability

Patrick Fénichel

Groupe de Recherche sur l'Interaction Gamétique, Faculté de Médecine, 06107 Nice Cedex 02, France

ABSTRACT

Evaluation of acrosomal status is a useful approach of sperm fertilizing ability. Acrosomal dysfunctions (abnormal forms, high spontaneous acrosome reaction (AR) and low induced AR, defectuous enzymatic activity) are associated with a decreased fertilizing ability. Such dysfunctions have been found in case of unexplained fertilization failures, or when the classical parameters were modified (asthenospermia, polyzoospermia, teratospermaia or frozen-thawed sperm). Inducible AR (induced minus spontaneous AR) seems to be the most informative test. Evaluation of acrosomal function can be of clinical interest to predict IVF results, to understand repeated fertilization failures, to evaluate male infertility and to choose therapies: pharmacological enhancement (follicular fluid, pentoxyfiline, adenosine) of capacitation or microinjection rather than conventional IVF.

L'évaluation du statut acrosomique représente une approche fonctionnelle et dynamique du pouvoir fécondant des spermatozoïdes. Ses anomalies (dysmorphie, taux élevé de réaction acrosomique (RA) spontanée et faible réponse de RA induite, activité enzymatique défectueuse) paraissent associées à une fécondance diminuée. Mais les milieux d'incubation, les inducteurs et les tests utilisés restent pour l'instant d'une telle diversité qu'il est parfois difficile de comparer entre eux les résultats. Ces anomalies sont retrouvées aussi bien dans les échecs inexpliqués de fécondation in vitro (FIV) qu'en cas d'altérations des paramètres classsiques (asthénospermie, polyzoospermie, tératospermie, congélation/ décongélation). Le taux de RA inductible (RA induite moins RA spontanée) en utilisant A23187, le liquide folliculaire, ou d'autres inducteurs, semble être le paramètre le plus informatif. En pratique l'appréciation de la fonction acrosomique est susceptible d'apporter un élément pronostique, de compréhension des échecs à répétition, et d'appréciation de la gravité d'une hypofertilité masculine. Elle permet d'envisager enfin dans certains cas une amélioration de la fécondance des spermatozoïdes in vitro par des agents pharmacologiques (liquide folliculaire, adénosine, pentoxyfiline) voire d'aider à l'abandon des tentatives de FIV classique pour les remplacer par des cycles de fécondation assistée.

ACROSOMAL FUNCTION AND MALE INFERTILITY

In all species from sea invertebrates to primates, fertilization includes an activation step at the contact with the egg's vestments. This calcium-dependent step called "acrosome reaction" (AR) stimulates the secretory granule which recovers the anterior part of the sperm head. This event allows the progression of the spermatozoa through the egg barriers (cumulus, zona pellucida, oolemma) by the action of specific receptors and/or hydrolases and proteases (1). In fact AR is an essential fertilization step as illustrated by male infertility associated with marked acrosome abnormalities (2). Patients with a majority of acrosomeless round-headed spermatozoa cannot conceive (3). Even sub-zonal insemination does not allow fusion. The only solution is to microinject directly this acrosomeless spermatozoon into the cytoplasma of the oocyte.

Evaluation of acrosomal function may be useful to accuretely appreciate male fertility and to understand apparent unexplained infertility and/or unsuccessfull IVF. This evaluation must be associated with a specific analysis of the other sperm functions (motility, capacitation, sperm-zona binding, sperm-oocyte fusion and nucleus decondensation). As mentionned before, AR is related to capacitation and to gametic interaction (zona and oolemma) but does not seem to be directly related to motility or to nucleus decondensation.

HOW TO EXPLORE ACROSOMAL FUNCTION?

This exploration implies morphological, dynamic and biochemical aspects. Capacitation which is a prerequest for AR has to be appreciated as well although the lack of simple tests (4). Morphological screening of the sperm acrosome can be done by classical staining. However fluorescent probes make it easier to appreciate some minor abnormalities (5-6) concerning the size, shape, regularity or density of the acrosome. Electronic microscopy has shown that even in normal fertile donors the frequency of acrosome modifications is high (7). The spontaneous acrosome reaction rate during incubation in a defined medium is physiologically low (8). Premature spontaneous AR prevents from binding to the zona pellucida. Induced AR rate has been proposed by many authors (9) as a good approach of acrosome function. Many inducers, culture media and times of incubation have been proposed. Ionophore calcum has been frequently used although far from physiological way. It by-passes part of the transductive mechanisms (1) involved in AR before calcium influx but it is a strong inducer with a good intraindividual reproductibility (Fig.1). Follicular fluid, progesterone, zona pellucida, phorbol esters, low temperature, freezing/thawing were also experimented (9-10). The most physiological approach will be the use of ZP3 recombinant as reported by Barratt et al. (11).

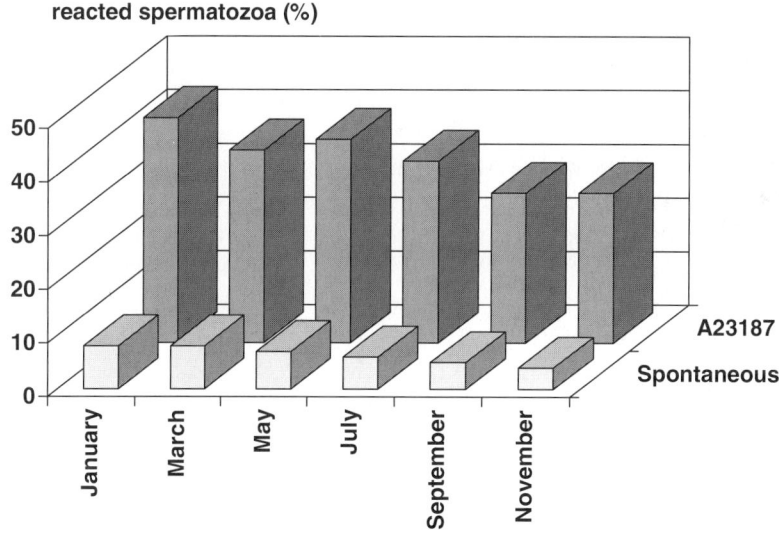

Figure 1: **Response to ionophore calcium: intra-individual variation**
Response to A23187 (10µM in B2 medium, 1 hour after 6 hours preincubation) has been reevaluated every two months during one year for the same fertile donor.

The method of quantification of AR is also important to consider as shown by Parinaud et al. (12) who compared PNA and GB24 mab (13). It is likely that all these methods do not screen exactly the same subpopulations. Enzymatic activity can be appreciated with a predetermined substrate as for acrosin (14). Physiological AR occurs after capacitation which has no morphogical substratum. Capacitation has been for a long time mesured by the rate of fertilization in a homo- or heterospecific test (15). A better knowledge of the biochemical mechanisms led to new ways of evaluation. The AR response to an inducer such as A23187 has been shown to be related to the state of capacitation (8,16). Fluorescent probes (mabs, lectins) may reflect the membrane's modifications. Chlortetracyclin becomes fluorescent when binding to the sperm membrane and can serve to differentiate the stages of capacitation (17). At least protein phosphorylation represents an other approach of capacitation (4). The heterospecific hamster test depends on several sperm functions (capacitation, AR, fusion and nucleus decondensation). Its results are indirectly dependent with capacitation and AR levels. Analysis of sperm specific proteins involved in the binding or in the transductive pathway will allow isolation of specific abnormalities as reported by Tesarik et al. (18) for the sperm progesterone receptor.

RELATION BETWEEN ACROSOMAL STATUS AND SPERM FERTILIZING ABILITY

Acrosome reaction and in vitro fertilization

In vitro fertilization represents a useful situation to evaluate the place of acrosome reaction in assessing fertilizing ability. Several groups have been able to differentiate the pattern of AR in relation with IVF as represented on table I. Although Plachot et al. (19) did not find any correlation with spontaneous AR after 17 h incubation in B2 medium, an exaggerated spontaneous premature AR seems to be deletereous (8, 20-21). The inducible sperm subpopulation (induced minus spontaneous AR) can be even more discriminative as reported by Cummins et al. (22), Fénichel et al. (8) or Henkel et al. (23). Neverthereless when considering an individual case can these acrosome tests be predictive? and are they more useful than the classical sperm parameters ? Several authors have pointed on the minimal inducible subpopulation using mostly A23187. For Pampiglione et al.(24) stimulated AR (A23187) < 31% increase in the number of reacted spermatozoa predicts fertilization failure in 100%. Cummins et al. (22) give the threshold to predict poor fertilization outcome in vitro 90% for I-S<5%. Henkel et al. (23) conclude that an inducibility (low temperature) < 7.5 % is indicative of subfertility. In a progressive discriminant analysis Parinaud et al. (21) reported that it was possible to predict up to 83 % of IVF results when associating spontaneous AR and acrosome response to TPA, to some parameters of motility and morphology. In this study A23187 induced AR did not seem however to have an additive predictive value.

Authors	Medium (incubation time)	Inducer	Acrosome reaction: spontaneous S induced I	Correlation
Plachot (19)	B2		S	No
Takahashi (20)	Tubal fluid (24h)		S	3 patterns
Fénichel (8)	B2 (6h)		S	P < 0.005
	B2 (6h)	A23187	I	P<0.05
	B2 (6h)	A23187	I-S	P<0.05
Cummins (22)	Tyrode (24h)		S	No
	Tyrode (24h)	A23187	I	P<0.01
	Tyrode (24h)	A23187	I-S	P<0.01
Henkel (23)	BWW (3h)	low tps	I	No
	BWW (3h)	low tps	I-S	P<0.05
Parinaud (21)	B2 (24h)		S	P<0.05
	B2 (24h)	A23187	I-S	P<0.001
	B2 (24h)	TPA	I-S	P<0.05

Table I: **Relation between acrosome reaction and in vitro fertilization**

Unexplained infertility or fertilizing failures

Acrosome function in case of unexplained infertility or failure of IVF has been studied by several groups . Calvo et al. (25) reported a low response of AR to follicular fluid in 12 cases out of 15 unexplained infertility. Koukoulis et al. (14) showed a decrease activity of acrosin in case of unexplained infertility. Fénichel et al. (8) found a subgroup of 5 out of 8 cases of repetitive unexplained failure of in vitro fertilization with a low response to ionophore calcium (Fig.2) and 8 out of 16 for Pampiglione et al. (24). Morphological or ultrastructural acrosomal abnormalities have been found in unexplained failures of IVF (26).

Acrosomal status and sperm abnormalities

Low induced AR found in cases of failure of IVF, suggests the responsability of acrosomal dysfunction although normal clinical sperm parameters are present. When sperm parameters are abnormal relation have been established with acrosomal function. In polyzoospermia Töpfer-Pedersen et al. (27) found an absence of spontaneous AR in vitro. Pillikian et al. (28) reported a decreased induced AR in asthenospermia. Moreover Oehninger et al. (29) described in male infertility with severe teratospermia a defective calcium influx and spontaneous and progesterone-induced AR. One of the most interesting predictive factor associated with IVF success in case of severe teratospermia (>70% abnormal forms) was found by Liu and Baker (6) to be the percentage of normal acrosomes monitored by fluorescent lectins.

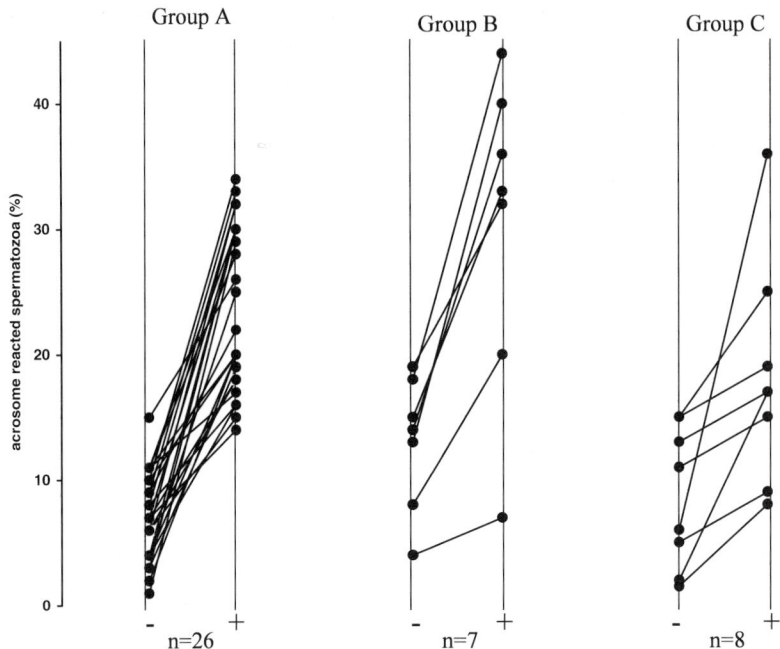

Figure 2: **Acrosome reaction and in vitro fertilization**
Spontaneous (-) and A23187-induced (+) acrosome loss have been evaluated after 6 hours incubation in B2 medium on the same sperm sample prepared for IVF. The results are expressed in percentages of positive acrosome-reacted spermatozoa. Three groups have been separated following the fertilization rate: group A>50% fertilization rate; group B<50%; group C, no fertilized oocytes.

Sperm donors and cryopreservation
Examination of fertility rates of semen donors with normal classical semen quality represents a very useful situation to evaluate the relation between sperm parmeters and fertilizing ability. Inseminations are usually performed in women who have no known infertility factors. Such a study has been reported by Marshburn et al. (30) who found a correlation between pregnancy rates and motility (P<0.04), abnormal forms (P<0.05) and AR induced by follicular fluid or progesterone(p<0.05). Several works in animals (31) and in humans (32-35) have pointed on the membrane damages associated to sperm freeezing/thawing with premature breakdown of the acrosome, thus explaining the reduced fertility potential of cryopreserved sperm.

Evaluation of acrosomal function
Screening for acrosome function (morphology, spontaneous and induced AR, enzymatic activity) gives useful informations about sperm fertilizing ability. However these exploration is associated with some difficulties such as the lack of standardization concerning culture media, inducers and the mode of evaluation of AR. The results are therefore difficult to compare. Centrifugations can also be very different from one protocol to another and be associated with sperm dammage. Acrosomal exploration must also be associated and integrated to the other sperm parameters. An inducer more physiological than A23187 must be choosen like progesterone or recombinant of ZP3.

THERAPEUTIC CONSEQUENCES

If evaluation of acrosomal function represents indeed an interesting approach of male infertility, does it realy help in therapeutic decisions? This evaluation does not seem to be useful before the first cycle of IVF because of its low individual predictive value but in case of unexplained failure it can suggest the pathological mechanism, contribute to make a prognosis and lead to a pharmacological improvement of sperm fertilizing ability. If acrosome abnormal forms are too predominant IVF has to be stopped and assisted fertilization can be proposed.
Fertile sperm donors include a low spontaneous AR rate and a high dynamic response. Induced minus spontaneous AR has a good predictive value in relation with physiological knowledge (8,36). Premature acrosome reacted spermatozoa can not bind to the zona pellucida. They must only be capacitated. Lipidic peroxydation can be evocated and in this case centrifugation must be very soft and protective agents can be tested. Two different causes may explain the absence of induced AR response: capacitation may be too slow or the transductive mechanisms leading to AR are abnormal. In the first case of slow capacitation, several physiological or pharmacological agents (follicular fluid, progesterone, pentoxyfiline, analogues of adénosine) have been proposed (37-38) which stimulate the membraneous or cytoplasmic mechanisms without inducing AR as shown on Fig3 . It is obviously necessary to demonstrate such an effect in vitro not only in a group of patients but in a specific individual case before its use in vivo. Tesarik et al. (37) have reported such an improvement by pentoxyfiline in a group of patients with low A2317 induced AR. With the same goal Tasdemir et al. (38) obtained an improvement in IVF rate after demonstrating that pretreatment with pentoxyfiline was usefull to enhance the induced response to A23187. When capacitation is not concerned and

AR cannot be induced, assisted fertilization(ICSI) must be preferred. AR assessment can be used to monitore damages induced by sperm freezing-thawing. This test can modulate the individual prognosis of pegnancy and techniques which try to protect the sperm membranes can be developped.

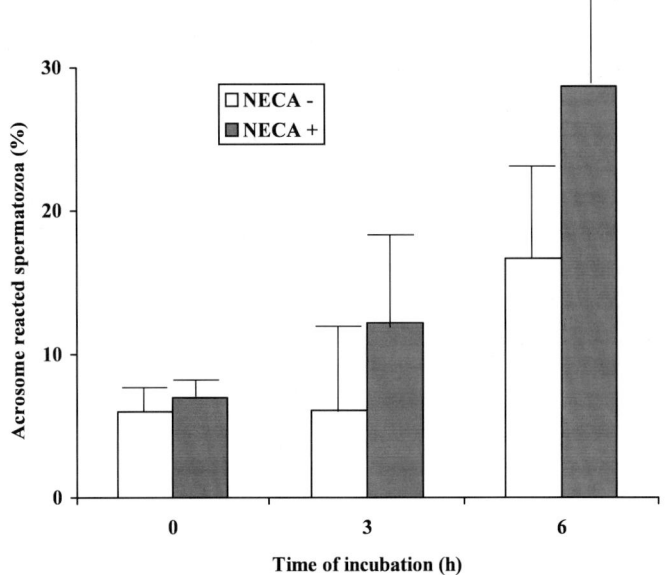

Figure 3: **Stimulation of capacitation in vitro by NECA an agonist of A2 adenosine receptors**
A23187-induced acrosome reaction (10 μM in B2 medium during 10 min) after 0, 3 or 6 h preincubation in B2. NECA (100 μM) has been added during the last 30 min of incubation in B2. N=10. Acrosome reaction has been evaluated by double staining (GB24-ethidium homodimere) and flow cytometry.

At least what are the goals of acrosomal evaluation ? In a practical point of view AR evaluation may give a predicive indication on the fertilizing ability, suggest an explanation in case of unexplained infertilities, help to improve capacitation by pharmacological agents and decide when prefer an assisted fertilization.

REFERENCES

1. Zanefeld L.J.D., Anderson R.A., Mack S.R., De Jonge C.J. Mechanism and control of the human sperm acrosome. Human Reprod 1993, 8:2007-2008

2. Schill WB Some disturbances of acrosomal development and function in human permatozoa. Human Reprod 1991, 8:969-978.
3. Jeyendran RS, Van Der Ven HH, Kennedy WP, Heath E, Perez-Pelaez M, Sobrero AJ, Zanefeld LJD: Acrosomeless sperm, a cause of primary male infertility. Andrologia 1976,17:31-35.
4. Fénichel P. Pourquoi et comment améliorer la capacitation sans induire la réaction acrosomique. Contracep Fertil Sex 1994, 22:321-326.
5. Cross NL, Meizel S: Methods for evaluating the acrosomal status of mammalian sperm. Biol Reprod 1989,41:635-640.
6. Liu DY, Baker GHW. The proportion of human sperm with poor morphology but normal intact acrosomes detected with pisum sativum agglutinin correlates wuth fertilization in vitro. Fertil Steril 1988, 50:288-293.
7. Bisson JP, David G, Magnin C. Etude ultrastructurale des anomalies de l'acrosome dans les spermatozoïdes à têtes irrégulière. Bull Ass Anatom 1975,
8. Fénichel P, Donzeau M, Farahifar D, Basteris B, Ayraud N, Hsi B. Dynamics of human sperm acrosome reaction: relation with in vitro fertilization. Fertil Steril 1991;55:994-999.
9. Wolf DP. Acrosomaal status quaantification in human sperm. Am J Reprod Immunol Microbiol 199, 20:106-111.
10. Tesarik J. Comparison of acrosome reaction-inducing activities of human cumulus oophorus, follicular fluid and ionophore A23187 in human sperm populations of proven fertilizing ability in vitro. J Reprod Fert 1985;74:383-388.
11. Barratt C.L.R. Modulation of human sperm function by follicular fluid, oviductal fluid and recombinant human ZP3, British Aandrology Society, London, 24th and 25th September 1993.
12. Parinaud J, Labal B, Vieitez G, Richoilley G, Grandjean H, Comparison between fluorescent peanut agglutinin lectin and GB24 antibody techniques for the assessment of the acrosomal status; Hum Reprod 1993, 8:1685-1689.
13. Fénichel P., Hsi B.L., Farahifar D., Donzeau M., Barrier-Delpech D., Yeh C.J.G.: Evaluation of the human sperm acrosome reaction using a monoclonal antibody, GB24, and fluorescence-activated cell sorter. J Reprod Fertil 1989, 87:699-706
14. Koukoulis G.N., Vantman D., Dennison L, Banks S.M., Sherins R.J. Low acrosin in a subgroup of men with idiopathic infertility does nor t correlate with sperm density, percent motility, curvilinearity. Fertil Steril 1989, 52:120-127.
15. Perreault SD, Rogers BJ. Capacitation pattern of human spermatozoa. Fertil Steril 1982, 38:258-263.

16. Byrd W, Wolf DP. Acrosomal status in fresh and capacitated human ejaculated sperm. Biol Reprod 1986, 34: 859-869.
17. Lee MA, Trucco GS, Bechtol KB, Wummer N, Kopf GS, Blasco L, Storey BT. Capacitation and acrosome reaction in huaman spermatozoa monitored by a chlortetracycline fluorescence assay. Fertil Steril 1987, 48: 649-658.
18. Tesarik J, Mendoza C. Defective function of a non genomic progesterone receptors as a sole anomaly in infertile patients. Fertil Steril 1992, 38:793-797.
19. Plachot M, Mandelbaum J, Junca AM. Acrosome reaction of human sperm used for in vitro fertilization. Fertil Steril 1984, 42:418-423.
20. Takahashi K, Wetzels AMM, Bastiaans BA, Janssen HJG, Rolland R. The kinetics of the acrosome reaction of human spermatozoa and its correlation with in vitro fertilization. Fertil Steril 1992;57:889-8894.
21. Parinaud J., Moutaffian H., Vieitez G., Richoiley G., Labal B. Relevance of acrosome function in the evaluation of semen in vitro fertilizing ability. Fertil Steril 1995; 63:598-603.
22. Cummins JM, Pember SM, Jequier AM, Yovitch JL, Hartmann PE. A test of the human sperm acrosome reaction following ionophore challenge; Relationship to fertility and other seminal parameters. J Androl 1991, 2:98-103.
23. Henkel R., Müller C., Miska W., Gips H., Schill W.B. Determination of the acrosome reaction in huamn spermatozoa is predictive of fertilization in vitro. Hum Reprod 1993, 8:2128-2132.
24. Pampiglione J.S., Tan S.L., Campbell S. The use of the stimulated acrosome test as a test of fertilizing ability in human spermatozoa. Fertil Steril 1993, 59:1280-84.
25. Calvo L, Vantman D, Banks SM, Tezon J, Koukoulis GN, Dennison L, Sherins RJ: Follicular fluid-induced acrosome reaction distinguishes a subgroup of men with unexplained infertility not identified by semen analysis. Fertil Steril 1989, 52:1048.
26. Jeulin C, Feneux D, Serres C, Jouannet P, Guillet-Rosso F, Belaisch-Allart J, Frydman R, Testart J: Sperm factors related to failure of human in vitro fertilization. J Reprod Fertil 1986, 76:1.
27. Töpfer-Pedersen E, Heissler E, Schill WB: The kinetic of acrosome reaction: an additional sperm parameter. Andrologia 1985, 17:224.
28. Pillikian S., Guérin J.F., Adeleine P., Ecochard R. Czyba J.C. Spontaneous and ionophore induced acrosome reaction in asthenozoospermic infertile semen. Human Reprod 1992, 7:991-992.
29. Oehninger S., Blackmore P., Morshedi M., Sueldo C., Acosta A.A., Alexander N.J. Defective calcium influx and acrosome reaction

(spontaneous and progesterone-induced) in spermatozoa of infertile men with severe teratospermia. Fertil Steril 1994, 61:349-354.
30. Marshburn PB, Stovall DW, Hammond MG, talbert LM, Shabanowitz RB. Fertility rates in men with normal semen characteristics: spermatozoal testing by induction of the acrosome reaction and Wright-Giemsa staining for subtle abnormal forms. Obstet Gynecol 1991, 77:250-255.
31. Farlin ME, Jasko DJ, Graham JK, Squires EL. Assessment of pisum sativum agglutinin in identifying acrosomal damage in stallion spermatozoa. Mol Reprod Dev 1992, 32:23-27.
32. Centola GM, Mattox JH, Burde S, Leary JF. Assessment of the viability and acrosome status of fresh and frozen-thawed human opermatozoa using single-wavelength fluorescence microscopy. Mol Reprod Dev 1990, 27:130-135.
33. Cross NL, Hanks SE. Effects of cryopreservation in human sperm acrosomes Human Reprod 1991, 6:1279-1283.
34. Emiliozzi C, Vittori Ch, Donzeau M, Samson M, Fehlmann M, Fénichel P. Evaluation par double marquage de la réaction acrosomique (RA) spontanée et de la viabilité des spermatozoïdes après congélation-décongélation. Communication aux 6ième Journées Nationales de Périconceptologie: Lyon, 14-16 Mai 1992.
35. Mc Laughlin EA, Ford WCL, Hill MGR. Effects of cryopreservation on the human sperm acrosome and its response to A23187. J Reprod Fertil 1993, 99:71-76.
36. Tesarik J: Appropriate timing of the acrosome reaction is a major requirement for the fertilizing spermatozoon. Hum Reprod 1989, 4:95.
37. Tesarik J., Mendoza C. Sperm treatment with pentoxifylline improves the fertilizing ability in patients with acrosome reaction insufficiency; Fertil Steril 1993, 60:141-148.
38. Tasdemir M, Tasdemir I, Kodama H, Tanaka T. Pentoxifyline-enhanced acrosome reaction correlates with fertil ization in vitro Hum Reprod 1993, 8:2102-2107.

Physiopathology of acrosome dysfunctions

F.M. Köhn, R. Henkel, K.F. El-Mulla, W.B. Schill

Department of Dermatology and Andrology, Justus Liebig University, Giessen, Germany

Abstract

Human sperm acrosome dysfunctions include acrosomal malformations, pathological spontaneous or induced acrosome reaction, and decreased acrosin activity. Examples of specific acrosomal defects are the syndrome of round-headed spermatozoa (globozoospermia), the crater defect syndrome, the syndrome of decapitated spermatozoa and the "miniacrosome" sperm defect syndrome. Non-specific alterations show a variety of acrosomal malformations, often in combination with other morphological disorders of the spermatozoon. The inducibility of the acrosome reaction, which is of predictive value for the fertilizing capacity of spermatozoa, depends on the stimuli used and may by influenced by sperm malformations or environmental factors. Acrosin activity may be reduced in semen samples from patients with severe teratozoospermia, polyzoospermia or varicoceles.

Les dysfonctions de l'acrosome de spermatozoïde humain peuvent être des malformations de l'acrosome, une réaction acrosomique spontanée ou induite pathologique, ou encore une baisse de l'activité acrosine. Il existe des pathologies de l'acrosome spécifiques telles que le syndrome des têtes rondes (globozoospermies), les syndromes du cratère ou des spermatozoïdes décapités ou encore celui des miniacrosomes. D'autre part des altérations non spécifiques sont variées et souvent associées à d'autres altérations morphologiques des spermatozoïdes. L'inductibilité de la réaction acrosomique, paramètre prédictif de la capacité fécondante du spermatozoïde, dépend des stimuli utilisés et peut être influencée par des anomalies du spermatozoïde ou par des facteurs environnementaux.

L'activité acrosine peut être diminuée chez les patients atteints de tératozoospermie ou de polyspermie ou porteurs de varicocèle.

INTRODUCTION

The human sperm acrosome reaction is an exocytotic process which leads to the release of the acrosomal content after fusions of the plasma and outer acrosomal membranes (1). Since physiological fertilization of the oocyte requires acrosome reacted spermatozoa, the assessment of acrosomal morphology, spontaneous and induced acrosome reaction and the detection of acrosin provide important information about human sperm functions. Before intracytoplasmic sperm injection (ICSI) was established, acrosome or acrosin defects caused definitive male infertility.

MORPHOLOGICAL ACROSOME DEFECTS

Acrosomal defects become manifest as specific defects with complete absence of the acrosome or as non-specific alterations showing a variety of acrosomal malformations which are often associated with other morphological disorders of the spermatozoon (2). Examples of specific acrosomal defects (3) are the syndrome of round-headed spermatozoa (globozoospermia), the crater defect syndrome, the syndrome of decapitated spermatozoa and the "miniacrosome" sperm defect (4).

The occurrence of exclusively round-headed spermatozoa was first discussed by Meyhöfer (5). This specific acrosomal defect is caused by a disturbed differentiation of the nuclear-perinuclear skeletal complex (6) during spermatohistogenesis, when the acrosomal vesicle originating from the Golgi region differentiates independently from the nucleus (7). Spermatozoa without acrosomes contain no acrosin (8) or only traces (9) and are unable to fuse with zona-free hamster oocytes (9) or human oocytes after subzonal injection (10). In addition, they are incapable of binding to the human zona pellucida (11). However, round-headed spermatozoa are able to decondense (12).

Recent studies reported pregnancies achieved after microinjection with spermatozoa from patients with globozoospermia (13).

The crater defect syndrome is characterized by nuclear and acrosomal invaginations of all spermatozoa with normal tail structures (14). During spermatohistogenesis, the development and elongation of the sperm head seem to be disturbed. Due to the missing equatorial segment infertility is likely.

Decapitated spermatozoa can easily be identified under the light microscope, because the region where the head is expected shows only cytoplasmic thickenings which correpond to midpieces and mitochondria (2). Although decapitated spermatozoa usually have good progressive motility, they are not able to fertilize oocytes. This defect is caused by a dissociation between the proximal and distal centrioles during the first step of spermatid differentiation (15). It demonstrates that the sperm tail can differentiate independently of the nuclear development.

The "miniacrosome" sperm defect (4) was described in two infertile brothers. All spermatozoa of the ejaculates were devoid of equatorial segments and postacrosomal sheaths, whereas the acrosome was small and cup-like or absent in some cases. These spermatozoa are not able to bind to the oolemma or to fuse with zona-free hamster oocytes.

While specific acrosomal defects are rarely observed in andrological patients, non-specific acrosomal sperm disorders are of greater clinical importance. Atypical acrosomes have also been reported to occur during aging spermatogenesis (16). The majority of spermatozoa that are bound to the human zona pellucida and oolemma are morphologically normal (17).
Spermatozoa with minor acrosomal disturbances show good penetration rates in the zona-free hamster oocyte penetration test, whereas severe acrosomal malformations cause a significant reduction of oocyte penetration (18). Sperm morphology and the proportion of spermatozoa with normal intact acrosomes were demonstrated to be of prognostic value for the outcome of in vitro fertilization (19, 20). Oehninger et al. (21) concluded that patients with severe head abnormalities have a lower ability to achieve successful pregnancies in IVF programs. This may be due to the fact that spermatozoa with acrosomal defects have decreased rates of spontaneous, progesterone- or human follicular fluid-induced acrosome reaction (22-24). In contrast, acrosome reacted spermatozoa in samples with severe acrosomal malformations showed normal acrosomal regions. Using a monoclonal antibody against human pro-acrosin to stain the acrosomal principal region of human spermatozoa, Albert et al. (25) found IVF failures to be correlated with an increased number of acrosomes showing reduced size of this region which is involved in the acrosome reaction. However, since even severe sperm malformations do not influence fertilization and pregnancy rates after ICSI (26), this procedure can be recommended in cases of male infertility related to morphological disorders.

SPONTANEOUS AND INDUCED HUMAN SPERM ACROSOME REACTION

A variety of artificial and physiological stimuli have been reported to induce the human sperm acrosome reaction in vitro (1). While the spontaneous acrosome reaction does not correlate with the fertilization rates in IVF programs (27), the inducibility of acrosome reaction (i.e. difference between induced and spontaneous acrosome reaction) by calcium ionophore A 23187 (28-30), human follicular fluid (31) and low-temperature (32) is of prognostic value for sperm fertilization capacity.

Henkel et al. (32) demonstrated that patients with less than 13.0% acrosome reacted spermatozoa and less than 7.5% inducible acrosome reaction have significant lower fertilization rates in IVF programs (Fig.1, Table 1). The inducibility of acrosome reaction, however, depends on the stimulus used.

	LIMITING VALUE			
	2.5%	**5%**	**7.5%**	**10%**
Sensitivity	8.3%	25.0%	50.0%	70.8%
Specificity	98.0%	92.0%	86.0%	66.0%
Pos. pred. value	66.6%	60.0%	63.1%	50.0%
neg. pred. value	69.0%	71.8%	78.2%	82.5%

Table 1: **Various limiting values of the inducibility of the AR** *(difference between test value of AR after low temperature induction and the spontaneous AR) to predict the fertilizing capacity of spermatozoa from different patients*

Table 2 demonstrates that spermatozoa from andrological patients (n=50) do not respond uniformly to different acrosome reaction inducers after capacitation for 18 hours at 37°C. The numbers (mean±SEM) of acrosome reacted spermatozoa in PBS- and DMSO-treated controls were similar.

Treatment with ionophore, progesterone, phorbolmyristate acetate (PMA), pentoxifylline (Ptx), dbcAMP and low temperature markedly increased the percentages of acrosome reacted spermatozoa. Significant positive correlations were found among the numbers of acrosome reacted spermatozoa after induction by the various stimuli (Table 3). Highest correlations were found between progesterone and ionophore, progesterone and PMA, Progesterone and dbcAMP, dbcAMP and PMA, dbcAMP and ionophore, Ptx and cold-treatment, Ptx and PMA. However, only 18 of 50 patients (36%) responded uniformly to all inducers with an increase of acrosome reaction of at least 5%. Best responses were found after treatment with ionophore and cold. Most non-responders were observed after incubation with progesterone (14/50=28%), dbcAMP (16/50=32%) and PMA (9/50=18%).

FIG 1A

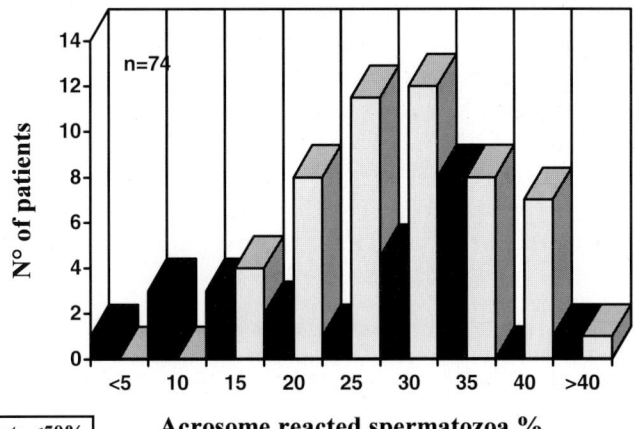

■ Fert. rate <50%
□ Fert. rate >50%

FIG 1B

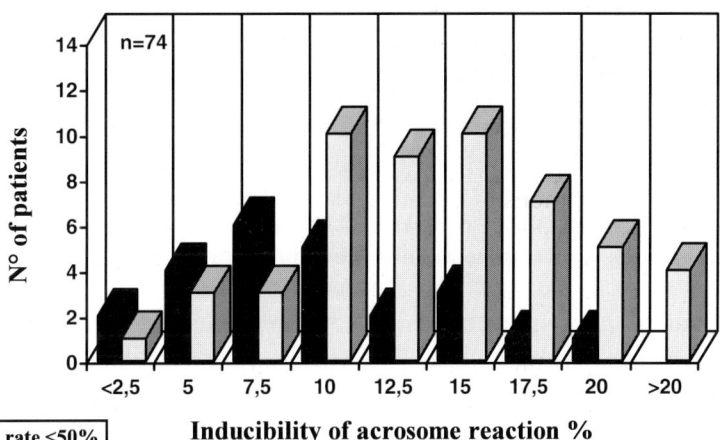

■ Fert. rate <50%
□ Fert. rate >50%

Figure 1: **Correlation of the number of patients to the percentage of acrosome reacted spermatozoa after low temperature induction (A) and to the inducibility of AR (B)**

All studies about the inducibility of acrosome reaction should consider the high degree of inter- and intrasubject variability of acrosome reaction in both patients and fertile donors; the time of sexual abstinence does not seem to have a significant effect (33).

INDUCTION	DOSAGE	N	LIVING ACROSOME REACTED SP (% MEAN ± SEM)
Control (PBS)	-	50	13.2 ± 1.0
Control (DMSO)	0.1%	50	12.8 ± 0.9
Progesterone	10 µM	50	21.0 ± 1.3
PMA	10 µM	50	21.7 ± 1.4
dbcAMP	1 mM	50	21.1 ± 1.3
Cold	-	50	24.9 ± 1.1
Ptx	1 mg/ml	50	25.0 ± 1.2
A23187	10 µM	50	28.1 ± 1.3

Table 2: **Induction of acrosome reaction by different inducers.**
Compared to the corresponding controls, the numbers of acrosome reacted spermatozoa (p<0.001) higher after treatment with the inducers. The differences between progesterone and A23187, PMA and A23187 and dbcAMP and A23187 were statistically significant (p<0.05)

	PROGESTERONE	PMA	DBCAMP	COLD	PTX
A 23187	r = 0.67	r = 0.58	r = 0.69	r = 0.52	r = 0.47
Ptx	r = 0.44	r = 0.62	r = 0.44	r = 0.85	
Cold	r = 0.38	r = 0.58	r = 0.48		
dbcAMP	r = 0.63	r = 0.72			
PMA	r = 0.70				

Table 3: **Spearman rank correlations between the percentages of living acrosome reacted spermatozoa after induction by various stimuli.**

Pathological inducibility (< 7.5%) of acrosome reaction after cold treatment (32) is reproducible in the majority of tests. When semen samples of 29 andrological patients with reduced inducibility were investigated a second time, inducibility of acrosome reaction was found reproducibly decreased in 86.2% (25/29).

As mentioned previously, human sperm acrosome reaction may be affected in spermatozoa with head malformations. Acrosome reaction and acrosin activity seem also to be decreased in polyzoospermic patients (34). In addition, other factors such as smoking or environmental toxins may impair human sperm acrosome reaction (35,36). Whereas the percentages of spontaneously acrosome reacted spermatozoa do not show significant differences between fertile men (n=20, 9.5±2.7%) and smokers (n=30, 10.3

± 3.2%), the inducibility of acrosome reaction was markedly lower in spermatozoa from smokers (7.1 ± 3.2% vs 11.5 ± 4.4%, p<0.05, Fig.2). Even after exclusion of all smokers with oligozoospermia (n=10), the differences of inducible AR between smokers and fertile men were still obvious (7.6 ± 3.0% vs 11.5 ± 4.4%, p<0.05).

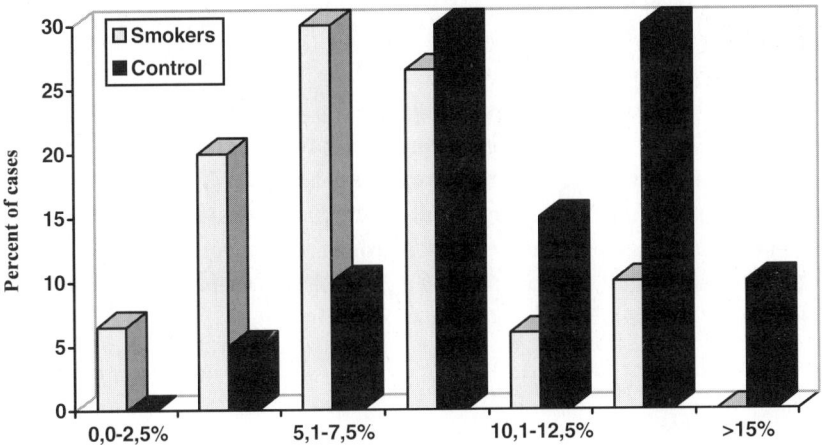

Figure 2: **Inducibility of acrosome reaction (AR):** *AR was induced by 10µM ionophore A23187 (1h, 37°C) after 3 h capacitation at 37°C. The percentages of induced acrosome reaction were calculated by substrating the percentages of spontaneous AR from that obtained after incubation with ionophore.*

Environmental factors may also affect human sperm acrosome reaction. Spermatozoa from healthy donors (n=7) were exposed to 0.5 µM, 5 µM, 50 µM, 500 µM and 1 mM platinic chloride (35). After 3 and 6 hours at 37°C, viability, membrane integrity and acrosome reaction were examined by trypan blue, hypoosmotic swelling test and fluoresceinated pisum sativum agglutinin, respectively (Table 4). While sperm motility, viability and membrane integrity were not affected after 3 hours, acrosome reaction increased from 16.0±6.4% (control, mean±SEM) to 22.3±4.3% (5 µM), 28.0±4.3% (50 µM, p<0.01), 29.3±3.9% (500 µM, p<0.01) and 43.9±7.4% (1mM, p<0.001).

In summary, platinic chloride induces human sperm acrosome reaction after 3 hours before cytotoxic effects are measurable and, therefore, seems to induce exocytotic processes in human spermatozoa.

H_2PtCL_6 (μM)	MOTILITY (%)	DEAD SPERMATOZOA (%)	HOST TEST POSITIVE (%)	ACROSOME REACTION (%)
1000	60.1 ± 6.5	25.1 ± 4.5	90.6 ± 2.3	43.9 ± 7.4 [a]
500	62.0 ± 7.2	18.4 ± 4.7	89.9 ± 2.8	29.3 ± 3.9 [b]
50	68.7 ± 4.7	14.9 ± 4.4	87.6 ± 4.2	28.0 ± 4.3 [b]
5	70.0 ± 4.9	15.7 ± 4.5	90.9 ± 2.9	22.3 ± 4.3 [b,c]
0.5	70.3 ± 6.2	13.4 ± 3.7	91.4 ± 2.9	21.0 ± 3.3 [b,c]
Control	69.1 ± 5.8	15.4 ± 4.3	91.0 ± 3.1	16.0 ± 2.4 [c]

Table 4: **Effect of hydrogen hexachlroplatinate (H_2PTCL_6) on motility, viability, membrane integrity and acrosome reaction of human spermatozoa in seminal plasma after 3 hours of incubation.** *Ejaculates of semen donors (n=7) were mixed (1:50) with various stock of hydrogen hexachlroplatinate to obtain final concentrations of 1000, 500, 50, 5 and 0.5 μM. Values (mean ± SEM) with the same superscript in each column do not differ significantly.*

ACROSIN ACTIVITY

Acrosin, a serine proteinase, is essential for binding to and penetration through the zona pellucida and seems to be involved in capacitation and acrosome reaction (37). Acrosin activity is correlated with the IVF outcome (38,39). No acrosin activity or only traces can be measured in men with round-headed spermatozoa (8,9). The acrosin activity is also reduced in semen samples with polyzoospermia and severe teratozoospermia, including the syndrome of decapitated spermatozoa (40). In most other sperm populations, acrosin activity is normal. However, a wide overlap of the range of acrosin levels is seen in most andrological groups (3). Factors that may affect acrosin activity are the time of sexual abstinence (40) and varicoceles (36). When gelatinolysis was used for measurement of acrosin activity, the mean diameters of halos were found to be significantly smaller in patients with varicoceles (16.1±6.6μM vs 26.1±17.7, $p<0.05$); a lower number of spermatozoa in this group showed halos (53.5±20.0% vs 75.2±13.5%, $p<0.01$) than those in semen samples from fertile donors.

CONCLUSION

Male sperm acrosomal dysfunctions include different defects of the acrosome morphology and special acrosomal functions such as acrosome reaction and acrosin activity. The detection of these disorders helps to discriminate between fertile and infertile patients and provides important information for diagnostic and therapeutic procedures.

REFERENCES

1. Zaneveld LJD, De Jonge CJ, Anderson RA, Mack SR. Human sperm capacitation and the acrosome reaction. Hum Reprod 1991;6:1265-75.
2. Schill WB. Acrosomal disturbances causing male infertility. In: Holstein AF, Leidenberger F, Hölzer KH, Bettendorf G, eds. Carl Schirren Symposium: Advances in andrology. Berlin: Diesbach, 1988:35-46.
3. Schill WB. Some disturbances of acrosomal development and function in human spermatozoa. Hum Reprod 1991;6:969-78.
4. Baccetti B, Burrini AG, Collodel G, Magnano AR, Piomboni P, Renieri T. A "miniacrosome" sperm defect causing infertility in two brothers. J.Androl 1991;12:104-11.
5. Meyhöfer W. Beiträge zur cytophotometrischen Beurteilung pathogenetisch veränderter Samenzellen unter besonderer Berücksichtigung der Rundkopf spermatozoen nach Feulgen und Fastgreenfärbung. Z Haut Geschlechtskr 1965;39:174-82.
6. Escalier D. Failure of differentiation of the nuclear-perinuclear skeletal complex in the round-headed human spermatozoa. Int J Dev Biol 1990;34:287-90.
7. Holstein AF, Schirren C, Schirren CG. Human spermatids and spermatozoa lacking acrosomes. J Reprod Fertil 1973;35:289-91.
8. Schill WB. Quantitative determination of acrosin activity in human spermatozoa. Fertil Steril 1974;25:703-12.
9. Jeyendran RS, van der Ven HH, Kennedy WP, Heath E, Perez-Pelaez M, Sobrero AJ, Zaneveld LJD. Acrosomeless sperm. A case of primary male infertility. Andrologia 1985;17:31-6.
10. Dale B, Iaccarino M, Fortunato A, Gragnaniello G, Kyozuka K, Tosti E. A morphological and functional study of fusibility in round-headed spermatozoa in the human. Fertil Steril 1994;61:336-40.
11. Aitken RJ, Kerr L, Bolton V, Hargreave T. Analysis of sperm function in globozoospermia: implications for the mechanism of sperm-zona interaction. Fertil Steril 1990;54:701-7.

12. Lanzendorf S, Maloney M, Ackerman S, Acosta A, Hodgen G. Fertilizing potential of acrosome-defective sperm following microsurgical injection into eggs. Gamete Res 1988;19:329-37.
13. Liu J, Nagy Z, Joris H, Tournaye H, Devroey P, Van Steirteghem A. Successful fertilization and establishment of pregnancies after intracytoplasmic sperm injection in patients with globozoospermia. Hum Reprod 1995;10:626-9.
14. Baccetti B, Burrini AG, Collodel G, Magnano AR, Piomboni P, Renieri T, Sensini C. Crater defect in human spermatozoa. Gamete Res 1989;22:249-55.
15. Holstein AF, Schill WB, Breucker H. Dissociated centriole development as a cause of spermatid malformation in man. J Reprod Fertil 1986;78:719-25.
16. Holstein AF. Spermatogenese im Alter - ein Grenzgebiet zwischen normaler und pathologischer Anatomie. Urologe A 1986;25:130-7.
17. Liu DY, Baker HWG. Acrosome status and morphology of human spermatozoa bound to the zona pellucida and oolemma determined using oocytes that failed to fertilize in vitro. Hum Reprod 1994;9:673-9.
18. Heywinkel E. Kapazitierung und Oozytenpenetration der Spermatozoen. Gynäkologe 1985;18:92-7.
19. Kruger TF, Acosta AA, Simmons KF, Swanson RJ, Matta JF, Oehninger S. Predictive value of abnormal sperm morphology in in vitro fertilization. Fertil Steril 1988;49:112-7.
20. Liu DY, Baker HWG. Relationships between human sperm acrosin, acrosomes, morphology and fertilization in vitro. Hum Reprod 1990;5:298-303.
21. Oehninger S, Acosta AA, Morshedi M, Veeck L, Swanson RJ, Simmons K, Rosenwaks Z. Corrective measures and pregnancy outcome in in vitro fertilization in patients with severe morphology abnormalities. Fertil Steril 1988;50:283-7.
22. Fukuda M, Morales P, Overstreet JW. Acrosomal function of human spermatozoa with normal and abnormal head morphology. Gamete Res 1989;24:59-65.
23. Heywinkel E, Freundl G, Hofmann N. Acrosome reaction of spermatozoa with different morphology. Andrologia 1993;25:137-9.
24. Oehninger S, Blackmore P, Morshedi M, Sueldo C, Acosta AA, Alexander NJ. Defective calcium influx and acrosome reaction (spontaneous and progesterone-induced) in spermatozoa of infertile men with severe teratozoospermia. Fertil Steril 1994;61:349-54.
25. Albert M, Gallo JM, Escalier D, Parseghian N, Jouannet P, Schrevel J, David G. Unexplained in-vitro fertilization failure: implication of

acrosomes with a small reacting region, as revealed by a monoclonal antibody. Hum Reprod 1992;7:1249-56.
26. Nagy ZP, Liu J, Joris H, Verheyen G, Tournaye H, Camus M, Derde MP, Devroey P, Van Steirteghem AC. The result of intracytoplasmic sperm injection is not related to any of the three basic sperm parameters. Hum Reprod 1995;10:1123-9.
27. Plachot M, Mandelbaum J, Junca AM. Acrosome reaction of human sperm used for in vitro fertilization. Fertil Steril 1984;42:418-23.
28. Fénichel P, Donzeau M, Farahifar D, Basteris B, Ayraud N, Hsi BL. Dynamics of human sperm acrosome reaction: relation with in vitro fertilization. Fertil Steril 1991;55:994-9.
29. Cummins JM, Pember SM, Jequier AM, Yovich JL, Hartmann PE. A test of the human sperm acrosome reaction following ionophore challenge. J Androl 1991;12:98-103.
30. Sukcharoen N, Keith J, Irvine DS, Aitken RJ. Predicting the fertilizing potential of human sperm suspensions in vitro: importance of sperm morphology and leucocyte contamination. Fertil Steril 1995;63:1293-1300.
31. Calvo L, Vantman D, Banks SM, Tezon J, Koukoulis GN, Dennison L, Sherins RJ. Follicular fluid-induced acrosome reaction distinguishes a subgroup of men with unexplained infertility not identified by semen analysis. Fertil Steril 1989;52:1048-54.
32. Henkel R, Müller C, Miska W, Gips H, Schill WB. Determination of the acrosome reaction in human spermatozoa is predictive of fertilization in vitro. Hum Reprod 1993;8:2128-32.
33. Troup SA, Lieberman BA, Matson PL. The acrosome reaction to ionophore challenge test: assay reproducibility, effect of sexual abstinence and results of fertile men. Hum Reprod 1994;9:2079-83.
34. Töpfer-Petersen E, Völcker C, Heissler E, Schill WB. Absence of acrosome reaction in polyzoospermia. Andrologia 1987;19:225-8.
35. Köhn FM, Schill WB, Schuppe HC, Jeyendran RS. Hydrogen hexachloroplatinate induces human sperm acrosome reaction. Int J Androl; in press.
36. El-Mulla KF, Köhn FM, El-Beheiry AH, Schill WB. The effect of smoking and varicoceles on human sperm acrosin activity and acrosome reaction. Hum Reprod (Abstract Book 2) 1995;10:10.
37. De Jonge CJ, Mack SR, Zaneveld LJD. Inhibition of the human sperm acrosome reaction by proteinase inhibitors. Gamete Res 1989;23:387-97.
38. Bielfeld P, Krüssel JS, von Eckardstein S, Mikat-Drodzynski B, Moustafa M, Fenkes G, Schuppe HC. Does the total acrosin activity of

human spermatozoa add additional information regarding IVF outcome? Hum Reprod (Abstract Book 2) 1995;10:96-7.
39. Henkel R, Müller C, Miska W, Schill WB, Kleinstein J, Gips H. Determination of the acrosin activity of human spermatozoa by means of a gelatinolytic technique. A simple, predictive method useful for IVF. J Androl 1995; 16:272-7.
40. Schill WB. Determination of active, non-zymogen acrosin, proacrosin and total acrosin in different andrological patients. Arch Dermatol Res 1990;282:335-42.

Human sperm acrosome reaction. Eds P. Fénichel, J. Parinaud.
Colloque INSERM/John Libbey Eurotext Ltd © 1995. Vol. 236, pp. 339-353.

Mechanisms and prevention of lipid peroxidation in human spermatozoa

John Aitken

MRC Reproductive Biology Unit, 37 Chalmers Street, Edinburgh EH3 9EW, Scotland

Abstract

Human spermatozoa are extremely susceptible to oxidative stress because of their high polyunsaturated fatty acid content and relative lack of antioxidant protection. In addition, these cells are constantly subjected to oxidative attack originating from without, in the case of leucocytes, or from within, in view of the spermatozoon's innate capacity to generate reactive oxygen species, including superoxide anion and hydrogen peroxide. The endogenous production of such molecules appears to reflect their role in the capacitation of human spermatozoa, via mechanisms including the stimulation of tyrosine phosphorylation. In this context, the induction of sperm capacitation appears to involve the low, steady-state production of reactive oxygen intermediates at a level that does not induce peroxidative damage. However, should exposure to such molecules be enhanced, then the limited antioxidant defences of the spermatozoa will be overwhelmed, leading to a loss of membrane integrity and a collapse of sperm function. Such oxidative stress can arise as a result of leucocytic infiltration into the ejaculate or as a result of defects in the spermatozoa that increase the endogenous output of toxic oxygen metabolites. The latter may, in part, involve the retention of excess residual cytoplasm during the terminal stages of spermatogenesis and the increased generation of the substrate for reactive oxygen species generation, NADPH. However, other mechanisms, such as the premature activation of the putative oxidase complex, are also a possibility. These studies have been effective in demonstrating a defined biochemical mechanism by which human sperm function can be compromised and hold implications for the management of male infertility as well as insights into the possible aetiology of this complex pathology.

Les spermatozoïdes humains sont extrêmement sensibles aux stress oxydatifs en raison d'une part de leur contenu important en acides gras polyinsaturés et, d'autre part, de leur manque relatif en protecteurs antioxydants. De plus ces cellules sont soumises sans arrêt à des attaques oxydantes venant de l'extérieur dans le cas des leucocytes ou de l'intérieur lorsque l'on considère la capacité innée des spermatozoïdes à générer des radicaux libres tels que les anions superoxydes ou les peroxydes d'hydrogène. La production endogène de ces molécules traduit leur rôle dans la capacitation des spermatozoïdes humains, par l'intermédiaire de mécanismes impliquant la stimulation de la phosphorylation sur tyrosines. Dans ce contexte, l'induction de la capacitation du sperme semble impliquer la production faible et constante de radicaux libres intermédiaires à un niveau tel qu'elle n'entraîne pas de péroxydation. Cependant si l'exposition à ces molécules augmentait, les défenses du spermatozoïde seraient alors rapidement submergées et cela conduirait à une perte de l'intégrité membranaire et à une disparition des fonctions spermatiques. Un tel stress oxydant peut provenir d'une infiltration leucocytaire dans l'éjaculat ou bien de défauts structurels qui pourraient augmenter l'excrétion endogène de radicaux libres oxygénés toxiques. Ce dernier cas peut impliquer en partie la rétention de l'excès de cytoplasme résiduel durant les phases terminales de la spermiogenèse et l'augmentation de la génération de substrats pour la formation de radicaux libres oxygénés, NADPH. Cependant d'autres mécanismes tels que l'activation prématurée d'un hypothétique complexe oxydase sont également une possibilité. Ces études ont permis de démontrer un mécanisme biochimique précis au cours duquel les fonctions du spermatozoïde peuvent être remises en cause, ont des conséquences pour la prise en charge de l'infertilité masculine et amènent un éclairage nouveau sur les étiologies possibles de cette pathologie complexe.

INTRODUCTION

Male infertility is a highly prevalent condition, the incidence of which may be increasing (1,2). Although genetic factors have been identified in a minority of cases exhibiting severe oligo- or azoospermia (3), in the main, the aetiology of male infertility is not understood. In the absence of such information, the development of improved techniques to diagnose and treat the infertile male is not possible. More importantly, until the causes of male reproductive dysfunction are resolved, it will not be possible to identify those who are susceptible and, where feasible, explore the possibility of prevention. In order to address these important clinical issues, it is essential that andrological research is focused on the aetiology of defective sperm function.

This is a difficult task because male infertility is not one condition but a collection of many different pathologies each with a different spectrum of functional defects and each caused by a different mix of aetiological factors. Thus, before the biochemistry of impaired sperm function can be addressed, it will be necessary to classify individual cases in terms of the precise nature of the biological defects responsible for the loss of fertilizing potential. This endeavour has involved the development of a wide range of different functional bioassays to permit assessment of the various biological properties that human spermatozoa must express if they are to fertilize the ovum in vivo. To this end, assays of sperm-cervical mucus interaction, sperm transport to the site of fertilization, movement characteristics, sperm-zona interaction and sperm-oocyte fusion, have been developed and evaluated in a variety of different clinical contexts (4, 5). The purpose of these bioassays is not so much to act as diagnostic tests in their own right, but to serve as a means of defining the precise nature of the functional defects present in the spermatozoa . It is only when the true nature of defective sperm function has been defined, that the important task of unraveling the biochemical basis male infertility can begin and light shed on the possible aetiological factors involved.

It was in this context that assays of sperm-oocyte fusion were first developed, refined and validated in terms of their capacity to predict the fertility of male subjects in vivo and in vitro (6). In the course of these studies, it was discovered that a common attribute of male infertility is that the spermatozoa fail to fuse with the vitelline membrane of the oocyte even after the spermatozoa have been stimulated with the divalent cation ionophore, A23187. This functional defect was found to be associated with failed fertilization in vivo and in vitro and was observed in both oligozoospermic individuals and men exhibiting idiopathic infertility whose semen profile was apparently normal (7-10). The importance of these studies lay in the implication that, *whatever the nature of the defects present in the spermatozoa of such patients, they lay downstream from the calcium influx that normally triggers sperm activation.* Thus, even after increases in intracellular calcium and pH had been induced in the spermatozoa of such patients by A23187, sperm-oocyte fusion was still impaired. This biological information focused attention on the nature of the damage that the plasma membrane might have sustained, that would have prevented such responses from taking place. It was in this context, that lipid peroxidation was considered as a possible factor in the aetiology of male infertility.

GENERATION OF REACTIVE OXYGEN SPECIES BY HUMAN SPERM SUSPENSIONS

The possible involvement of lipid peroxidation as a cause of defective sperm function was first suggested by John MacLeod in 1943 (11) but later elaborated by Thaddeus Mann and colleagues in a series of publications in the late 1970's (12, 13). The clinical importance of this pathophysiological mechanism became apparent when it was discovered that the functional defect discussed above, characterized by a failure to exhibit sperm-oocyte fusion following ionophore challenge, was associated with the excessive generation of reactive oxygen species by the sperm suspensions (14, 15). This negative association between reactive oxygen species generation and impaired sperm function has since been confirmed in many independent laboratories (16-20) and firmly establishes oxidative stress as a significant factor in the aetiology of male infertility. This conclusion has, in turn, raised a number of important questions concerning the source and nature of the reactive oxygen species responsible for initiating peroxidative damage in the spermatozoa, the nature of the damage induced and the effectiveness of antioxidants in preventing such damage in vivo and in vitro. In addition, the discovery of a free radical-generating system in human spermatozoa raises fundamental questions about the physiological function of reactive oxygen species in normal spermatozoa and the cell and species specificity of such activity. In this brief review we shall address some of these issues beginning with the nature and source of reactive oxygen metabolites in the human ejaculate.

REACTIVE OXYGEN SPECIES AND LEUKOCYTES

Every human semen sample is contaminated with leukocytes and, in general, it is the polymorph that predominates (21, 22). The presence of polymorphonuclear leukocytes is significant because these cells are potent producers of reactive oxygen species and in the human ejaculate appear to be spontaneously active. Thus, if a small volume of luminol is added directly to unprocessed human semen samples, a chemoluminescent signal is generated that exhibits a high correlation with the concentration of seminal leukocytes (Figure 1). However, despite the presence of activated leukocytes in concentrations that range from 10^4 to more than 10^6/ml, there does not appear to be an overt relationship between the presence of these cells and any aspect of the semen profile, or even fertility (23, 24). This conclusion is based on 2 patient populations sampled in different parts of the United Kingdom and featuring median leukocyte concentrations of 1.3 and 3.4 x 10^4/ml, and leukocytospermia frequencies of 2.7 and 7.8% respectively. In an independent patient population sampled in the United States (25), the median leukocyte concentration, and the incidence of leukocytospermia, were both approximately 10 fold higher (28 x10^4 / ml and 23%) and negative correlations with different aspects of the semen profile were noted. These observations suggest that seminal leukocyte concentrations up to 1-2 x 10^6/ml can be tolerated extremely well by the spermatozoa; it is only when the level of leukocyte contamination considerably exceeds this limit, that sperm quality is impaired.

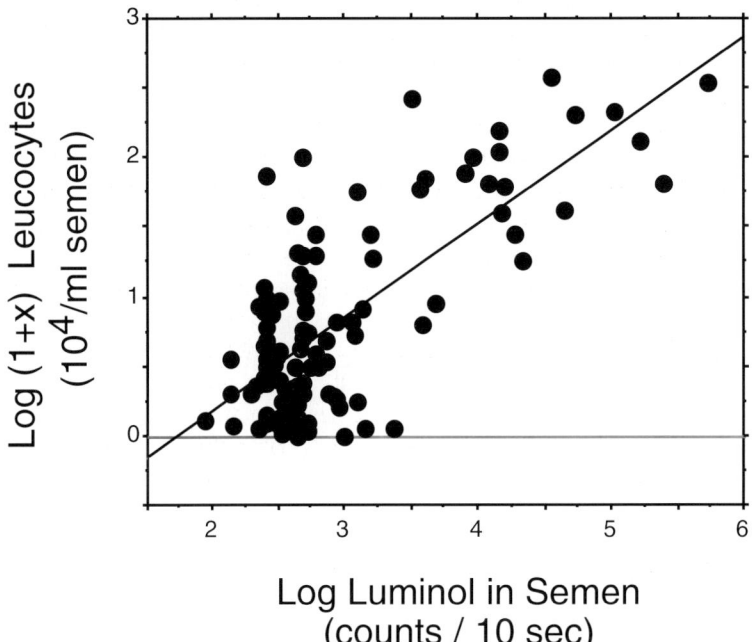

Figure 1. *The leukocytes present in human sperm suspensions are spontaneously active in the generation of reactive oxygen species, producing chemiluminescent signals on addition of luminol (24).*

This relative tolerance of high levels of leukocyte contamination in the original semen samples contrasts with the situation in washed sperm preparations, where even low numbers of leukocytes appear to damage sperm function (26-29). The susceptibility of the spermatozoa to leukocyte attack in washed culture media, compared with their relative resistance to attack in semen, can be explained in terms of the antioxidant protection offered by seminal plasma (13). The latter is extremely well endowed with antioxidant enzymes including catalase- and superoxide dismutase- like activities, as well as a range of small molecular weight scavengers such as uric acid and vitamin†C (13, 29). While the spermatozoa are bathed in seminal plasma they are well protected from extracellular sources of oxidative stress including infiltrating leukocytes. However in washed sperm preparations, the spermatozoa are deprived of such protection and are extremely vulnerable to attack by the cytotoxic oxygen metabolites released by activated leukocytes. Possibly the only extracellular protection offered by most conventional IVF media is albumin and, if serum is used, the iron- and copper- binding properties of transferrin and caeruloplasmin respectively. However, certain media, particularly Hams F10, contain milligram amounts of copper and ion salts and, as a consequence, actually promote peroxidative damage in both gametes and embryos.

LEUKOCYTE DETECTION

Given the importance of leukocyte contamination as a source of oxidative stress in vitro, it is clearly important to devise strategies for detecting these cells and, if necessary, either eliminating them from the sperm suspension or neutralizing their cytotoxic influence. In terms of detection, the methods devised must be sensitive, accurate and extremely rapid. In this context, the most accurate technique for quantifying leukocyte numbers is probably immunocytochemistry, employing monoclonal antibodies against leukocyte specific markers, such as CD45. The problem with this procedure is that it is insensitive, because the sampling volume is normally only 10 µl and the limits of detection of the method in the order of 10^3 - 10^4 leukocytes/ml. Immunocytochemistry is also too time consuming for a routine IVF laboratory wishing to effect on-line screening of all sperm preparations for leukocyte contamination. The answer to this problem is to use a chemical method for detecting leukocytes based on the fact that these cells possess receptors on their surface for the peptide, formyl-methionyl-leucyl-phenylalanine (FMLP) (30). Leukocytes respond to the presence of this reagent with a rapid burst of reactive oxygen species generation (Figure 2) that can be detected very readily using chemiluminescence techniques. Experiments with radiolabelled FMLP indicate that the receptor for this peptide is not expressed by spermatozoa and so the signal obtained provides a specific indication of the level of leukocyte contamination (30). Studies with the FMLP provocation test emphasize just how difficult it is to produce leukocyte-free sperm preparations using the conventional swim-up and Percoll gradient procedures (30). Even when Percoll concentrations in excess of 90% are employed, small numbers of leukocytes will still be found in the sperm pellet following centrifugation.

Although the numbers of leukocytes penetrating the high density Percoll layers may be small, they are still potentially harmful. The impact of contaminating leukocytes on sperm function is usually assessed by adding activated leukocytes directly to washed suspensions of human spermatozoa.

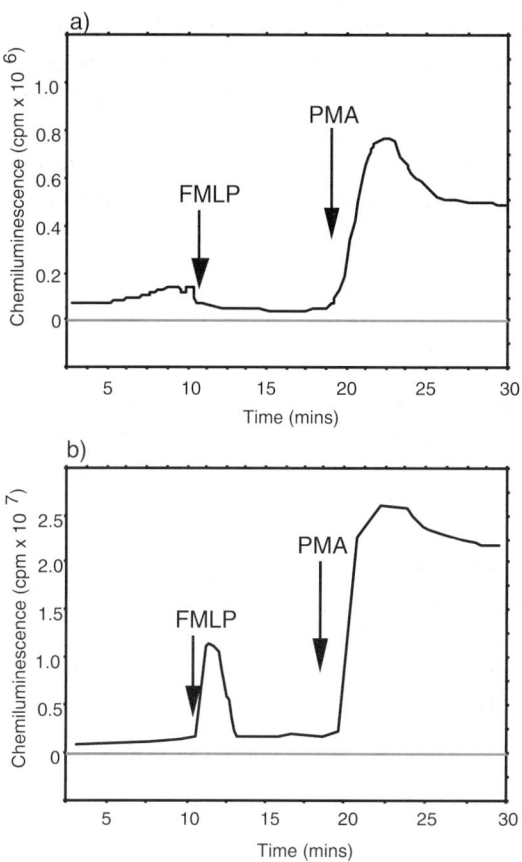

Figure 2.: **Chemiluminescent analyses of hydrogen peroxide generation by human sperm suspensions.** *In sample (a) no response to the leukocyte-specific probe, FMLP, was observed so the subsequent surge of reactive oxygen species generation elicited by PMA must have emanated from the spermatozoa. Alternatively in (b) an FMLP signal was observed, indicating that the following PMA response was, at least partly, due to the presence of contaminating leukocytes.*

Although this approach has generated important data, it is does not give a true reflection of the consequences of mild leukocytospermia, because it does not take account of the damage induced in spermatozoa as they are compacted with leukocytes during the sperm preparation procedure. Centrifugation times of 20 or 30 minutes are commonly used in sperm preparation protocols and during this period of time not only will the spermatozoa be compacted together with free radical generating leukocytes but the act of centrifugation will itself stimulate an increase in reactive oxygen species generation (31). Added to this the presence of ferrous and cuprous ion supplements in certain IVF media and ideal conditions are created for the induction of peroxidative damage in the pelleted sperm population.

The interactions that take place between spermatozoa and activated leukocytes in washed sperm pellets are probably clinically important, since negative correlations have recently been observed between the outcome of the FMLP provocation test and fertilization rates in two independent IVF-ET programs (26, 27). Moreover, a causal association between leukocyte contamination and impaired fertilization is indicated by experiments in which a significant improvement in the fertilizing capacity of human spermatozoa was observed following the selective removal of contaminating leukocytes from the sperm suspensions(28). For these reasons, the development of efficient techniques for counteracting the damaging effects of leukocyte contamination could be important for improving fertilization and pregnancy rates in a clinical context.

COUNTREACTING LEUKOCYTE CONTAMINATION

Once leukocytes have been identified in human sperm preparations, they should either be removed and /or their toxic influence neutralized. Leukocyte removal can best be achieved by use of paramagnetic beads or ferrofluids coated with an antibody against a leukocyte specific antigen such as CD 45 (30). In terms of neutralizing the oxidative stress created by these cells, a variety of reagents have been screened for their ability to suppress the peroxidative damage induced by contaminating leukocytes. The most effective reagents appear to be hypotaurine or thiols such as glutathione, which have been shown to protect human spermatozoa very effectively from the loss of motility induced by co-incubation with high concentrations (5×10^6/ml) of activated leukocytes (Figure 3). In contrast, mixtures of vitamins E and C were largely ineffective in protecting spermatozoa from leukocyte attack. Since the effective reagents are all potential scavengers of hydroxyl radicals, the acute damage induced on exposure of human spermatozoa to activated leukocytes may be largely due to the first chain initiation of peroxidative damage rather than the propagation of this process.

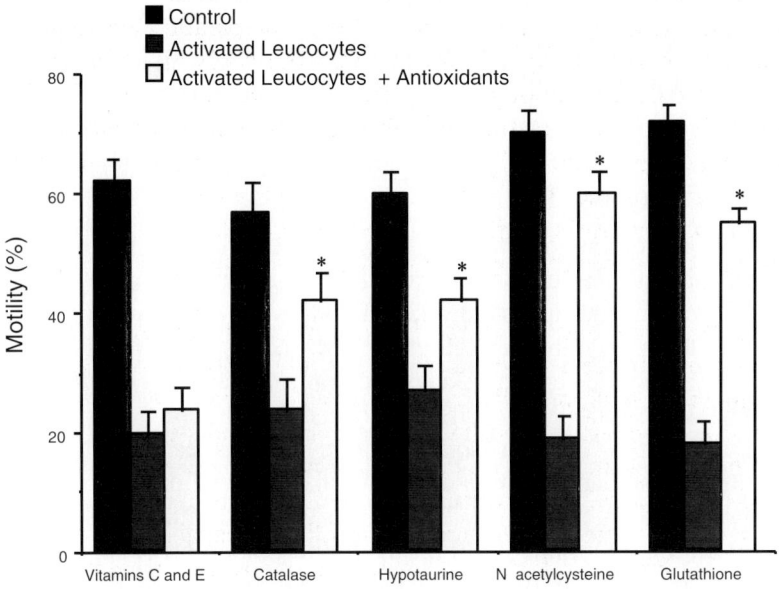

Figure 3. **Influence of antioxidants on the loss of motility induced on exposure of human spermatozoa to 5 x 10^6 activated leukocytes/ml (32).**

SPERMATOZOA AND REACTIVE OXYGEN SPECIES

The possibility that human spermatozoa might generate reactive oxygen species was first put forward by John MacLeod (11). In view of the protective effect that catalase exerted on the motility of human spermatozoa incubated in oxygenated media, he hypothesized that these cells could generate hydrogen peroxide from oxygen and that the former could impair human sperm function. He was correct on both counts. Human spermatozoa exhibit a capacity for reactive oxygen species generation that is independent of the mitochondrial electron transport chain. The primary product of this free radical generating system appears to be superoxide anion which then dismutates to hydrogen peroxide under the influence of superoxide dismutase (33). The mechanism by which human spermatozoa manufacture reactive oxygen species is uncertain although NADPH is readily used by these cells as a substrate for superoxide anion generation. The production of superoxide in response to NADPH is suppressed by the presence of diphenylene iodonium, an inhibitor of NADPH oxidase activity in many cell types including macrophages, B-cells and neutrophils. Although this observation may suggest a similarity between the NADPH oxidase of phagocytic leukocytes and the free radical generating system present in human spermatozoa, monoclonal antibodies against key constituents of the neutrophil oxidase do not cross react with human spermatozoa. Thus, differences between the NAPDH oxidase-like activities in human spermatozoa and leukocytes, undoubtedly exist.

PATHOLOGICAL REACTIVE OXYGEN SPECIES PRODUCTION

Clinically, it is important to determine why defective human spermatozoa from infertile patients increase their capacity for reactive oxygen species generation in both the steady state and following PMA stimulation. This could be due to premature activation of the oxidase and/or increased availability of substrate to an oxidase complex that is constitutively activated. The latter possibility is strengthened by the fact that simply supplying spermatozoa, or even isolated sperm membranes, with NADPH results in the dose-dependent induction of reactive oxygen species generation without the need for any kind of activation stimulus. If substrate availability is an important rate limiting step in the generation of superoxide, then this must be coupled to an increase in the activity of the hexose monophosphate shunt, which is the major pathway for NADPH generation in the cell. Some evidence in support of this hypothesis has been obtained. The enzyme that controls the rate of glucose flux through the hexose monophosphate shunt is glucose-6-phosphate dehydrogenase (G-6-PDH). The cellular content of this enzyme appears to be elevated in spermatozoa exhibiting high rates of reactive oxygen species generation (34). Moreover the G-6-PDH content of human spermatozoa is highly correlated with the content of other cytoplasmic enzymes such as creatine phosphokinase (CPK) which is, in turn, associated with peroxidative damage to the spermatozoa and a loss of function (35).

Such results have led to the hypothesis that one of the features of spermatozoa exhibiting high rates of reactive oxygen species generation is the retention of excess residual cytoplasm during the terminal stages of spermiogenesis. As a consequence of this enhanced cytoplasmic space, the spermatozoa exhibit high cellular contents of a variety of cytoplasmic enzymes, including lactic acid dehydrogenase (LDH), CPK and G-6-PDH, all of which have been associated with defective sperm function in independent studies (34-36). Since enzymes such as LDH and CPK perform valuable cellular functions, they should not be directly harmful to the spermatozoa in high amounts. The cellular damage is probably induced by the G-6-PDH which, by stimulating the generation of NADPH, fuels the excessive production of reactive oxygen species that initiates the lipid peroxidation cascade through which sperm function is lost (Figure 4).

Although the retention of excess residual cytoplasm is a significant factor in regulating the output of reactive oxygen species by human spermatozoa, it cannot be the only factor. If spermatozoa are treated with a phorbol ester, then there is an extremely rapid induction of hydrogen peroxide generation (Figure 2), which is augmented in cases of male infertility, and which must reflect an activation event presumably mediated by protein kinase C.

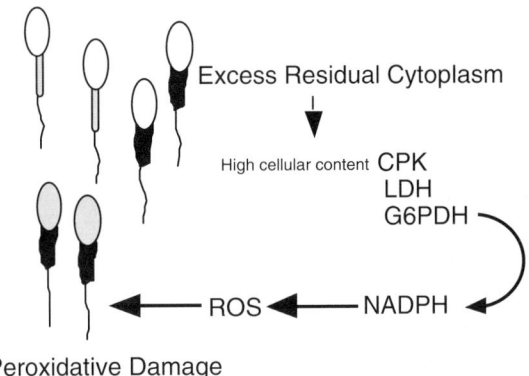

Figure 4. **Proposed mechanism by which errors in spermiogenesis lead to the retention of excess residual cytoplasm and elevated levels of cytoplasmic enzymes such as LDH, CPK and G-6-PDH.** *The latter then precipitates a loss of sperm function, by stimulating the generation of NADPH which then fuels the production of reactive oxygen species and initiation of a lipid peroxidation cascade.*

PHYSIOLOGICAL PRODUCTION OF REACTIVE OXYGEN SPECIES

Human spermatozoa are extremely vulnerable to oxidative stress because they are rich in polyunsaturated fatty acids, such as decosahexaenoic acid, which are very susceptible to free radical attack and the initiation of a lipid peroxidation cascade. Moreover the spermatozoon is, compared with most somatic cells, poorly endowed with antioxidant defense enzymes by virtue of the lack of cytoplasmic space. Given the inherent vulnerability of this cell-type to oxidative stress it is remarkable that the spermatozoon has evolved a highly specialized capacity to generate reactive oxygen species. The fact that this has occurred, suggests that such molecules are of importance in the control of normal sperm function. Evidence has already been obtained to suggest that hydrogen peroxide generation is involved in the induction of sperm capacitation in both human and hamster spermatozoa (37-39). Moreover, it has been demonstrated in the case of human spermatozoa that the importance of hydrogen peroxide lies in the stimulation of tyrosine phosphorylation (37). Incubation of human spermatozoa with catalase inhibits the functional responses of human spermatozoa to both A23187 and physiologically-meaningful agonists such as progesterone and recombinant ZP3, in association with a dramatic decline in the level of tyrosine phosphorylation (37). Conversely, the stimulation of reactive oxygen species production with NADPH is associated with a significant enhancement in the capacity of the spermatozoa for fusion with the oocyte in concert with a marked increase in the levels of tyrosine phophorylation. The redox regulation of tyrosine phophorylation may be of general significance as a regulatory mechanism, not just a unique feature of sperm cell biology. Similar redox regulated processes have been suggested for the control of phosphorylation in other types of tyrosine kinase receptor, as well as the activation pathway for the transcription factor NF-kB in T-cells (40-42).

The positive role of hydrogen peroxide in stimulating tyrosine phophorylation is not the only way in which reactive oxygen species can stimulate human sperm function. The superoxide anion also promotes the appearance of hyperactivated motility through mechanisms that are still to be resolved (43). So powerful is this effect that spermatozoa will even hyperactivate in seminal plasma if the levels of superoxide dismutase in semen are not sufficient to scavenge this radical species (44). In other cell types, superoxide anion has been shown to induce changes of a kind that are normally associated with capacitation, including increases in intracellular calcium, intracellular pH and the activation of phospholipase A_2 (45). In this respect the spermatozoon's use of superoxide anion to control of cell function is not unique, but reflective of the general importance of reactive oxygen species in signal transduction phenomena.

REFERENCES

1. Auger J, Kunstmann JM, Czyglik F, Jouannet P Decline in semen quality among fertile men in Paris during the past 20 years. New Eng J Med 1995; 332 : 281-5.
2. Carlsen E, Giwercman A, Keiding N, Skakkebaeck NE Evidence for decreasing quality of semen during past 50 years. Brit. Med. J. 1992; 305: 609-13.
3. Chandley AC. The genetic basis of male infertility. Reprod Med Rev 1995; 4 : 1-8.

4. Aitken RJ. Assessment of sperm function for IVF. Human Reprod 1986; 3 : 89-95.
5. Irvine DS, Aitken RJ. Seminal fluid analysis and sperm function testing. In: Bremner WJ, ed. Clinical Andrology. Clinics of North America. Philadelphia : Saunders, 1994 : 725-48.
6. Aitken RJ. The zona free hamster oocyte penetration test and the diagnosis of male inpfertility. Int. J. Androl. Suppl. 1986 ; 6: 1-199.
7. Aitken RJ, Ross A, Hargreave T, Richardson D, Best F. Analysis of human sperm function following exposure to the ionophore A23187: comparison of normospermic and oligozoospermic men. J Androl 1984; 5: 321-9.
8. Irvine DS, Aitken RJ. Predictive value of in vitro sperm function tests in the context of an AID Service. Human Reprod 1987; 1 : 539-45.
9. Aitken RJ, Thatcher S, Glasier AF, Clarkson JS, Wu FCW, Baird DT. Relative ability of modified versions of the hamster oocyte penetration test, incorporating hyperosmotic medium or the ionophore A23187, to predict IVF outcome. Human Reprod 1987; 2 : 227-31.
10. Aitken RJ, Irvine DS, Wu FC. (1991) Prospective analysis of sperm-oocyte fusion and reactive oxygen species generation as criteria for the diagnosis of infertility. Am J Obstet Gynec 1991; 64 : 542-51.
11. MacLeod J. The role of oxygen in the metabolism and motility of human spermatozoa. Am J Physiol 1943; 138 : 512-8.
12. Aitken RJ. A free radical theory of male infertility. Reprod Fertil Dev 1994; 6 : 19-24.
13. Jones R, Mann T, Sherins RJ. Peroxidative breakdown of phospholipids in human spermatozoa: spermicidal effects of fatty acid peroxides and protective action of seminal plasma. Fertil Steril 1979; 31 : 531-7.
14. Aitken RJ, Clarkson JS. Cellular basis of defective sperm function and its association with the genesis of reactive oxygen species by human spermatozoa. J Reprod Fertil 1987; 83 : 459-69.
15. Aitken RJ, Clarkson JS, Hargreave TB, Irvine DS, Wu FCW. Analysis of the relationship between defective sperm function and the generation of reactive oxygen species in cases of oligozoospermia. J Androl 1989; 10: 214-20.
16. Zalata A, Hafez T, Comhaire F. Evaluation of the role of reactive oxygen species in male infertility. Human Reprod 1995 (in press)
17. Weese DL, Peaster ML, Himsl KK, Leach GE, Lad PM, Zimmern PE. Stimulated reactive oxygen species generation in the spermatozoa of infertile men. J Urol 1993; 149 : 64-7
18. Mazzilli F, Rossi T, Marchesini M, Ronconi C, Dondero F. Superoxide anion in human semen related to seminal parameters and clinical aspects. Fertil Steril 1994; 62 : 862-8

19. Iwasaki A, Gagnon C. Formation of reactive oxygen species in spermatozoa of infertile patients. Fertil Steril 1992; 57 : 409-16.
20. D'Agata R, Vicari E, Moncada ML, Sidoti G, Calogero AE, Fornito MC, Minacapilli G, Mongioi A, Polosa P Generation of reactive oxygen species in subgroups infertile men. Int J Androl 1990; 13 : 344-51
21. Aitken RJ, West K, Buckingham D. Leukocytic infiltration into the human ejaculate and its association with semen quality, oxidative stress and sperm function. J Androl 1994; 15 : 343-52
22. Wolff H, Anderson DJ. Immunohistologic characterization and quantification of leukocyte subpopulations in human semen. Fertil Steril 1988; 49 : 497-504.
23. Tomlinson MJ, Barratt CLR, Cooke ID. Prospective study of leukocytes and leukocyte subpopulations in semen suggests that they are not a cause of male infertility. Fertil Steril 1993; 60 : 1069-75.
24. Aitken RJ, Buckingham DW, Brindle J, Gomez E, Baker HWG, Irvine DS. Analysis of sperm movement in relation to the oxidative stress created by leucocytes in washed sperm preparations and seminal plasma. Human Reprod 1995 (in press).
25. Wolff H, Politch JA, Martinez A, Haimovici F, Hill JA, Anderson DJ. Leukocytospermia is associated with poor semen quality. Fertil Steril 1990; 53 : 528-36.
26. Sukcharoen N, Keith J, Irvine DS, Aitken RJ. Analysis of sperm function tests in the prediction if in vitro fertilization rates. Fertil Steril 1994 (in press).
27. Krausz C, Mills C, Rogers S, Tan SL, Aitken RJ. Stimulation of oxidant generation by human sperm suspensions using phorbol esters and formyl peptides: relationship with motility and fertilization in vitro. Fertil Steril 1994; 62 : 599-605.
28. Aitken RJ, Buckingham DW, West K, Brindle J. On the use of paramagnetic beads and ferrofluids to assess and eliminate the leukocytic contribution to oxygen radical generation by human sperm suspensions. Am J Reprod Immunol 1995 (in press)
29. Zini A, de Lamirande E, Gagnon C. Reactive oxygen species in semen of infertile patients: levels of superoxide dismutase-and catalase-like activities in seminal plasma and spermatozoa. Int J Androl 1993; 16 : 183-8.
30. Krausz C, West K, Buckingham D, Aitken RJ. Development of a technique for monitoring the contamination of human semen samples with leucocytes. Fertil Steril 1992; 57 : 1317-25.
31. Aitken RJ, Clarkson JS. Significance of reactive oxygen species and antioxidants in defining the efficacy of sperm preparation techniques. J Androl 1988; 9 : 367-76.

32. Baker HWG, Brindle J, Irvine DS, Aitken RJ. Protective effect of antioxidants on the impairment of sperm motility by activated polymorphonuclear leucocytes. Fertil Steril 1995 (in press).
33. Alvarez JG, Touchstone JC, Blasco L, Storey BT. Spontaneous lipid peroxidation and production of hydrogen peroxide and superoxide in human spermatozoa. J Androl 1987; 8 : 338-48.
34. Aitken RJ, Krausz C, Buckingham D. Relationships between biochemical markers for residual sperm cytoplasm, reactive oxygen species generation, and the presence of leukocytes and precursor germ cells in human sperm suspensions. Molec Reprod Dev 1994; 39 : 268-79.
35. Huszar G, Vigue L Correlation between the rate of lipid peroxidation and cellular maturity as measured by creatine kinase activity in human spermatozoa. J Androl 1994; 15 : 71-7.
36. Casano R, Orlando C, Serio M, Forti G. LDH and LDH-X activity in sperm from normospermic and oligozoospermic men. Int J Androl 1991; 14 : 257-63.
37. Aitken RJ, Paterson M, Fisher H, Buckingham DW, van Duin M. Redox regulation of tyrosine phosphorylation in human spermatozoa is involved in the control of human sperm function. J Cell Sci 1995 (in press).
38. Bize I, Santander G, Cabello P, Driscoll D, Sharpe C. Hydrogen peroxide is involved in hamster sperm capacitation in vitro. Biol Reprod 1991; 44 : 398-403.
39. Griveau JF, Renard P, Le Lannou D. An in vitro promoting role for hydrogen peroxide in human sperm capacitation. Int J Androl 1994; 17: 300-7.
40. Anderson MT, Staal FJT, Gitler C, Herzenberg LA, Herzenberg LA. Separation of oxidant-initiated and redox regulated steps in the NF-kB signal transduction pathway. Proc Nat Acad Sci USA 1994; 921: 11527-31.
41. Gamou S, Shimizu N. Hydrogen peroxide preferentially enhances the tyrosine phosphorylation of epidermal growth factor receptor. FEBS Lett 1995; 357 : 161-5.
42. Koshio O, Akanuma Y, Kasuga M. Hydrogen peroxide stimulates yrosine phosphorylation of the insulin receptor and its tyrosine kinase activity in intact cells. Biochem J 1988; 250 : 95-101.
43. Ikebuchi Y, Masumoto N, Tasaka K, Koike K, Kasahara K, Miyake A, Tanizawa O. Superoxide anion increases intracellular pH, intracellular free calcium, and arachidonate release in human amnion cells. J Biol Chem 1991; 266: 13233-7.

The acrosome and intracytoplasmic sperm injection

André Van Steirteghem, Zsolt Nagy, Jiaen Liu, Hubert Joris and Paul Devroey

Centre for Reproductive Medicine, University Hospital and Medical School, Brussels Free University (Vrije Universiteit Brussel), Laarbeeklaan 101, B-1090 Brussels, Belgium

ABSTRACT

In order to obtain fusion and penetration of the sperm head into the oocyte, the spermatozoon must be acrosome-reacted. The present report examines the relationship between the acrosomal status of the spermatozoon and its influence on the outcome of two recently introduced procedures of assisted fertilization i.e. subzonal insemination and intracytoplasmic sperm injection as well as the outcome of intracytoplasmic injection of round headed spermatozoa.

Avant de fusionner avec la membrane plasmique et de pénétrer dans l'ovocyte, le spermatozoïde doit avoir fait sa réaction acrosomique. Nous examinons ici les relations entre le statut acrosomique et les résultats des deux nouvelles techniques de fécondation assistée, l'insémination subzonale et l'injection intracytoplasmique ainsi que les résultats de l'injection intracytoplasmique dans les cas de globozoospermie.

ENHANCEMENT OF ACROSOME REACTION AND SUBZONAL INSEMINATION OF A SINGLE SPERMATOZOON IN MOUSE EGGS (1)

The acrosome reaction was induced by various means. These were 1) varying incubation time (between 30 and 150min) in T6, a glucose-containing medium (2), 2) incubation in T6 medium with added calcium ionophore A23187 (3), 3) incubation in T6 medium added dbcGMP and imidazole (4), 4) exposure to an electric field (between 750 and 1500 V/cm for 2.5 msec), and 5) a combination of incubation in a medium with dbcGMP and imidazole and electrporation (1). Two methods were used to determine whether the spermatozoa had intact acrosomes or not.: the Bryan stain procedure and immunolocalisation by FITC-labeled monoclonal antibodies (6). The mean percentages of acrosome-free spermatozoa obtained increased by steps from 36ù to 67%, 73%, 86% and 92%.

Individual spermatozoa from various treatments were afterwards microinjected under the zona pellucida of a mouse oocyte. The fertilization rate for eggs microinjected with a spermatozoon treated with A23187, dbcGMP and imidazole, by electroporation and by a combination of the last two methods also increased by steps from 17% to 34%, 36% and 70%, respectively.

Ninety-five percent if the fertilized oocytes reached the early blastocyst stage, thirty-eight percent of these blastocysts implanted in pseudopregnant mice, and twenty-eight percent developed to term. These results indicated the varying degrees of success of different ways of inducing acrosomal loss in spermatozoa. The highest percentage of acrosome-free spermatozoa was obtained by combining the incubation in medium containing dbcGMP and imidazole with electroporation. By using these treated spermatozoa it was possible to achieve fertilization and further development once inserted in the perivitelline space by micromanipulation procedure.

INDUCTION OF ACROSOME REACTION IN HUMAN SPERMATOZOA USED FOR SUBZONAL INSEMINATION (SUZI) AND INTRACYTOPLASMIC SPERM INJECTION (ICSI) (7, 8)

The results of the experimental study of SUZI (1) in the mouse led us to adopt a similar approach in clinical SUZI: human spermatozoa were treated in order to increase the acrosome reaction rate prior to the injection into the perivitelline space. In a first series of 44 treatment cycles, up to three spermatozoa were injected into the perivitelline space of oocytes from 43 couples in whom fertilization had failed in conventional IVF (7). The selected spermatozoa were treated to enhance the percentage of acrosome-free spermatozoa either by incubation for 24h in T6 medium with 50% follicular fluid (v/v) (9) or by incubation for 24h in T6 medium followed by electroporation (5) and incubation for a few hours in T6 medium with 3.5 mM pentoxifylline. After two procedures, the mean percentage of acrosome-free spermatozoa increased from less than 10% to 35.5% and 53.9% respectively. Real and degenerative acrosome-reacted spermatozoa were assessed by labeling with the fluorescent isothiocyanate-conjugated Concanavalin A and incubation in PBS with Hoechst 3358 (10). After microinjection of up to three spermatozoa into the perivitelline space of metaphase-II oocytes, 6.7% of the oocytes were damaged by the injection procedure. The overall 2-PN fertilization rate was 19.6%; 6.5% of the injected oocytes had only one pronucleus and 2.8% three or more pronuclei. The normal fertilization rate was not different for the two treatment procedures used to enhance the acrosomal loss; The further development of the 2-PN oocytes was also similar for the two sperm treatments, i.e. 86% of the 2-PN oocytes developed to cleaved embryos which were suitable for embryo transfer or cryopreservation. One, two or three embryos were replace in 34 cycles and seven patients became pregnant (7).

Meanwhile the first pregnancies and births had been described after transfer of embryos obtained after microinjection of a single spermatozoon into the ooplasm of a metaphase-II oocyte (11). This novel procedure of assisted fertilization, i.e. intracytoplasmic sperm injection -ICSI- was applied together with SUZI in the first 300 cycles of assisted fertilization carried out at the Centre for Reproductive Medicine of the Dutch-speaking Brussels Free University (8). These 300 cycles included the 44 SUZI cycles mentioned before. The 200 infertile couples had had unsuccessful IVF cycles (151 couples) or too poor semen characteristics to carry out conventional IVF (49 couples). Sperm selected after Percoll was treated to enhance acrosomal loss by incubation in medium with follicular fluid or by electroporation. In 45 cycles it was possible to assess the acrosomal status of spermatozoa used for injection procedure. After exposure for 24h to follicular fluid the mean acrosomal reaction rate of living spermatozoa was 13.9% 'range, 4 to 23); after electroporation the mean acrosomal reaction rate was 18.0% (range, 4 to 44). The damage rate after SUZI (9% of the injected oocytes) was significantly lower than after ICSI (23% of the injected oocytes). However the 2-PN fertilization was significantly higher after ICSI (33.5% of the 716 injected oocytes) than after SUZI (13.1% of the 2214 injected oocytes). Only in the protocol in which electroporation was applied after 24 hours' incubation did the acrosome reaction correlate with the fertilization rate after SUZI (r=0.50; P=0.018). With the same treatment, the score real acrosome reacted (%) x concentration after sperm selection $(x10^6/ml)x10^{-2}$ was clearly linked to the fertilization rate (r=0.64; P=0.001) obtained after SUZI. A significant better fertilization rate was observed after the injection of spermatozoa treated to induce the acrosome reaction than with oocytes injected with untreated spermatozoa. Pregnancies and births were obtained after transfer of SUZI-embryos and ICSI-embryos and after a mixture of SUZI- and ICSI-embryos.

The higher fertilization rate after ICSI than after SUZI became even more evident in the subsequent 300 cycles where both ICSI and SUZI were applied (12). The much higher fertilization rate after ICSI and the similar cleavage rate for both procedures led to the availability of many more morphological good-quality embryos after ICSI. Many of these embryos implanted after transfer and developed into healthy children. These results as well as a controlled comparison between SUZI and ICSI on sibling oocytes indicated the much superior efficacy of ICSI. This had as a consequence that as of August 1992 ICSI was the sole procedure of assisted fertilization at the Brussels Free University Centre of Reproductive Medicine (13).

TREATMENT OF SPERMATOZOA FOR ICSI (14)

In our Centre the ICSI procedure was developed together with SUZI and the same sperm treatments, such as electroporation or incubation of sperm with pentoxifylline (PTX) and 2-deoxyadenosine (DOA) were initially also used prior to ICSI (7, 8, 12, 13). Since in ICSI a single spermatozoon is directly injected into the ooplasm, the zona pellucida and oocyte membrane are bypassed. Controlled studies were carried out to establish whether the sperm treatments that were assumed to enhance the motility of spermatozoa or to induce the acrosome reaction had any effect on the results of ICSI. Firstly, we used two controlled studies to compare fertilization and embryo cleavage after ICSI using spermatozoa treated by three different methods: in a first study PTX + DOA (method A) was compared with electroporation (method B) in 21 patients and, secondly, method A was compared with no specific treatment (method C) in 32 patients. There was no difference in the rates of fertilization and embryo cleavage when ICSI was done with spermatozoa treated by procedures A, B or C.

Spermatozoa were exposed to a higher Ca^{++} concentration (5 mM $CaCl_2$, $2H_2O$) in the final step of our initial sperm preparation in order to provide more acrosome-reacted spermatozoa (9). The hypothesis was subsequently put forward that this high Ca^{++} concentration might be the factor responsible for our high success rate after ICSI (15). In a second study, therefore, we compared the ICSI results for sibling oocytes from 12 patients using either spermatozoa treated with T6 medium containing 1.78 mM $CaCl_2$, $2H_2O$ and 5 mM $CaCl_2$, $2H_2O$ or spermatozoa prepared in

Earle's medium containing 1.78 mM $CaCl_2$, $2H_2O$. There was no difference in the fertilization and embryo cleavage rates between the two different media used during sperm selection; These two studies led to the conclusion that it is not necessary to carry out specific treatment of spermatozoa prior to ICSI. High fertilization and pregnancy rates can be obtained by ICSI in patients with severe male-factor infertility by using spermatozoa with no special treatment.

ICSI AND GLOBOZOOSPERMIA (16)

Patients with globozoospermia or round-head spermatozoa in the semen are considered sterile. This condition consists of spermatozoa without acrosome or post-acrosomal sheet and with several other ultrastructural anomalies: round or abnormally shaped nuclei, abnormal mitochondria and sometimes abnormal midpieces and tails (17, 18); Several studies have indicated that round-headed spermatozoa are unable to bind to the zona pellucida or to penetrate the oocyte in a zona-free hamster test, and similar results have been reported in human oocytes: no normal fertilization has been observed in IVF after insemination of human oocytes with round-headed spermatozoa (19-23). The fertilization capacity of round-headed spermatozoa after ICSI into human oocytes has been examined. In pre-clinical experiments, 45 oocytes were injected; 41 oocytes were intact after injection, 15 oocytes were fertilized normally, and 13 of these 15 oocytes developed further in vitro. ICSI was carried out in 11 treatments cycles of seven infertile couples with globozoospermia. Normal fertilization and embryo transfer occurred in four cycles (three patients). Positive serum human chorionic gonadotrophin was observed in three cycles (two patients): one patient had a pre-clinical abortion and the other became pregnant twice: the first pregnancy was ectopic and the second pregnancy is a twin pregnancy which ended in the birth of two healthy children.

Acknowledgments:
We are indebted to the clinical, scientific, technical, nursing and secretariat staff of the Centre for Reproductive Medicine. This work was supported by grants from the Belgian Fund for Medical Research.

REFERENCES

1. Palermo G, Van Steirteghem A. Enhacement of acrosome reaction and subzonal insemination of a single spermatozoon in mouse eggs. Mol Reprod Dev 1991; 30:339-345.
2. Fraser LR. Dibutyryl cyclic AMP decreases capacitation time in vitro in mouse spermatozoa. J reprod Fertil 1981; 62:63-72.
3. Green DPL. Induction of the acrosome reaction in guinea pig spermatozoa in vitro by the Ca ionophore A23187. J Physiol 1976; 260:18-19.
4. Talansky BE, Barg PE, Gordon JW. Ion pump ATPase inhibitors block the fertilization of zona-free mouse oocytes by acrosome-reacted spermatozoa. J Reprod fertil 1987; 79:447-455.
5. Tomkins PT, Houghton JA. The rapid induction of the acrosome reaction of human spermatozoa by electropermeabilization. Fertil Steril 1988; 40:329-336.
6. Moore HDM, Smith CA, Hartman TD, Bye AP. Visualization and characterization of the acrosome reaction of human spermatozoa by immunolocalization with monoclonal antibody. Gamete Res 1987; 17:245-259.
7. Palermo G, Joris H, Devroey P, Van Steirteghem AC. Induction of acrosome reaction in human spermatozoa used for subzonal insemination. Hum Reprod 1992;7:248-254.
8. Palermo G, Joris H, Derde M-P, Camus M, Devroey P, Van Steirteghem AC. Sperm characterstistics and outcome of human assisted fertilization by subzonal insemination and intracytoplasmic sperm injection. Fertil Steril 1993;59:826-835.
9. Stock CE, Bates R, Lindsay KS, Edmonds DK, Fraser LR. Extended exposure to follicular fluid is required for significant stimulation of the acrosome reaction in human spermatozoa. J Reprod Fertil 1989;86:401-411.
10. Holden CA, Hyne RV, Sathananthan AH, Trounson AO. Assessment of the human sperm acrosome reaction using concanavalin A lectin. Mol Reprod Dev 1990;25:247-257.
11. Palermo G, Joris H, Devroey P, Van Steirteghem AC. Pregnancies after intracytoplasmic injection of a single spermatozoon into an oocyte. Lancet 1992; 340:17-18.
12. Van Steirteghem AC, Liu J, Joris H, Nagy Z, Janssenswillen C, Tournaye H, Derde M-P, Van Assche E, Devroey P. Higher success rate by intracytoplasmic sperm injection than by subzonal insemination. Report of a second series of 300 consecutive treatment cycles. Hum Reprod 1993; 8:1055-1060.

13. Van Steirteghem AC, Nagy Z, Joris H, Liu J, Staessen C, Smitz J, Wisanto A, Devroey P. High fertilization and implantation rates after intracytoplasmic sperm injection. Hum Reprod 1993; 8:1061-1066.
14. Liu J, Nagy Z, Joris H, Tournaye H, Devroey P, Van Steirteghem AC. Intracytoplasmic sperm injection does not require special treatment of the spermatozoa. Hum Reprod 1994;9:1127-1130.
15. Edwards RG, Van Steirteghem AC. Intracytoplasmic sperm injections (ICSI) and human fertilization: does calcium hold the key to success? Hum Reprod 1993;8:988-989.
16. Liu U, Nagy Z, Joris H, Tournaye H, Devroey P, Van Steirteghem A. Successful fertilization and establishment of pregnancies after intracytoplasmic sperm injection in patients with globozoospermia. Hum reprod 1995; 10:626-629.
17. Holstein AF, Schirren C, Schirren CG. Human spermatids and spermatozoa lcking acrosomes. J Reprod Fertil 1973; 35:489-491.
18. Pedersen H, Rebbe H. Fine structure of round-headed human spermatozoa. J Reprod Fertil 1974; 37:51-54.
19. Weissenberg R, Eshkol A, Rudak E, Lunenfeld B. Inability of round acrosomeless spermatozoa to pentrate zona-free hamster ova. Arch Androl 1983;11:167-169.
20. Syms AJ, Johnson AR, Lipshutz LI, Smith RG. Studies on human spermatozoa with round head syndrome. Fertil Steril 1984; 42:431-435.
21. Lanzendorf S, Mahoney A, Ackerman S, Acosta A, Hodgen G. Fertilizing potential of acrosome-defective sperm following microsurgical injection into eggs. Gamete Res 1988; 19:329-337.
22. Aitken RJ, Kerr L, Bolton V, Hargreave T. Analysis of sperm function in globozoospermia: implications for the mechanism of sperm-zona interaction. Fertil Steril 1990;54:701-707.
23. Dale B, Iaccarino M, Fortunato A, Gragnaniello G, Kyozuka K, Tosti E. A Morphological and Functional Study of Fusibility in Round-Headed Spermatozoa in the Human. Fertil Steril 1994;61:336-340.

Selection of acrosome reacted spermatozoa

Jean Parinaud and Hélène Moutaffian

Laboratoire de Fécondation, CHU La Grave, 31052 Toulouse, France

ABSTRACT

Acrosome reaction occurs only in a small percentage of spermatozoa, which represents the potentially fertile subpopulation of sperm cells. Therefore the selection of these cells is of great interest for the study of gamete interaction and for enhancement of micromanipulation methods. The selection methods use immunobeads coated with antibodies directed against the inner acrosomal membrane (GB24 or MH61), on which the human acrosome reacted spermatozoa get fixed. The detachment can be done either mechanically one by one or immunologically using anti-Fab'2 antibody, which allows to recover enough acrosome reacted spermatozoa to perform morphological and meabolical studies. Using this method we have shown that acrosome reaction occurs in the most morphologically normal spermatozoa and is followed by a loss of motility and a decrease in longevity. Moreover, when injected in the perivitelline space of hamster oocytes, the selected spermatozoa had a higher fertilization rate than unselected spermatozoa, confirming that acrosome reaction is necessary for the fusion with the oocyte plasma membrane and that the selection method does not alter the fertilizing ability of the spermatozoa. Therefore, these methods represent a new way for understanding the sperm functions.

Seule une faible proportion de spermatozoïdes est apte à faire la réaction acrosomique et constitue la sous-population fertile des spermatozoïdes. Leur sélection présente donc un intérêt à la fois pour étudier l'interaction gamétique et pour améliorer les techniques de micro-injection. Les techniques sont basées sur l'utilisation d'immunobilles recouvertes d'un anticorps spécifique de la membrane acrosomique interne (GB24 ou MH61) sur lesquelles vont se fixer les spermatozoïdes ayant fait la réaction acrosomique. Le décrochage peut ensuite se faire soit mécaniquement un par un, soit en utilisant un anticorps anti-Fab'2 qui va permettre de décrocher suffisamment de spermatozoïdes pour pouvoir faire des études morphologiques et métaboliques. Avec cette dernière méthode, nous avons pu montrer que la réaction acrosomique se produit au niveau des spermatozoïdes les plus normaux et qu'elle induit une chute de la mobilité et de la longévité des spermatozoïdes. De plus, lorsqu'ils sont injectés dans l'espace péri-vitellin d'ovocytes de hamster, ces spermatozoïdes sélectionnés donnent des taux de fécondation plus élevés que les spermatozoïdes pris au hasard. Ceci confirme le rôle essentiel de la réaction acrosomique dans la capacité de fusion avec la membrane plasmique ovocytaire, et montre que la technique de sélection n'altère pas le pouvoir fécondant. Ces méthodes, efficaces et ne lésant pas les cellules, ouvrent de nouvelles voies d'étude de l'interaction gamétique.

INTRODUCTION

Acrosome reaction can be induced by various physiological or pharmacological stimuli. However only few spermatozoa are able to undergo acrosome reaction. Indeed, Biefeld et al. (1) have obtained 16% of acrosome reacted cells after induction by zona-pellucida, Siegel et al. (2) 46% with follicular fluid and our group (3) 48% with progesterone. Since acrosome reaction is an essential step in fertilization events, these reacting sperm cells represent the potentially fertile subpopulation of sperm cells. Its relative low proportion in semen does not allow to characterize this subpopulation and to evaluate the metabolic changes induced by acrosome reaction. Therefore, the isolation of such a cell subpopulation is of great interest for understanding gamete unteraction processes. Moreover, it has been shown that acrosome reaction is necessary for the fusion with oocyte plasma membrane. Therefore, the obtention of suspension containing only acrosome reacted spermatozoa could be useful for enhancing the results of subzonal inseminations (4-5).

COLLECTION OF ACROSOME REACTED SPERMATOZOA

Since acrosome reaction doesn't induce significant changes in the physical characteristics of the spermatozoa, no physical method can be used to separate acrosome intact and acrosome reacted spermatozoa. On the opposite, acrosome reaction induces the exposure of the inner acrosomal membrane and thus of the antigens which are present on the surface of this membrane. Therefore, monoclonal antibodies, directed against these antigens, can be used to select reacted spermatozoa.

The antibodies can be fixed on paramagnetic polystyrene beads coated with sheep antimouse IgG. Okabe et al. (6) have fixed MH61 antibody, directed against the inner acrosomal, on such beads. After a preincubation period in the presence of an acrosome reaction inducer, spermatozoa were incubated with the beads. Acrosome reacted spermatozoa got fixed on the beads, which were then collected with a magnet. Using this method they have shown that $83.7\% \pm 4.3\%$ of bound sperms were acrosome reacted versus $13.7\% \pm 4.2\%$ in the initial suspension. The efficiency of the method, expressed as the percentage of the recovered acrosome reacted spermatozoa, ranged from 27% to 90%(7).

DETACHING BOUND SPERMATOZOA FROM IMMUNOBEADS

Two kinds of techniques have been used for detaching bound spermatozoa from immunobeads: mechanical and immunological ones.

The mechanical detachment consists in aspirating bound spermatozoa with a micropipette with a hole larger than the sperm head and smaller than the beads, so that it is pull of the bead. This method has been successfully used by Ying et al. (8) and by our team (9). The detached sperms keep their fertilizing ability and thus their main function. However, this technique necessitates to detach spermatozoa one by one from the beads which makes impossible any morphological and functional studies on the subpopulation of acrosome reacted spermatozoa. Moreover, nothing can be known on the fate of the antisperm antibody (remaining on the bead or on the spermatozoa?) and on the integrity of the membrane after such a manipulation.

The immunological method is adapted from the one described by Rasmussen et al. for lymphocytes (11). The principle is related to the use of an anti-Fab'2 antibody which reacted with the antibody fixed on the cells and thus decrease its affinity for the cells surface antigen. Therefore the cells are pulled of the beads and remain free of antibody. We have adapted this technic to the selection of acrosome reacted spermatozoa. Indeed, Moutaffian and Parinaud (12) have used GB24 coated beads to select spermatozoa after induction of acrosome reaction by follicular fluid.

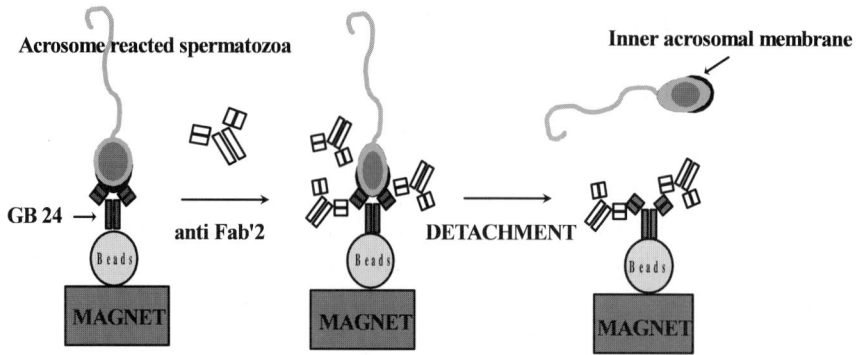

Figure 1. **Method to select acrosome-reacted spermatozoa.**
Spermatozoa were incubated in the presence of immunobeads coated with GB24, an antibody specific of the inner acrosomal membrane. Acrosome reacted spermatozoa bound to the beads and non reacted cells were eliminated by washes. Bound spermatozoa were then detached from the beads using anti mouse Fab'2 antibody. Reacted spermatozoa were then recovered in the supernatant.

This method allowed to recover $170 \pm 48 \times 10^3$ spermatozoa, that was a yield of $6.2\% \pm 0.9\%$ in the recovery of acrosome reacted spermatozoa. The percentage of acrosome reacted spermatozoa in the selected population was $88\% \pm 3\%$ versus $32\% \pm 6\%$ in the whole sperm population ($P<0.01$). This increase concerned fully reacted spermatozoa as well as equatorial segment (table 1), since the ratio of equatorial segment to whole reacted cells was not changed (0.27 ± 0.05 versus 0.30 ± 0.05; NS). Moreover, the selected population was enriched only in live reacted spermatozoa, the percentage of dead reacted spermatozoa remaining unchanged.

	WHOLE SPERM POPULATION	SELECTED SPERMATOZOA
Live fully reacted (%)	8.8 ± 1.8^a	51.8 ± 4.9
Live equatorial segment (%)	9.4 ± 3.3^a	18.6 ± 4.3
Live unreacted (%)	60.1 ± 5.7^a	8.7 ± 1.8
Dead fully reacted (%)	11.1 ± 3.2	12.7 ± 2.2
Dead equatorial segment (%)	2.9 ± 0.6	5.2 ± 1.5
Dead unreacted (%)	6.2 ± 1.4^b	3.1 ± 1.7
Whole reacted (%)	32.3 ± 5.5^a	88.2 ± 3.0

Table 1: **Acrosomal status in the whole and selected sperm populations***
* Data are mean $\pm$ SEM from 20 experiments; $^a P < 0.01$; $^b P < 0.05$

When incubated with FITC-rabbit anti-mouse antibody, no cell was labelled, indicating that all molecules of GB24 were detached from the sperm heads. Moreover, the method did not affect cell viability since $83.7\% \pm 3.1\%$

were still alive after selection (versus 80.3% ± 3.7% in the whole sperm cells; NS).

However, the yield of this method remained low. Indeed, 13,106 ± 4,022 x10^3 reacted spermatozoa were incubated with the beads and only 152 ± 42 x10^3 reacted spermatozoa were recovered. This was partialy due to the difficulties to obtain an homogeneous repartition of the magnetic beads on the flask, since they tended to cluster together, reducing the chances of interaction between spermatozoa and beads. On the other hand, the selected population was not 100% acrosome reacted (88% ± 3%). The contamination by acrosome intact spermatozoa could be explained by a partial efficiency of washes, some non reacted spermatozoa remaining trapped between beads.

CHARACTERISTICS OF SELECTED SPERMATOZOA

Despite no difference in viability at the end of the 4 hour incubation in 50% follicular fluid (table 2), the acrosome reacted spermatozoa had a dramatically reduced longevity since quite none of them were still alive after a 18 hour incubation in B2 medium (0.9% ± 0.4% versus 45.9% ± 5.1% in the whole population; $P < 0.01$).

This observation question the idea of degenerative acrosomal loss applied to dead reacted spermatozoa (12-13). Indeed, as reported by Mortimer et al. (14), « there were no evidence that dead reacted spermatozoa had undergone a true acrosome reaction before senescence and death, rather than having suffered post-mortem degeneration ». Our data indicate that acrosome reaction induces sperm death and that, even degenerative acrosome loss cannot be excluded in few spermatozoa, the whole reacted sperm population (live and dead) must be taken into account when studying induced acrosome reaction. However, we cannot exclude a deleterious effect of the selection method.

Almost all the acrosome reacted spermatozoa were immotile at the time of selection (table 2). Moreover, when studying the motile reacted sperm cells, all the parameters (mean progressive velocity, mean path velocity, curvilinear velocity, mean linearity, mean amplitude of lateral head displacement) were reduced. This drop of motility in the selected population could be due to the influx of calcium inside the cells which can have a detrimental effect on motility (15-16). Theses changes in intracellular calcium concentrations are an essential step of acrosome reaction (17), which can explain the diminution of motility observed after induction of acrosome loss (16,18). In our experiments, calcium influx has been triggered by the progesterone contained in the follicular fluids (19). Moreover, Tesarik and Mendoza (20) have shown that spermatozoa able to swim out a microinjection needle, i.e. having progressive motility, are enriched in equatorial segment pattern of acrosome reaction, i.e. freshly reacted (21), and depleted of fully reacted cells, suggesting that after acrosome reaction the spermatozoa become progressively immotile. In the fertilization events, motility is not necessary after zona crossing, since, using sub-zonal sperm insemination, it has been shown that immotile spermatozoa are able to fuse with the oocyte membrane (22).

	WHOLE SPERM CELLS	SELECTED SPERMATOZOA
Viability (%)	80.3 ± 3.7	83.7 ± 3.1
Viability after a 18 hour incubation (%)	45.9 ± 5.1 [a]	0.9 ± 0.4
Motility (%)	52.7 ± 7.1 [a]	6.7 ± 3.3
Progressive motility (%)	30.2 ± 5.3 [a]	2.6 ± 1.7
Mean path velocity (μ/s)	50.3 ± 11.5 [a]	11.4 ± 5.1
Rapid motility (%)	36.7 ± 8.4 [a]	3.6 ± 2.1
Mean amplitude of head displacement (μ)	4.1 ± 0.5 [a]	0.9 ± 0.4
Mean curvilinear velocity (μ/s)	65.5 ± 7.7 [a]	15.1 ± 6.0
Mean progressive velocity (μ/s)	45.3 ± 5.6 [a]	10.1 ± 4.9
Linearity (%)	61.8 ± 3.8 [a]	18.9 ± 7
Hyperactive motility (%)	5.9 ± 1.9 [a]	0.7 ± 0.7
Normal forms (%)	51.8 ± 4.8	58.5 ± 6.3
Head abnormalities (%)	20.3 ± 3.2 [b]	14.9 ± 2.6
Midpiece abnormalities (%)	5.7 ± 1.3	3.4 ± 1.3
Tail abnormalities (%)	15.9 ± 5.8	21.0 ± 7.4

Table 2: **Comparison of whole and selected sperm populations***
* *Data are mean ± SEM from 20 experiments for viability, 19 for motility and 13 for morphology.* [a] *$P < 0.01$;* [b] *$P < 0.05$*

Despite no significant difference in the percentage of morphologically normal spermatozoa between the selected population and the whole one, there was a significantly lower percentage of head abnormalities; this reduction concerned mostly thin heads (1.8% ± 1.0% versus 5.6% ± 0.9%; P < 0.01). The midpiece abnormalities were slightly but the percentage of bent tails was significantly lower (1.0% ± 0.5% versus 3.8% ± 1.1%; P < 0.01). On the opposite, the percentage of tail abnormalities was slightly but none of the specific abnormalities (absent, short, coiled or double tails) was significantly enhanced. The multiple anomalies index was identical in the selected and the whole population (1.24 ± 0.34 versus 1.30 ± 0.04; NS). These findings are consistent with those of Liu and Baker (23), who found that 84% of acrosome reacted spermatozoa, bound to zona-pellucida, were normal as compared to only 38% in the culture medium. This difference is higher than that observed in our study, likely due to the fact that Liu and Baker (23) used zona-pellucida for acrosome reaction induction, which is probably more selective than follicular fluid. Moreover, Carrell et al. (24) have reported that sperms with head abnormalities have lower spontaneous acrosome reaction and lower response to A23187 than normal sperms. Since spermatozoa able to undergo acrosome reaction represent the fertile sperm subpopulation, these data are in good agreement to those of Mashiach et al. (25) and of Kaskar et al. (26), who reported sperm morphology as the best semen predictive parameter of in vitro fertilization.

EFFECTS OF ACROSOME REACTED SPERM SELECTION ON THE FERTILIZATION RATE AFTER SUB-ZONAL INSEMINATION

The results of sub-zonal insemination (SUZI) are greatly enhanced by induction of acrosome reaction (AR) (4-5). However, the techniques used to induce AR, either incubation with follicular fluid or electroporation, do not allow to obtain more than 30% of live reacted sperm. Since acrosome reaction can not be observed without staining, spermatozoa are randomly choosen for microinjection. In order to increase the chances of injecting at least one acrosome reacted sperm, up to 6 spermatozoa are injected, leading to fertilization rate enhancement but also to an increase in the number of polyspermic zygotes (27).Therefore, the injection of selected acrosome reacted spermatozoa could allow to increase the number of obtained diploid zygotes.

To verify this hypothesis, we have injected either randomly choosen or selected human spermatozoa in the perivitelline space of hamster oocytes (9). The acrosome reaction was previously induced by a 4 hour incubation in presence of 20% follicular fluid.

Table 3 shows that the percentage of spermatozoa having fertilized a hamster egg is significantly higher in the selected than in the whole population.

This results are close to those of Ying et al. (8) who reported a fertilization rate 7.3% with bead-selected spermatozoa versus 2.8% with randomly selected spermatozoa ($P < 0.05$).

	UNSELECTED SPERMATOZOA	SELECTED SPERMATOZOA
No of injected spermatozoa	70	68
No of decondensated heads or male pronuclei	5 (7%)	16 (24%)[a]

[a] $P < 0.01$

Table 3. **Fertilization of hamster oocytes after subzonal insemination with unselected and selected human spermatozoa (9).**

These data suggest that this method could allow an increase in the diploidic fertilization in SUZI and thus the number of transferable embryos. However, this study was performed with normal sperms and hamster eggs. Further sudies must be done to confirm these results with abnormal sperms and with human oocytes.

CONCLUSION

The selection of acrosome reacted spermatozoa in order to optimize the results of microinjections procedures is now of poor interest since it has been widely shown that intra cytoplasmic sperm injection (ICSI) has a greater efficiency than SUZI (28) and that it does not require acrosome reaction (29).
On the opposite, these methods allows to separate a sub population of human sperm in which the fertilizing one is included. Therefore they represent a new way for the study of gamete interaction and specially of behavior of the spermatozoa after acrosome reaction.

REFERENCES

1. Bielfeld P, Faridi A, Zaneveld LJD, De Jonge CJ. The zona pellucida induced acrosome reaction of human spermatozoa is mediated by protein kinases. Fertil Steril 1994;61:536-541.
2. Siegel MS, Paulson RJ, Graczykowski JW. The influence of human follicular fluid on the acrosome reaction, fertilizing capacity and proteinase activity of human spermatozoa. Hum Reprod 1990;5:975-980.
3. Parinaud J, Labal B, Vieitez G. High progesterone concentrations induce acrosome reaction with a low cytotoxic effect. Fertil Steril 1992;58:599-602.

4. Fishel S, Jackson P, Antinori S, Johnson J, Grossi S, Versaci C. Sub-zonal insemination for the allevation of infertility. Fertil Steril 1990;54:828-835.
5. Palermo G, Joris H, Devroey P, Van Steirteghem AC. Induction of acrosome reaction in human spermatozoa used for sub-zonal insemination. Hum Reprod 1992;7:248-254.
6. Okabe M, Matzno S, Nagira M, Ying X, Kohama Y, Mimura T. Collection of acrosome-reacted human sperm using monoclonal antibody-coated paramagnetic beads. Mol Reprod Dev 1992;32:389-393.
7. Ohashi K, Saji F, Wakimoto A, Tsutsui T, Nakazawa T, Okabe M, et al. Selection of acrosome-reacted sperm with MH61-immunobeads. J Androl 1994;15:78-82.
8. Ying X, Okabe M, Mimura T. Selection of acrosome-reacted human spermatozoa and their fusing ability by micro-injection into the perivitelline space of hamster eggs. Hum Reprod 1993;8:1074-1078.
9. Parinaud J, Vieitez G, Labal B, Richoilley G. Selection and micro-injection of acrosome-reacted human spermatozoa. Hum Reprod 1994;9:128-129.
10. Rasmussen AM, Smeland. EB, Eriksen BK, Caignault L, Funderud S. A new method for detachment of dynabeads from positively selected B lymphocytes. J Immunol Methods 1992;146:195-202.
11. Moutaffian H, Parinaud J. Selection and characterization of human acrosome reacted spermatozoa. Hum Reprod, in press.
12. Talbot P, Chacon RS. A triple-stain technique for evaluating normal acrosome reactions of human sperm. Journal of Experimental Zoology 1981;215:201-208.
13. Mendoza C, Carreras A, Moos J, Tesarik J. Distinction between true acrosome reaction and degenerative acrosome loss by a one-step staining method using Pisum sativum agglutinin. J Reprod Fert 1992;95:755-763.
14. Mortimer D, Curtis EF, Camenzind AR. Combined use of fluorescent peanut agglutinin lectin and Hoechst 33258 to monitor the acrosomal status and vitality of human spermatozoa. Hum Reprod 1990;5:99-103.
15. Fraser LR. Minimum and maximum extracellular Ca2+ requirements during mouse sperm capacitation and fertilization in vitro. J Reprod Fert 1987;81:77-89.
16. Byrd W, Tsu J, Wolf DP. Kinetics of spontaneous and induced acrosomal loss in human sperm incubated under capacitating and noncapacitating conditions. Gamete Res 1989;22:109-122.
17. Fraser LR. Calcium channels play a pivotal role in the sequence of ionic changes involved in the initiation of mouse sperm acrosomal exocytosis. Mol Reprod Dev 1993;36:368-376.

18. Fleming AD, Yanagimachi R. Fertile life of acrosome-reacted guinea pig spermatozoa. Journal of Experimental Zoology 1982;220:109-115.
19. Blackmore PF, Beebe SJ, Danforth DR, Alexander N. Progesterone and 17a-hydroxyprogesterone: novel stimulators of calcium influx in human sperm. J Biol Chem 1990;265:1376-1380.
20. Tesarik J, Mendoza C. Most living acrosome-reacted spermatozoa do not fuse with the oocyte when inserted into the perivitelline space. Fertil Steril 1994;61:529-535.
21. Tesarik J, Mendoza C, Carreras A. Fast acrosome reaction measure: a highly sensitive method for evaluating stimulus-induced acrosome reaction. Fertil Steril 1993;59:424-430.
22. Terriou P, Giorgetti C, Hans E, Spach JL, Salzmann J, Carlon N, et al. Subzonal sperm insemination and total or extreme asthenozoospermia - An effective technique for an uncommon cause of male infertility. Fertil Steril 1993;60:1057-1061.
23. Liu DY, Baker HWG. Acrosome status and morphology of human spermatozoa bound to the zona pellucida and oolemma determined using oocytes that failed to fertilize in vitro. Hum Reprod 1994;9:673-679.
24. Carrell DT, Zobell RL, Middleton RG, Urry RL. A functional analysis and the potential clinical significance of 7 categories of sperm morphology. Journal of Urology 1994;151:376-380.
25. Mashiach R, Fish B, Eltes F, Tadir Y, Ovadia J, Bartoov B. The relationship between sperm ultrastructural features and fertilizing capacity in vitro. Fertil Steril 1992;57:1052-1057.
26. Kaskar K, Franken DR, Vanderhorst G, Oehninger S, Kruger TF, Hodgen GD. The relationship between morphology, motility and zona pellucida binding potential of human spermatozoa. Andrologia 1994;26:1-4.
27. Sakkas D, Lacham O, Gianaroli L, Trounson A. Subzonal sperm microinjection in cases of severe male factor infertility and repeated in vitro fertilization failure. Fertil Steril 1992;57:1279-1288.
28. Palermo G, Joris H, Derde M-P, Camus M, Devroey P, Van Steirteghem AC. Sperm charactersistics and outcome of human assisted fertilization by subzonal insemination and intracytoplasmic sperm injection. Fertil Steril 1993;59:826-835.
29. Liu J, Nagy Z, Joris H, Tournaye H, Devroey P, Van Steirteghem AC. Intracytoplasmic sperm injection does not require special treatment of the spermatozoa. Hum Reprod 1994;9:1127-1130.

The use of acrosomal antigens as contraceptive immunogens: studies on the intra-acrosomal antigen SP-10

John C.R Herr

Department of Cell Biology and the Center for Recombinant Gamete Contraceptive Vaccinogens, University of Virginia, Charlottesville, Virginia 22908, USA

Abstract

SP-10 is an intra-acrosomal protein consisting, in humans, of 265 amino acids. Human SP-10 is encoded by a four exon, single copy gene located on chromosome 11 at band q23-24. Within the acrosome SP-10 shows considerable microheterogeneity, consisting of a group of proteins from 18-34 kDa. These forms of SP-10 are generated through alternative splicing and likely, the action of endoproteases of acrosomal origin. The SP-10 protein is expressed only in the testis, and is first detected postmeiotically in round spermatids where it is packaged in the acrosomal vesicle. In mature sperm SP-10 has been localized to the principal segment and posterior bulb of the equiortial segment. Following the acrosome reaction, SP-10 is found on the inner acrosomal membrane, in the equatorial segment, and associated with hybrid vesicles.

Antibodies to SP-10 significantly inhibit fertilization in vitro by preventing tight binding of sperm to the zona pellucida. These antibodies to SP-10 affect sperm motility and the ability of sperm to complete the acrosome reaction.

Recombinant forms of SP-10 have been injected into female primates and have elicited strong immune responses. The antibodies generated to recombinant SP-10 recognize the native SP-10 protein from human sperm and localize to the acrosome.

To date, contraceptive effects in vivo have not yet been demonstrated for SP-10 nor for any other protein in the category of intra-acrosomal proteins which are restricted only to the acrosomal compartment. Acrosomal antigens which reside solely within the membranes and matrix of the acrosome have the advantage of offering a precise staging of immunocontraceptive vaccine action to the cascade of events occurring after sperm-zona binding. Conceptually, this targeted timing of vaccine action offers an attractive model for a prefertilization contraceptive vaccine. The disadvantage of such intra-acrosomal antigens is that in order for inhibition of fertilization to occur in vivo, antibody to such intraacrosomal antigens must be generated at sufficient levels in the oviduct and/or zona pellucida to contact these antigens at the egg surface within the narrow window of time when these antigens "decloak" and are accessible. Antibody levels generated to intra-acrosomal antigens must be sufficient to block one or several stages in the cascade of events involving primary and secondary binding to the zona, induction of the acrosome reaction, shedding of the acrosomal ghost, penetration of the zona pellucida, and binding to the oolemma.

SP10 est une protéine intra-acrosomique constituée chez l'humain de 265 acides aminés. Chez l'homme, SP10 est codée par un gène unique quadri exonique localisé sur la bande q23-24 du chromosome 11. A l'intérieur de l'acrosome SP10 montre une importante micro-hétérogénéité structurale avec des protéines dont le PM varie entre 18 et 34 kD. Les différentes isoformes de SP10 sont le résultat d'un épissage alternatif et de l'action probable d'endoprotéases acrosomiques. La protéine SP10 est exprimée exclusivement dans le testicule et est détectée à partir du stade des spermatides rondes, au moment de la formation de l'acrosome. Dans le spermatozoïde, SP10 a été localisée dans le segment principal et la portion postérieure du segment équatorial. Après la réaction acrosomique, SP10 est retrouvée sur la membrane acrosomique interne, sur le segment équatorial et dans les vésicules membranaires.

Les anticorps anti-SP10 inhibent la fécondation in vitro de façon significative en bloquant la fixation des spermatozoïdes sur la zone pellucide. Ces anticorps diminuent la mobilité des spermatozoïdes et leur capacité à faire la réaction acrosomique.

Des formes recombinantes de SP10 ont été injectées à des primates femelles et ont induit de fortes réponses immunitaires. Les anticorps induits reconnaissent la SP10 native du spermatozoïde humain et se fixent sur l'acrosome.

Actuellement, des effets contraceptifs in vivo n'ont été démontrés ni pour SP10 ni pour aucune autre protéine purement intra-acrosomique. Les antigènes acrosomiques, présents uniquement dans les membranes et la matrice de l'acrosome ont l'avantage d'offrir un effet vaccinal sur une étape précise des événements qui suivent l'interaction gamétique. Conceptuellement, cette vaccination très ciblée dans le temps procure un modèle intéressant dans la contraception vaccinale pré-fécondation. L'inconvénient est que, pour obtenir une inhibition de la fécondation in vivo, il est nécessaire d'obtenir des taux élevés d'anticorps dans l'oviducte et/ou la zone pellucide pour qu'ils puissent se fixer sur les antigènes dans le très court laps de temps où ceux-ci sont démasqués et accessibles.

Les taux d'anticorps doivent être suffisants pour bloquer une ou plusieurs étapes de la cascade événementielle impliquée dans la fixation sur la zona, l'induction de la RA, la perte de l'acrosome, la traversée de la zone pellucide et la fixation à la membrane plasmique.

INTRODUCTION

This paper will discuss the potential use of intra-acrosomal sperm proteins as contraceptive vaccine immunogens. There will be three themes: First, general consideration will be given to the criteria used to identify contraceptive vaccine candidates. Second, special problems associated with the use of intra-acrosomal antigens as contraceptive immunogens will be highlighted and two categories of acrosomal antigens will be distinguished. Third, recent data regarding the intra-acrosomal antigen SP-10 will be discussed in order to emphasize the generic issues surrounding the development of intraacrosomal antigens for contraceptive testing.

PRE-FERTILIZATION VACCINE FOR FEMALES.

The principal focus will be on a vaccination model in which the vaccine recipient is a female and the objective of immunization is to induce infertility at a stage prior to completion of fertilization. This type of vaccine, in contrast to vaccines which are directed against antigens of the trophoblast or early embryo [eg. HCG], has been termed a "pre-fertilization vaccine".

INTRODUCTION TO THE SP-10 PROTEIN

SP-10 is a intra-acrosomal acrosomal protein known to be conserved across various mammalian species including humans, baboons, macaques, pigs, foxes, and mice (1). In humans, the protein is 265 amino acids in length and contains a typical signal sequence of 17 amino acids at its amino terminis (3). Human SP-10 is encoded by a single copy gene consisting of four exons located on human chromosome 11 at band q23-24. Western blots have shown the human SP-10 protein consists of a series of protein isoforms ranging from 18-34 kDa (7). At least four of the SP10 isoforms are generated by alternative splicing of the SP-10 transcript and there is indirect evidence that other SP-10 isoforms are generated by endoproteolytic hydrolysis by acrosomal enzymes (3-5). In mature human sperm SP-10 is localized to the acrosomal matrix and is also associated with acrosomal membranes (6). The World Health Organization Taskforce on Contraceptive Vaccines has designated SP-10 as a "primary vaccine candidate" (9). The discussion below will highlight several features of the SP-10 protein that have led to its consideration as a contraceptive vaccine immunogen.

THE CRITERIA OF TISSUE SPECIFICITY.

The sperm molecules for inclusion in a contraceptive vaccine must be testis specific proteins in order to reduce the chance of autoimmunity, which may arise if antigens common to many tissues were utilized in a vaccine formulation. The acrosome represents a major organelle unique to spermiogenesis and as such, holds considerable promise as a structure comprised of at least some gene products expressed only in the testis. The acrosome possesses features similar to both secretory granules and lysosomes and some proteins common to secretory granules and lysosomes in other tissues have been demonstrated in the acrosome. However, unique proteins of the acrosomal membranes and matrix, if they can be definitively demonstrated to be testis specific gene products, meet the important criteria of tissue specificity and can continue on the contraceptive vaccine development pathway.

SP-10 AS A MODEL TESTIS-SPECIFIC GENE PRODUCT.

The intra-acrosomal protein, SP-10, is an example of a protein which has met the criteria of testis specificity. Following cloning of the human SP-10 cDNAs, a baboon model was developed by cloning and sequencing baboon SP-10 cDNAs. The tissue specificity of the intra-acrosomal protein SP-10 was then examined by Northern blot and PCR analysis using baboon tissues. Messenger RNA from 36 tissues in the female baboon (Papio papio) was isolated, separated on agarose gels, transferred to nylon, and probed with either an SP-10, ,β-actin, or cyclophilin cDNA. Northern blots, which were processed at both low and high stringency, showed SP-10 to be expressed exclusively in the testis. The mRNA from each tissue was also reverse transcribed and both SP-10 and, β-actin were amplified by PCR from the resulting cDNA. Ethidium bromide stained agarose gels of the SP-10 PCR products showed three clear bands from the testis, but no co-migrating bands from the other tissues. Southern blots of the PCR products showed that only the 3 bands in the testis were related to SP-10. The data demonstrated that the SP-10 gene products are testis specific; an essential characteristic for a contraceptive vaccine candidate molecule. This study, which employed the most sensitive methods for detecting low abundance messages, represents one of the more extensive examinations of the testis specificity of a primate gene (1).

SP-10 IS A POST-MEIOTIC GENE PRODUCT.

In situ hybridization for the SP-10 message was also performed on human testis sections with biotin and ^{35}S labeled riboprobes. The SP10 message was observed to be expressed in round spermatids found in stages 1, 11, and 111 of the seminiferous cycle (13). Qualitative evaluation, using both detection systems, suggested that there was an increase in transcription as spermatids developed from the Golgi phase in stages I and 11 to cap phase in stage 111. Quantitative analysis of silver grains with the ^{35}S-labeled probe confirmed these observations. Very little SP-10 mRNA was detected in spermatids at stages IV, V, and Vl, and rarely were silver grains found in spermatogonia or spermatocytes.

LOCALIZATION IN THE TESTIS.

Probing immunohistochemically for the SP-10 protein at light and electron microscopic levels also gave evidence of tissue specificity. At the light microscopic level, the SP-10 protein was observed only in the seminiferous epithelium and not in any other tissue. EM immunohistochemistry showed a precise onset of the SP-10 protien in round spermatids (14). The SP-10 protein was first detected in Golgi phase spermatids and then remained associated with the membranes and matrix of the acrosome in all subsequent stages. Taken together, the evidence indicates that the SP-10 protein is a testis specific gene product expressed post-meiotically.

IMMUNOGENICITY.

In order for a sperm antigen to be potentially useful as a contraceptive vaccine agent, the antigen must be a strong immunogen capable of inducing antibody mediated [humoral, B cell] and/or cell mediated immune responses [eg: T helper cells, macrophages, natural killer cells]. Because sperm represent cells that do not normally differentiate in the female body, sperm specific proteins, may prove to be powerful immunogens in female animals. Intra-acrosomal antigens which are testis specific may be particularly good immunogens in female recipients.

IMMUNOGENICITY OF RECOMBINANT SP-10 IN FEMALE PRIMATES.

The intra-acrosomal protein SP-10 is an example of a strong immunogen in female animals. Recombinant SP10 molecules of both human and baboon SP-10 have been made in the pET vector system.

The full length open reading frames for human and baboon SP-10 were placed under the inducible T7 bacteriophage RNA polymerase/promoter system (11). The recombinant protein contains a pel B signal sequence of 27 amino acids and the entire SP-10 coding region, minus the endogenous SP-10 signal sequence of 17 amino acids. An in-frame fusion was made such that a stretch of six histidine residues were produced at the carboxy terminus of SP-10. Upon induction of gene expression, large amounts of SP-10 were synthesized and the recombinant protein segregated into an insoluble fraction. The protein was then solubilized in 6 M guanidine HCl and purified by immobilized metal affinity chromatography (IMAC). The yield of purified protein preparation was approximately 10 milligrams per one liter of culture. Immunoreactivity of the purified recombinant SP-10 with: a) MHS-10, a monoclonal antibody specific to SP-10; and b) rabbit polyclonal sera raised against SP-10, indicated that the synthesized antigen was suitable for immunization studies. Four female baboons were then immunized with the recombinant baboon SP-10 antigen. Immunoblots using pre-immune and immune sera from these animals indicated that all four baboons produced antibodies that reacted with native SP-10 protein extracted from human sperm in a manner identical to that of MHS-10, the positive control. Immune sera also stained the acrosome region of human and baboon sperm head by immunofluorescence. These results demonstrated that the full length recombinant baboon SP-10 antigen was immunogenic in female baboons and generated an immune response which recognized the native antigen on the sperm head, indicating that the recombinant SP-10 antigen is a suitable vaccine immunogen (1 1).

THE IMPORTANCE OF SURFACE ACCESSIBILITY OF SPERM ANTIGENS CHOSEN FOR CONTRACEPTIVE VACCINE DEVELOPMENT.

In the case of antibody mediated events, the sperm antigen targets chosen for contraceptive development must be accessible on the sperm surface so that immune events such as sperm agglutination, sperm Iysis, antibody coating of surface antigens, or phagocytosis of opsonized sperm might proceed. Certain cell mediated processes, such as NK cell Iysis of targets, also require interactions between the NK cell and sperm surface antigens, although other cell mediated events, such as release of cytokines inhibitory to sperm function, do not necessarily require the target antigens to be exposed on the sperm surface. Whether B cell or T cell immune effectors are consider, delivery of antibodies, cytokines or phagocytic and Iytic cells will be through the vehicle of the secretions of the female reproductive tract [oviductal fluid, uterine fluid [milk], and cervical mucus].

MECHANISMS OF CONTRACEPTIVE ACTION IN VIVO.

As sperm progress through the female reproductive tract immune effectors in female secretions may exert contraceptive effects which act in various regions. Thus, anti-sperm antibodies present in cervical mucus might agglutinate or Iyse sperm in the vagina prior to sperm passage through the cervix. Sperm, coated with surface antibody, might be prevented from swimming through and penetrating cervical mucus, [a clinical condition often referred to as the "shaking phenomenon", well described in the literature on sperm-cervical mucus interaction interaction]. Sperm might be trapped or Iysed by antibodies present in uterine secretions and thus prevented from reaching the oviduct. Antibodies present in oviductal fluid might likewise bind to sperm antigens and prevent key steps in the fertilization process from occurring in the oviduct. For example, penetration of the cumulus mass, binding to the zona, capacitation, induction of the acrosome reaction, shedding of the acrosomal ghost, penetration of the zona pellucida, binding to the oolemma, or internalization of the spermatozoa represent stages of spermegg interaction where antibodies bound to sperm might inhibit key functions.

IMMUNOGLOBULINS EMBEDDED WITHIN THE ZONA PELLUCIDA.

In considering these possible immunocontraceptive events in the oviduct it is important to appreciate that the zona pellucida is itself permeable to immunoglobulins. Anti-sperm antibodies may become embedded in the zona pellucida during differentiation of the oocyte within the ovarian follicle, where the oocyte is bathed in follicular fluid which contains immunoglobulins. In addition, passage of the egg through the oviduct may also result in antibody equilibrating within the layers of the zona pellucida. If such antibody were directed against sperm antigens and sufficient antibody were present in the oviductal fluids and tissues surrounding the egg, fertilization might be blocked.

Two categories of acrosomal antigens may be distinguished based on surface accessibility.

It is useful to consider acrosomal antigens in two categories: 1) Antigens which are restricted in the mature sperm to the acrosomal membranes and matrix [eg. acrosin, SP10]; and 2) Antigens which have both a plasmamembrane form and an intra-acrosomal form [eg. PH-20 (hyaluronidase)]. Proteins with dual localizations both on the sperm plasmamembrane and within the acrosome are accessible to antibody at many stages of sperm transport within the female tract. However, proteins which are restricted to the acrosomal membranes and matrix afford a much narrower window for immunological interdiction and contraceptive action. Such antigens within the acrosomal compartment become accessible to antibody as the acrosome reaction is initiated, fusion pores form, hybrid vesicles develop, and the acrosomal membranes and matrix are exposed to the surrounding medium.

The blessing and the curse of acrosome restricted intra-acrosomal antigens as contraceptive vaccine immunogens.

Restricted localization of acrosomal proteins to the matrix and membranes of the acrosomal compartment may be both a blessing and a curse from the contraceptive development standpoint. As a blessing, intra-acrosomal proteins [which remain sequestered until initiation of the acrosome reaction] may afford precise staging of vaccine action to events occurring after sperm-zona binding. Conceptually, this targeted timing of action offers an attractive model for a prefertilization contraceptive vaccine. As a curse, it must be appreciated that in order for inhibition of fertilization to occur in vivo, antibody to such intra-acrosomal antigens must be generated at sufficient levels in the oviduct and/or zona pellucida to contact these antigens at the egg surface within the narrow window of time when these antigens "decloak" and are accessible. Antibody levels must be sufficient to block one or several stages in the cascade of events involving primary and secondary binding to the zona, induction of the acrosome reaction, shedding of the acrosomal ghost, penetration of the zona pellucida, and binding to the oolemma.

SP-10 IS EXPOSED ON THE SPERM SURFACE FOLLOWING THE ACROSOME REACTION

Electron microscopic immunocytochemical observations of epididymal, ejaculated and capacitated sperm have revealed colloidal gold labeling of SP-10 to be most abundant within the principal segment and posterior bulb of the equatorial segment of the acrosome, while the colloidal gold labeling of SP-10 was sparse in the anterior equatorial segment of the acrosome (6). Following a follicular fluid induced acrosome reaction SP-10 was detected on the inner acrosomal membrane, in the equatorial segment, and associated with hybrid vesicles. With completion of the acrosome reaction, the entire anterior portion of the sperm head becomes remodelled as the inner acrosomal membrane becomes the limiting membrane over the anterior portion of the sperm nucleus. The persistence of SP-10 on this inner acrosomal membrane makes it an attractive candidate for blocking interactions of the inner acrosomal membrane and the egg investments. The localization of SP-10 after the acrosome reaction is consistent with the hypothesis this protein is involved in sperm-zona binding or penetration (6). This latter hypothesis has been directly shown using bovine in vitro fertilization.

ANTIBODIES TO SP-10 INHIBIT BOVINE IN VITRO FERTILIZATION BY AFFECTING SPERM PRIOR TO SPERM-ZONA SECONDARY BINDING (12).

Anti-SP-10 antibodies are cross-reactive with bovine sperm and reduce bovine fertilization rates in vitro by affecting both sperm motility and the ability of sperm to complete the acrosome reaction. To characterize bovine SP-10, sonicated bovine sperm extracts were analyzed by Western blot using three monoclonal antibodies (mAbs) previously developed to human SP-10 and a polyclonal antibody to recombinant baboon SP-10 (rbSP-10). Under denaturing and reducing electrophoretic conditions, the 6C12 mAb reacted with proteins from 30-35 kDa and the polyclonal antibody reacted with numerous proteins from 18-35 kDa. Under non-denaturing and non-reducing (native) electrophoretic conditions, both the 6C12 and MHS-10 mAbs reacted with proteins from 3540 kDa and the polyclonal antibody reacted strongly to a single protein band from 33-38 kDa. The 3C12 mAb did not recognize proteins from bovine sperm extracts in Western blot analysis under either condition. Indirect immunofluorescence revealed that the MHS-10 mAb, 6C12 mAb, and polyclonal antibody were reactive with the acrosomal region of methanol-fixed bovine sperm while the 3C12 mAb did not stain the sperm. The first IVF experiment revealed that, fertilization rates of bovine oocytes were significantly reduced ($p < 0.01$) from 86.5% in the control lacking antibody and 83.2 % in the null ascites control to 47.7% and 7.5% in groups treated with a 1:20 and 1:10 dilution of a cocktail containing the three SP-10 mAbs. In the next experiment, MHS-10 mAb ascites was added to the fertilization medium followed by immediate absorption of the antibody using rbSP-10. The resulting fertilization rate (81.3%) was not different ($p > 0.10$) than either the control lacking antibody (85.3%) or the null ascites (87.6%). However, a unabsorbed MHS-10 mAb ascites reduced ($p < 0.01$) fertilization rates to 16%, thus demonstrating that the reduction in fertilization rates was due to SP-10 antibodies and not another component of the ascites. In the final IVF experiment, the addition of polyclonal antisera to SP-10 to the fertilization medium resulted in a 44.3% fertilization rate, which was significantly lower ($p < 0.01$) than that of the control lacking antibody (79%) and the pre-immune sera (84%). Functional assays were performed to study the possible stage of sperm-egg interaction at which the antibodies were exerting their effect. The SP-10 mAb cocktail was shown to significantly reduce ($p < 0.05$) sperm-zona secondary binding during IVF. The MHS-10 mAb significantly reduced ($p < 0.01$) the motility and rapid motility of capacitated sperm but did not reduce the motility parameters of noncapacitated sperm. The MHS-10 mAb also reduced the ability of capacitated sperm to undergo the acrosome reaction while having no effect ($p > 0.10$) on sperm viability. Together these data indicate that antibodies to SP-10 block sperm-egg interaction by preventing secondary binding. This blockage of bovine fertilization appears to be due to an effect of antibodies on sperm motility and the ability of sperm to complete the acrosome reaction (12).

FUTURE RESEARCH DIRECTIONS

It should be appreciated that little is known about how best to generate secretory immunoglobulins within the female reproductive to sperm antigens. There is a further need to know what levels of antibody within oviductal secretions will exert contraceptive effects. Because the progression of sperm through the female reproductive tract offers many opportunities for immunocontraceptive interdiction, the ultimate contraceptive vaccine will likely be comprised of several sperm specific antigens, localized both to the sperm plasmalemma and to the inner acrosomal membrane of the remodeled, acrosome reacted sperm.

THE RESEARCH OPPORTUNITY

No contraceptive vaccine is currently on the market in any country and development of a contraceptive vaccine has many hurdles to overcome, not the least of which is achieving efficacy which will match that of contraceptive products currently in the marketplace-products which deliver 95% efficacy or better [over the counter birth control pills]. A continuing need exists to define, characterize, clone and evaluate testis specific molecules on the sperm plasmalemma and acrosomal membranes as contaceptive vaccinogens.

Supported by NIH HD 23789, U54 HD 29099, a grant from the Andrew W. Mellon Foundation, and CSA-93-125 from the CONRAD program of USAID.

REFERENCES

1. Freemerman AL, Wright RM, Flickinger CJ, Herr JC. Tissue specificity of the acrosomal protein SP-10: a contraceptive vaccine molecule. Biol Reprod 1994; 50:615-621.
2. Herr JC, Wright RM, John E, Foster J, Kays T, Flickinger CJ. Identification of human acrosomal antigen SP-10 in primates and pigs. Biol Reprod 1990; 42:377-382.
3. Wright RM, John E, Klotz K, Flickinger CJ, Herr JC. Cloning and sequencing of cDNAs coding for the human intra-acrosomal antigen SP-10. Biol Reprod 1990; 42:693-701 .
4. Herr JC, Klotz K, Shannon J, Wright RM, Flickinger CJ. Purification and microsequencing of the intra-acrosomal protein SP-10. Evidence that SP-10 heterogeneity results from endoproteolytic processes. Biol Reprod 1992; 47 ~ 20.
5. Freemerman AJ, Flickinger CJ, HerrJC. Characterization of alternatively spliced human SP-10 mRNAs. Mol Reprod Devel 1994; (in press).
6. Foster JA, Herr JC. Interactions of human sperm acrosomal protein SP-10 with the acrosomal membranes. Biol Reprod 1992; 46:981-990.

7. Herr JC, Flickinger CJ, Homyk M, Klotz K, John E. Biochemical and morphological characterization of the intra-acrosomal antigen SP-10 from human sperm. Biol Reprod 1992; 42:181-193.
8. Foster JA, Klotz K, Flickinger CJ, Thomas TS, Wright RM, Castillo JR, Herr JC. Human SP-10: acrosomal distribution, processing, and fate after the acrosome reaction. Biol Reprod 1994; 51:1222-1231.
9. Anderson DJ, Johnson PM, Alexander NJ, Jones WR, Griffin PD. Monoclonal antibodies to human trophoblast and sperm antigens: report of two WHO-sponsored workshops. J Reprod Immunol 1987; 10:231-257.
10. Dubova-Mihailova M, Mollova M, Ivanova M, Kehayov 1, Kyurkchiev S. Identification and characterization of human acrosomal antigen defined by a monoclonal antibody with blocking effect on in vitro fertilization. J Reprod Immunol 1991; 1 9:251-268.
11. Reddi PP, Castillo JR, Klotz K, Flickinger CJ, Herr JC. Production in Escherichia coli, purification and immunogenicity of acrosomal protein SP-10, a candidate contraceptive vaccine. Gene 1994; 147:189-195.
12. Coonrod SA, Westhusin ME, Herr, JC. Antibodies to SP-10 Inhibit Bovine In Vitro Fertilization by Affecting Sperm Prior to Sperm-Zona Secondary Binding. Biol. Reprod. [submitted]
13. Kurth BE, Wright RM, Flickinger CJ, Herr JC. Stage-specific detection of mRNA for the sperm antigen SP-10 in human testis. Anat Rec 1993; 236:619-625.
14. Kurth BE, Klotz K, Flickinger CJ, HerrJC. Localization of sperm antigen SP-10 during the six stages of the cycle of the seminiferous epithelium in man. Biol Reprod 1992; 44:814-821.

Chapter V
Chapitre V

Posters
Posters

Fluidity changes in sperm membranes during capacitation

[1]Morros A., [2]Iborra A., [1]Alsina M., [2]Martinez P.

[1]Unitat de Biofísica & [2]Unitat d'Immunologia (I.B.F.) Universitat Autonoma de Barcelona. 08193 Bellaterra, Spain

OBJECTIVES:
Sperm capacitation is usually measured by sperm hyperactivation and by the percentage of acrosome reacted cells at the end of the process. Important changes in the lipidic bilayer composition and organization trigger sperm capacitation and acrosome reaction. The main objective of this study is to provide a method that allows us to characterize the fluidity of sperm membranes at different stages of capacitation. Cholesterol is one of the principal responsible for these fluidity changes; we have used cholesterol acceptors to mimic the initial stages methods of capacitation, and membrane fluidity was measured by fluorescence anisotropy.

MATERIALS AND METHODS:
Washed goat sperm were resuspended in PBS, pH 7.4 to a final concentration of 5×10^7 cells/ml. In parallel two types of liposomes were prepared: dipalmitoyl phosphatidylcholine (DPPC), a pure saturated phospholipid, and egg phosphatidylcholine (EPC), a natural mixture of unsaturated phospholipids. Sperm was incubated in presence of liposomes or bovine serum albumin to allow cholesterol efflux and membrane fluidification. For the incorporation of the fluorescent probe (1, 6 -diphenylhexatriene (DPH) or its derivative TMA-DPH) to sperm membrane, the cells were incubated with the fluorophore for 45 minutes at 37°C. Emission spectra were obtained in the range of 425-450 nm for an excitation wavelength of 367 nm using a SLM-8000 spectrofluorometer, in the L-format, and the corrected steadystate anisotropy was then calculated.

CONCLUSION:
Important changes in the lipidic thermotropic behavior appear after cholesterol release from sperm membranes at short incubation times. The efficiency of the two types of liposomes and albumin are compared. Both gel-liquid phase transition temperature (Tm) and transition cooperativity changes indicate sperm membrane fluidification after incubation with albumin or EPC liposomes. Undesirable bi-directional transfer of lipids is observed when sperm are incubated with DPPC liposomes.
Fluorescence anisotropy allows to characterize the physical state of sperm membranes at different conditions that could simulate the initial stages of capacitation.

Fluorescence techniques used to study sperm membrane lipid architecture during capacitation

Gadella B.M., Harrison R.A.P.

Department of Development & Signalling, The Babraham Institute, Cambridge CB2 4AT, United Kingdom

OBJECTIVES:
In recent years, the great advances in light-detecting technology coupled with rapid data handling and storage, and the associated tremendous increase in the availability of fluorescent biochemical markers, have presented exciting new possibilities for studying cellular processes in living cells. Here we present three different ways in which we have used fluorescent lipid analogs to detect changes in the plasma membrane architecture of capacitating spermatozoa

1. LATERAL REDISTRIBUTION OF GLYCOLIPIDS IN THE SPERM HEAD PLASMA MEMBRANE

Acyl-labelled fluorescent lipid analogues were transferred into the sperm plasma membrane by incorporating them into unilamellar vesicles of dioleoylphosphatidylcholine (DOPC) before co-incubating the vesicles with spermatozoa Such labeled spermatozoa were incubated under various conditions, and lateral distribution of the incorporated lipid labels was followed in situ by analyzing digitized images obtained via fluorescence microscopy.

Phospholipid analogues always distributed evenly over the plasma membrane surface whereas glycolipid analogues selectively incorporated in the apical subdomain of the sperm head plasma membrane. However, the glycolipids redistributed towards the equatorial subdomain during incubation with bicarbonate/CO_2 and Ca^{2+} (a capacitative treatment).

2. CHANGES IN TRANSVERSE DISTRIBUTION OF PHOSPHOLIPIDS ACROSS THE PLASMA MEMBRANE BILAYER.

DOPC vesicles containing NBD-acyl-labeled phospholipid analogues were incubated with spermatozoa, and the rate of fluorescence incorporation was monitored directly by flow cytometry. The membrane-impermeable reducing agent, dithionite, was used to destroy NBD fluorescence in the outer leaflet of the bilayer in order to allow quantitation of the proportion of incorporated label that had been translocated across the bilayer.

NBD-phosphatidylserine and to a lesser extent NBD-phosphatidylethanolamine were translocated rapidly and essentially completely; however, NBD-phosphatidylcholine was only slowly translocated (to a limit of 12%). Capacitative treatment caused a significant slowing of the rate of aminophospholipid translocation and an increase in the limit of translocated NBD-phosphatidylcholine (to 30 %).

3. INCREASE IN PLASMA MEMBRANE FUSOGENICITY.

If DOPC vesicles containing N-rhodamine-, and N-NBD- headgroup-conjugated phosphatidylethanolamines is illurminated so as to excite NBD (470 nm), little NBD fluorescence (530 nm) but considerable rhodamine fluorescence (585 nm) is observed; the rhodamine has been excited by absorbing the emission energy from the NBD (fluorescence resonance energy transfer or FRET). When the vesicles fuse with cell membranes, the dilution of the probes diminishes FRET greatly, and the NBD fluorescence increases while the rhodamine fluorescence decreases.

By monitoring FRET, it was found that fusion of DOPC vesicles with sperm cells only took place if the spermatozoa had been incubated under capacitating conditions. Fusion appeared to be restricted to the equatorial subdomain of the sperm head.

Extracellular calcium inihibits tyrosine kinase activity during capacitation of human spermatozoa

Luconi M., Krausz C.S., Forti G. , Baldi E.

Dipartimento di Fisiopatologia Clinica, Unita' di Andrologia, Universita' di Firenze

OBJECTIVES:
An increase of intracellular Ca^{2+} concentrations ($[Ca2+]i$) (Baldi et al., J. Androl., 12:323-330,1991) and protein tyrosine phosphorylation (Luconi et al, Molec Cell. Endocrinol., 108:35-42,1995) has previously been demonstrated by our group during "*in vitro*" capacitation of human spermatozoa. In the present study we investigated the relationship between these two phenomena by studying tyrosine phosphorylation of proteins, tyrosine kinase and phosphatase activities during "*in vitro*" sperm capacitation in the presence or absence of calcium in the extracellular medium.

MATERIALS AND METHODS:
Spermatozoa, obtained from male normospermic partners of infertile couples, were prepared by Percoll gradient, and capacitated in an appropriate medium in the presence of BSA for the indicated times. After capacitation in the different conditions, spermatozoa were lysed in SB2x, and proteins separated by SDS-PAGE. Phosphotyrosine residues of the different proteins were revealed by western blot analysis using a monoclonal anti-phosphotyrosine antibody.

RESULTS:
We found that tyrosine phosphorylation of three proteins, of respectively 52-55, 75 and 97 kDa molecular weight range, increases during sperm capacitation, confirming previous results. However, when capacitation was obtained in (nominally) Ca^{2+}-free medium, unexpectedly, tyrosine phosphorylation of these proteins was further enhanced. Moreover, the spontaneous increase of tyrosine phosphorylation was still present when capacitation was obtained in the presence of EGTA and the intracellular Ca^{2+} chelator BAPTA-AM, suggesting that activation of tyrosine kinases during capacitation is a Ca^{2+}-independent mechanisms and that the increase of Ca^{2+} during capacitation is limiting rather than promoting tyrosine phosphorylation increase To confirm that an increase of $[Ca^{2+}]i$ decreases tyrosine phosphorylation of proteins, spermatozoa were treated with the Ca^{2+} ionophore A23187 and the endoplasmic Ca^{2+}-ATPase inhibitor thapsigargin previously shown to mobilize Ca^{2+} in spermatozoa Both treatments reduced tyrosine phosphorylation of sperm proteins, further confirming Ca^{2+} dependent inhibition of this mechanism

To establish whether the increase of tyrosine phosphorylation observed in Ca^{2+}-free medium was due to activation of tyrosine kinase(s) or inhibition of tyrosine phosphatase(s), the activity of these enzymes was measured in the different experimental conditions. Tyrosine kinase activity was higher in spermatozoa capacitated in Ca^{2+}-free when compared to complete medium (average percentage increase: 154+14, n=4, p<0.05), while protein tyrosine phosphatase activity was uneffected in these conditions.

CONCLUSION:
These results suggest that capacitation of human sperm is regulated by complex interactions between Ca^{2+}-dependent and independent pathways leading to activation/inhibition of tyrosine kinases. In particular, we suggest that the increase of $[Ca^{2+}]i$ during capacitation might play a role in controlling the process of tyrosine phosphorylation to ensure appropriate timing of full capacitation in the proximity of the oocyte.

Protein phosphorylation on tyrosine during human sperm capacitation

Emiliozzi C., Philip P., Ciapa B., Fénichel P.

Groupe de Recherche sur l'Interaction Gamétique, Faculté de Médecine, Nice 06107 France

OBJECTIVES:
To study the evolution of protein tyrosine phosphorylation pattern during capacitation *in vitro* by comparing the potential role of non specific (albumin, culture media, seminal plasma) and specific factors (progesterone and NECA an adenosine analog, acting via the adenylate cyclase system).

MATERIALS AND METHODS:
Spermatozoa from donors with normal spermogram were separated by percoll gradient. The patterns were analyzed by western blot using antiphosphotyrosine monoclonal antibody (UBI) after SDS-PAGE of solubilized sperm proteins. Capacitation was indirectly evaluated by the calcium ionophore-induced acrosome reaction response (GB 24 mab-ethidium homodimer-flow cytometry).

RESULTS:
Sperm incubation in culture media containing HSA 3% induced progressive tyrosine phosphorylation of at least 4 proteins with an apparent molecular weight around 200, 100, 70 and 50 kDa in relation with the capacitation state (increasing response to ionophore). The kinetic of phosphorylation showed an inter individual variability. Phosphorylation was inhibited by the lack of albumin in the culture medium but not by addition of seminal plasma. Progesterone enhanced phosphorylation of the 100 kDa protein in capacitated sperm (4h incubation in BWW-HSA); NECA which stimulates the sperm cyclic AMP, had an opposite effect on phosphorylation depending on the capacitation state. Tyrosine phosphorylation of the 100 kDa protein was enhanced before any incubation but decreased when compared to control after 1 h incubation. In contrast phosphorylation of a 50 kDa protein was systematically enhanced by NECA after 1 h preincubation.

CONCLUSION:
Capacitation *in vitro* of human sperm is associated with phosphorylation/dephosphorylation of several proteins. These biochemical events are influenced by both non specific factors (albumin, time, seminal plasma) and specific factors such as progesterone and modulators of the adenylate cyclase.

Human sperm acrosome reaction. Eds P. Fénichel, J. Parinaud.
Colloque INSERM/John Libbey Eurotext Ltd © 1995. Vol. 236, pp.393-394

Fate of two novel human sperm antigens HE4 and HE5 during *in vitro* capacitation

Osterhoff C., Kirchhoff C., Ivell R.

Institute for Hormone and Fertility Research, Grandweg 64, 22529 Hamburg, Germany

OBJECTIVES:
Human epididymal gene products HE4 and HE5, originally cloned as tissue-specific cDNAs from a human epididymal cDNA library (1,2) have been detected immunohistochemically on the sperm surface within the epididymis. Genbank searches had revealed a HE4 homology with protease inhibitors, whereas HE5 was already known as a GPI-anchored leucocyte differentiation antigen (3). To investigate the possible function of HE4 and HE5 during fertilization we analyzed the fate of these antigens during *in vitro* capacitation.

MATERIALS AND METHODS:
Liquefied semen samples and "swim up" sperm were incubated at 37°C in the presence of 5% CO_2 in prewarmed Ham's F10 or "universal IVF-medium". Aliquots were taken hourly (0-8h), smeared on slides, air-dried, and postfixed in 4% paraformaldehyde. Polyclonal antibodies were raised against a 14mer HE4-oligopeptide of highest predicted antigenicity in chicken and a recombinantly expressed fusion protein of HE4 in rabbits. In the case of HE5 a CDw52 (CAMPATH-1) monoclonal antibody was used (3). Immunostaining was performed using Cy3 fluorescent-conjugated second antibodies (4).

RESULTS:
Employing polyclonal antibodies of different sources HE4 related antigen was identified on the sperm surface of ejaculated sperm smears and in the surrounding medium. After washing or "swim up" treatments the antigen was detectable solely within the medium, but not on the spermatozoa even after shortest "swim up" incubation time (15 min.).
On the contrary, the HE5-related antigen was detectable on the whole sperm surface throughout the time period of up to 8h either in ejaculates or "swim up" treated sperm exclusively on the sperm surface itself and not in the surrounding medium.

CONCLUSION:
The involvement of extracellular proteinases (like acrosin) and proteinase inhibitors (like HE4) in the fertilization process has long been suggested, and the removal of extracellular or seminal plasma 'acrosin-inhibitors' from ejaculated spermatozoa seems to be an essential part of the capacitation process. Our results suggest that HE4 might be a decapacitation factor that is probably removed during residence of sperm in uterine fluid. The HE5 antigen seems to remain on the sperm surface during *in vitro* capacitation, not surprisingly, as it is bound via a GPI-anchor in the outer leaflet of the sperm membrane. So the function of HE5 might be further 'downstream' during the fertilization process, e.g. during membrane fusion of the gametes as HE5 is an integral part of the sperm membrane.

1) Kirchhoff, C., Habben, I., Ivell,R., Krull, N. (1991) Biol. Reprod. 45, 350-357. 2) Kirchhoff, C., Krull, N., Pera, I., Ivell, R., (1993) Mol. Rep. Dev. 34, 8-15. 3) Hale, G., Rye, P.D., Warford, A., Lauder, I., Brito-Babapulle, A. (1993) J. Reprod. Immunol. 23, 189-205. 4) Osterhoff, C., Kirchhoff, C., Krull, N., Ivell, R. (1994) Biol. Reprod. 50, 516-525.

Quantification of energetic patterns of human spermatozoa during capacitation process by ^{31}P magnetic resonance spectroscopy (^{31}P-MRS)

Hamamah S., [2]Seguin F., [1]Barthélémy C., [1]Royere D., [1] Perrotin F., [1]Lansac J.

1 Unité de Biologie de la Reproduction, Dépt de Gynéco-Obstétrique, Faculté de Médecine, CHU Bretonneau, F-37044 Tours cedex, France
2 Labo de Bioph Cell & RMN-INSERM U316, Faculté de Médecine, F-37032, Tours cedex, France

OBJECTIVES:

It is well know that the energetic metabolites play important roles in the spermatozoa survival as well as motility. ^{31}P magnetic resonance spectroscopy (^{31}P MRS) was used to evaluate the changes in the metabolic status and determine some energetic markers such as Inorganic phosphate (Pi), Phosphomonoester (PM), Phosphodiester (PD), Phosphocreatine (Pcr) and Adenosinetriphosphate g,a, b (ATP) during in vitro capacitation of human spermatozoa.

MATERIALS AND METHODS:

Abnormal semen samples (n=15) were obtained from patients participating to our IVF program. The samples were washed twice with Locke balanced buffered solution containing glucose (10 mM). The pellets were resuspended in Locke medium, divided in 4 aliquots (400 µl) and incubated for 2h at 37°C in Locke medium (control), or Locke supplemented with lactate (5 mM), fructose (5 mM) or calcium ionophore A23187 (2 mM). For ^{31}P MRS analysis, a BRUKER AM 200 WB spectrometer (4.7 T) operating at 81 MHz and equipped with a 5 mm ^{1}H / ^{31}P probe thermostated at 37°C was used. The data are mean ± SEM corresponding to the peak intensity.

RESULTS:

Characteristic ^{31}P MRS of spermatozoa incubated with calcium ionophore revealed high PM and ATP in comparison to spermatozoa incubated with lactate or fructose (PM: 27.6 ±8.0, ATP: 19.6 ± 2.8 VS 19.9 ± 1.1 ,16.5 ± 2.9 and 14.1 ± 0.4, 16.8 ± 3.1 respectively). However, PD levels was variable between treatment and higher after fructose or Lactate treatment compared with calcium ionophore (18.5 ± 2.7, 10.7 ± 3.8 Vs O respectively). We have also observed that the intracellular pH in fructose, Lactate and calcium ionophore treatment were 7.03 ± 0.22, 6.77 ± 0.10 and

6.81 ± 0.18 respectively. The motility as well as morphology % are discussed with regard to the metabolic results.

CONCLUSION:
These results demonstrates different metabolic patterns of human spermatozoa. Such analysis may be used to elucidate the molecular basis of the metabolic sperm disturbances and to evaluate the stimulatory effect of certain molecules which are able to preserve the sperm motility.

Sperm capacitation in human is transient and correlates with chemotactic responsiveness

Cohen-Dayag A[1], Tur-Kaspa I.[2], Dor J.[2], Mashiach S.[2], Eisenbach M.[1]

[1]Dept. Membrane Res. & Biophysics, The Weizmann Inst. of Science, Rehovot, Israel; [2]Dept. Obstetrics & Gynecology, Sheba Medical Center, Tel Aviv Univ. Medical School, Tel Hashomer, Israel.

OBJECTIVES:

Mammalian spermatozoa cannot fertilize the egg immediately after ejaculation, but they rather require a period of incubation for acquiring this capacity and becoming "capacitated". Recently it was found that human spermatozoa are chemoattracted to follicular factors, that only a small fraction in each sperm population is chemotactically responsive, and that the identity of the spermatozoa which belong to this category is continuously changing by turnover [Cohen-Dayag et al. (1994) Biol. Reprod. 50, 786-790]. This chemoattraction was correlated with human egg fertilization. These findings raised the possibility that chemotactic responsiveness is restricted to capacitated spermatozoa. On the basis of the correlation between chemotaxis and fertilization, we suggested that the role of chemotaxis is to select capacitated spermatozoa able of fertilizing the egg, i.e., that only capacitated spermatozoa can be attracted to the egg. Therefore, we determined whether or not the chemotactic spermatozoa are capacitated.

MATERIALS AND METHODS:

Fractionation of spermatozoa according to their chemotactic responsiveness and determination of the percentage of capacitated spermatozoa in chemotactically-enriched and -deficient subpopulations.

RESULTS:

The percentage of capacitated spermatozoa was 13 ± 4 (mean $\pm$ SD) fold higher in the subpopulation enriched with chemotactic spermatozoa than in the rest of the population. Furthermore, there was a temporal correlation between the capacitated state and the chemotactic responsiveness; both were transient and synchronous. The fraction of capacitated and chemotactically-responsive spermatozoa in the total sperm population remained unchanged during this period.

CONCLUSION:

The capacitated state of individual spermatozoa is not static, as has been believed, but rather temporary with a life span of 2.5-4.5 h. Furthermore, the synchronously transient nature of the capacitated state and the chemotactic responsiveness raises the possibility that spermatozoa acquire chemotactic responsiveness only when they become capacitated and lose it when the capacitation state is terminated. It is suggested that, in vivo, the role of sperm chemotaxis is to select the capacitated cells out of the non-capacitated ones and by turnover of capacitation to ensure the availability of capacitated spermatozoa for an extended period of time.

Stimulation of human sperm during capacitation *in vitro* by an analog of adenosine

Fénichel P.*, Gharib N.°, Emiliozzi C.*, Donzeau M.*, Ménézo Y.°

*Groupe de Recherche sur l'Interaction Gamétique, Faculté de Médecine, Nice 06107 France
°INSA, Villeurbanne, France

OBJECTIVES:
The effects of an agonist of adenosine 5'N-Ethyl-Carboxamidoadenosine (NECA) has been investigated on human sperm prepared for *in vitro* fertilization to verify its physiological meaning and its possible pharmacological use.

MATERIALS AND METHODS:
Effects of NECA at 100 µM in B2 medium on motility has been studying by CASA and by comparing the rate of motile sperm recovered by percoll gradient. Capacitation was evaluated indirectly by the response to A23187 (10µM, 30 min.) measuring acrosome reaction by double staining (GB24 mab/ethidium homodimer) and flow cytometry. Changes in cytoplasmic sperm cAMP were determined by RIA Pasteur kit. Tyrosine phosphorylated proteins were analyzed by western blot using antiphosphotyrosine mab (UBI).

RESULTS:
NECA did not modify sperm motility but enhanced cAMP production in uncapacitated sperm after 10 and 20 minutes incubation. NECA did not induce spontaneous acrosome reaction, evaluated by double staining after 0, 3 and 5 hours incubation in B2 but increased the number of capacitated spermatozoa able to respond to A23187 (10 µM in B2); $p<0.05$ at 5 hours preincubation. At the same time NECA was able to modify completely phosphorylation on tyrosine of sperm proteins involved in capacitation. This phosphorylation was enhanced for a 95 kD protein on uncapacitated sperm and inhibited on capacitating sperm (4 to 5 hours incubation in B2) but systematically enhanced for a 45 kD protein whatever the preincubation time.

CONCLUSION:
Human spermatozoa express adenosine receptors. Adenosine activates human sperm capacitation via cAMP production and protein phosphorylation /dephosphorylation without inducing acrosome reaction nor influencing motility. cAMP-dependent protein kinase A may control protein phosphorylation involved in human capacitation. Use of NECA in sperm handling for IVF should be evaluated in case of male infertility to improve capacitation without increasing premature spontaneous acrosome reaction (RA).

Origin and nature of the acrosome reaction-inducing substance (ARIS) of human follicular fluid (hFF)

Baltes P.*, Sanchez R.*#, Schalles U.K.*, Villegas J.*#, Peña P.*#, Henkel R.*, Turley H.+, Miska W.*

*Department of Dermatology and Andrology, Justus-Liebig University, Giessen, Germany; #Universidad de la Frontera, Temuco, Chile; +Institute of Reproductive Medicine, Giessen, Germany

OBJECTIVES:

The biochemical and immunological characterization of the "acrosome reaction-inducing substance" (ARIS) of human follicular fluid (hFF), and localization of its synthesis. Moreover a model for the modulation of the sperm acrosome reaction (AR) by the oviductal environment in the female genital tract should be found.

MATERIALS AND METHODS:

Isolation of "ARIS" by differential ultrafiltration and gel filtration; biochemical characterization by determination of molecular weight, pH-optimum, temperature stability, by protease digestion, dextran-coated charcoal (DCC)-treatment, carbohydrate structure analysis by lectin binding, and ligand-exchange experiments with ^{3}H-labeled progesterone; immunological characterization by means of poly- and monoclonal antibodies against human Corticosteroid-binding globulin (CBG). Quantitative determination of the AR by the triple-stain technique. Evaluation of the origin of "ARIS" by temporary culture of human cumulus oophorus cells; treatment of the culture medium with monoclonal anti-CBG and AR-induction; pulse experiments with ^{3}H-labeled leucin to measure protein secretion; western-blot analysis of the culture-supernatant with polyclonal anti-CBG; immunocytochemical and immunoelectronmicroscopical evaluations of cumulus cells with poly- and monoclonal anti-CBG.

RESULTS:

Previous experiments performed here have yielded several indications on the protein character of "ARIS", and according to the current literature, steroids also seem to play an important role in AR-induction. Our current findings show that hFF, which has been stripped off proteins and/or steroids (protease-, DCC-treatment) cannot induce the AR. However, after the removal of steroids, the AR-inducing activity of hFF can be restored by exogenous progesterone, but only in the presence of intact protein. Furthermore in gel filtration experiments with ^{3}H-progesterone-labeled hFF an elution of the radioactive signal in the high molecular weight range, corresponding to bound progesterone, was found. Based on these results we suggest that the effect of "ARIS" is a synergistic action of progesterone and a progesterone-binding protein. The protein has been shown to be immunological identical with the corticosteroid-binding globulin (CBG), which has already been described and serves as a transport protein for progesterone and cortisole in the plasma. Our findings also show that the CBG-progesterone complex is able to induce the AR in nanomolar concentrations, where neither progesterone nor the protein alone is able to bring about an effect. In the culture medium of human cumulus oophorus cells AR-inducing activity could be detected. The immunological as well as the radiochemical investigations strongly indicate that human cumulus cells actively express and secrete a CBG-like progesterone-binding protein.

CONCLUSION:
CBG and thereby "ARIS" is a member of the superfamily of serine protease inhibitors (SERPINs). The SERPINs perform numerous regulatory functions by means of their inhibitory effects. In the case of transport proteins, to which CBG belongs, they have lost their inhibitory properties, but have retained the typical structure and functional characteristics of SERPINs. CBG is able to bind and transport small molecules and then to release them at specific targets after undergoing SERPIN-specific conformation changes in the CBG molecule through the activity of a serine protease. On the basis of this the following mechanism is proposed for the role of the CBG-progesterone complex in the induction of the AR: Progesterone is transported by CBG to the spermatozoon. CBG is cleaved there by a plasma membrane-bound protease, leading to conformational changes within the protein. This causes a local release of progesterone, which possibly stimulates a Ca^{2+}-channel, thereby leading to an influx of Ca^{2+}, and finally to the induction of the AR.

Preincubation in peritoneal fluid affects follicular fluid induced acrosomal reactivity *in vitro*

Revelli A., La Sala G.B.*, Modotti M., Miceli A., Balerna M., Massobrio M.

*Institute of Gynecology and Obstetrics, Physiopathology of Reproduction, University of Torino and *Dept. of Gynecology and Obstetrics, Reggio Emilia Hospital, Italy; §Locarno Hospital, Switzerland*

OBJECTIVES:

To determine the effects of preincubation in peritoneal fluid (PF) on follicular fluid (FF)-induced sperm acrosomal reactivity (AR) *in vitro*.

MATERIALS AND METHODS:

Eighteen women participating in a IVF-ET program were stimulated with GnRH-a, HP-FSH and hCG. Pfs and Ffs were obtained at pick-up laparoscopy, centrifuged (3000 X g), filtered (0.22 mcm) and freezed (-20 °C) until use. Twenty-five microliters of a swim-up suspension (about 70 MIO spz/ml) from normospermic semen specimens were incubated (37°C, air atmosphere) with 50 mcl of PF or a control medium for 3 hours, after which 50 mcl of FF (volumetric proportion 50/50 with PF) were added. The percentage of acrosomally-reacted sperm was evaluated using a FITC-conjugated lectin, counting 200 spz/ incubate, at time = 0, after 3 hours in PF or control medium, at the moment of FF addition, as well as 1 and 20 hours later.

RESULTS:

PF showed no stimulating effects on acrosomal reactivity, as reported in previous studies of our group. When compared to the control medium (Earle's sol.), PF moderately but significantly reduced FF-induced acrosomal reactivity . This effect was evident both soon after FF addition and after 1 or 20 hours of incubation in the presence of FF.

CONCLUSION:

PF seems able to play a role in maintaining an unreacted sperm status. Anyway, the FF-dependent stimulation of AR is almost completely preserved also in presence of PF.

Inhibition of zona binding using solubilized human zona pellucida

Franken D.R[1]., Henkel R[2]., Kaskar K.[1], Habenicht U.F.[3]

1.Department of Obstetrics & Gynaecology, University of Stellenbosch, Tygerberg Hospital, South Africa 2. Department Andrology, University of Justus Liebig, Giessen, Germany, 3.Ernst Schering Research Foundation, Berlin, Germany

OBJECTIVE:
To evaluate the influence of solubilized human zonae pellucidae on zona binding potential of spermatozoa from fertile men.

MATERIALS AND METHODS:
Sperm samples from 4 fertile sperm donors were prepared by a standard wash and swim up method. Semen analysis was performed using WHO guidelines. Sperm morphology assessments were recorded according to strict criteria for normal spermatozoa. Post mortem derived human prophase oocytes were used for zona pellucida binding assays as well as for preparing zonae pellucidae solutions. Solutions were prepared by dissolving zonae pellucidae in droplets of NaH_2PO_4 (pH 2.5) to obtain solutions containing 0.1 and 0.5 zonae pellucidae/µL Zona solutions were then prepared using a double strength human tubal fluid (HTF) culture medium to adjust for pH and osmolarity differences caused by the zona solvent. Sperm from fertile donors were added (sperm concentration; 4×10^6 cells/ml) to separate zona solutions and pre-incubated for 20 minutes at 37°C. After the pre-incubation period prophase oocytes were added (10-fold) to the zona droplets containing sperm. Zona exposed sperm were then co-incubated with oocytes for 2 hours and evaluated for zona binding. All oocytes were removed and pipette 5X with a small bore micropipette to dislodge closely bound sperm cells. The number of firmly bound sperm to zona pellucida were determined under phase contrast microscopy (200X). Control incubation droplets included sperm, HTF medium and zona solvent alone.

RESULTS:
Spermatozoa from fertile men that have been exposed to solubilized human zona pellucida significantly inhibited zona binding. The mean (±SE) number of sperm bound for control, 0.1 ZP/µl and 0.5 ZP/µl were 181.2±12, 79.6±5 and 38.8±3, respectively. Both zona concentrations inhibit sperm binding to the zona pellucida significantly ($p<0.0001$) compared to the control values.

CONCLUSION:
The data describes the practical utilization of solubilized human zona pellucida to manipulate zona pellucida binding potential of sperm from fertile men.

The production and purification of recombinant human ZP3 from *E.coli*

Chapman N. R.[1,2], Hornby D. P.[2], Barratt C. L. R.[1], Moore H.D.M.[1,2]

Departments of [1]Molecular Biology & Biotechnology and [2] Obstetrics and Gynaecology, The University of Sheffield, Sheffield. S10 2UH, U.K..

OBJECTIVES:

Studies into the involvement of ZP3 in the human fertilization pathway have, until recently been greatly hindered by the paucity of sufficient quantities of the individual molecules that contribute to this process. The production of recombinant mouse-ZP3, (Beebe et al (1992) Dev. Biol. 15l: 48-54) and more recently, recombinant human-ZP3, (Van Duin et al (1994) Biol. Reprod. 51: 607-617) in mammalian cell lines has rectified this situation. However, since it is not clear whether the glycosylation of these recombinant molecules is of a uniform pattern, we have chosen to express human-ZP3 as a fusion with glutathione-S-transferase, (GST-HuZP3) in E. coli. This facilitates one-step purification of the recombinant protein expressed in this organism. We believe this system gives a more defined recombinant molecule than that obtained from mammalian cell culture.

MATERIALS AND METHODS:.

The cDNA sequence encoding the human-ZP3 was ligated into pGEX-KG as a *Bam*Hl-*Eco*Rl fragment following polymerase chain reaction amplification of the original cDNA sequence. A single (positive) colony was selected and used to inoculate a one liter culture. Cells were grown until mid-log phase was attained, (Absorbance at OD_{595} = 0.7). The culture was induced for a period of three hours at 37 °C by the addition of IPTG to a final concentration of 0.5 mM. Cells were then harvested, the pellet resuspended in PBS, (150 mM NaCl, 16 mM Na_2HP0_4, 4 mM NaH_2P0_4) pH 7.4 and the cells lysed by sonication.

RESULTS:

In order to recover the fusion protein, (GST-HuZP3), the supernatant, after sonication, was applied to glutathione-agarose beads, (Sigma) that had been equilibrated in 20 column volumes of PBS. The fusion protein was then eluted from the column with four washes in elution buffer,(PBS, pH 7.4, 10 mM reduced glutathione). The wash fractions were analysed on 10% SDS-PAGE, followed by western blotting. Blots were probed for the presence of GST-HuZP3 with rabbit-anti-pig-ZP3 immunoglobulin, (this antibody was the kind gift of Prof. A. Sacco,

Univ. of Michigan, USA) and then detected with a donkey-anti-rabbit-Ig conjugated to Horseradish PeroNdase, (Amersham) which would facilitate detection by ECL^{TM}, (Amersham). A single band was detected on the blots that: 1) corresponded to a species of ~72 kDa on coomassie stained gels, and 2) was exclusive only to the supernatants of transformants, not controls.

Biological activity of GST-HuZP3 and native heat-solubilised human zonae was assessed with three separate assays: 1) Their ability to specifically induce changes in the pattern of phosphorylation of sperm membrane proteins, 2) Their effect on intracellular Ca^{2+} leveis and 3) Their ability to induce the acrosome reaction. (For greater details of these assays see the abstract of Brewis et al 1995).

CONCLUSION :
These data show the successful expression and purification of the human-ZP3 from E.coli. This source of HuZP3 will be a great asset in the further study of the involvement of the ZP3 polypeptide in human fertilization.

The authors greatly acknowledge the financial support of the Infertility Research Trust and Serono, U.K..

The use of antibodies raised against synthetic peptides to conserved and unconserved regions of human ZP3 for characterization of sperm-egg interactions

McCann C.T., Barratt C.L.R.[1], Moore H.D.M.[1,2]

Departments of Obstetrics & Gynaecology[1] and Molecular Institution Biology & Biotechnology[2], University of Sheffield, Sheffield, S10 2UH, UK.

OBJECTIVES:

We have used recombinant zona pellucida proteins (Barratt et al., 1994) to investigate specific epitopes in the sperm-egg recognition process. Peptides were synthesized from conserved (peptide 252, 329-344 amino acids) and unconserved (peptide 267, 54-75 amino acids) regions of the consensus amino acid sequence of human ZP3 and conjugated to keyhole limpet haemocyanin Polyclonal antisera were raised in rabbits using these preparations. Antibodies were isotyped and immunoaffinity purified. Immunofluorescence and immunohistochemical studies using the purified antibodies were then performed using oocytes, solubilised zonae, recombinant human ZP3, ovarian tissue and other tissues

MATERIALS AND METHODS:

Sera were semi-purified by ammonium sulfate precipitation. Both antisera were found to be IgG by isotyping and were then passed through a protein A column to purify the immunoglobulin. The IgG's were used for indirect immunofluorescence on mouse, pig and hamster oocytes. Immunohistochemical studies were undertaken using sections of ovary, kidney, liver, spleen, brain and lung from human, mouse and pig. Dot blotting was used with heat solubilised human, mouse, pig and hamster zonae and recombinant human ZP3 expressed Results by Chinese hamster ovary cells. Appropriate negative and positive controls were used

RESULTS:

Antibody titers were assessed as 1:20,000 (252) and 1:15,000 (267) at exsanguination and after purification titers were 1:30,000 (252) and 1:25,000 (267). From immunofluorecence studies both antibodies were shown to be cross reactive with pig, mouse and hamster oocytes. The antisera was also shown to detect ovarian material, solubilised human, pig, hamster and mouse zonae, and recombinant human ZP3 but none of the other tissues by dot blotting Immunohistochemical studies were also undertaken using ovarian and non ovarian tissue

CONCLUSION

Two antibodies were generated which could detect recombinant ZP3 and were ovary and zona specific As yet no differences have been found in the specificities of the antibodies for the conserved and unconserved regions. These antibodies are currently being used in functional studies, to assess the importance of these regions for inducing the acrosome reaction and/or sperm-zona binding of human sperm.

[This work was supported by the Infertility Research Trust, UK].

Human sperm acrosome reaction. Eds P. Fénichel, J. Parinaud.

Calcium/progesterone mediated acrosome response and sperm maturity are not related in human spermatozoa

Huszar G. , Vigue L.

The Sperm Physiology Laboratory, Dept. OB/GYN, Yale Univ. Sch. of Med., New Haven CT, USA

OBJECTIVE:
We have demonstrated that sperm creatine kinase(CK) activity and the ratio of the CK-M vs. CK-B isoforms predict sperm maturity and the occurrence of pregnancies. Further, we have shown that high CK content immature sperm fail to bind to the oocyte, indicating surface membrane changes related to sperm maturation. In other studies focusing upon acrosome function, the sperm CK-parameters were not related to the results of zona-free hamster oocyte penetration assay or to the acrosome reaction to calcium-ionophore challenge test (ARIC). In this ongoing work we studied sperm CK-parameters and the rate of sperm capacitation and acrosome reaction under controlled exposure to calcium and progesterone.

MATERIALS AND METHODS:
The semen samples of 22 husbands of infertile couples (conc: 71.1 ± 9.7 x 10^6 sperm/ml, all data mean ± SEM), were washed at 500 x g for 18 minutes and the sperm were resuspended in HTF(Irvine Co.) containing 3% BSA and 5mM $CaCl_2$.

The sperm samples were incubated at 37°C for 3 hours and subsequently 3 µM progesterone was added. The rates of capacitation and acrosome reaction(AR) were determined with FITC-PSA (200 live sperm per time point) and with chlortetracycline at 0 time, at 3 hours (prior to addition of progesterone), and after two hour and overnight incubation in the presence of progesterone.

RESULTS:
The incidence of acrosome intact sperm at the 4 time points were: 87 ± 2%, 85 ± 2%, 76 ± 4% and 52 ± 6%, N=22). In order to gain further insight, we have analyzed the overnight AR rates in relation to factors that are associated with diminished fertility. There were no differences in oligospermic vs. normospermic samples (33.8 ± 12.7 vs. 56.2 ± 6.8%, p=0.22, N=4 and 18), in asthenospermic vs. normal motility samples (53 ± 0.9% vs. 51.8 ± 7.8%, p = 0.9, N=7 and 15), in samples with CK activity >0.25 IU/10^8 sperm or <10% CK-M/CK-B ratio vs.

mature CK value samples (64.9 ± 6.4% and 47.4 ± 8%, p=0.17, N=6 and 16). Most revealing was the analysis of the 9 samples in which all sperm parameters were normal: 5 samples showed high rates and 4 samples low rates of AR (overnight unreacted sperm: 20.3 ± 9.2% vs. 80.4 ± 2.2 %, p=0.003, N=5 and 4). The capacitated CTC pattern occurred at a similar rate in both groups, the difference was due to the loss of the acrosomal cap.

CONCLUSION:
1) In a defined environment there was a sample-to-sample variation in AR response following exposure to calcium/progesterone 2) There was no relationship between AR response and any semen parameters that are associated with diminished fertility. 3) As found previously with the hamster oocyte and ARIC studies, there is a subpopulation of men who may have mature sperm but show a defect in AR function. (Supported by HD-19505 and HD-32902).

Effect of lysophospholipids on the human sperm acrosome reaction

Llanos M.N., Morales P.*, Salgado A.M.*, Vigil P.*

INTA, university of Chile, P.O Box 138-11 and unit of Reproduction and Development, P. Catholic University of Chile, P.O Box 114-D Santiago, Chile

OBJECTIVES:
The acrosome reaction (AR) is a crucial step for mammalian fertilization. There is evidence that phospholipase A2 participates in the molecular mechanism of the mammalian sperm AR. For instance, phospholipase A2 inhibitors can block the hamster sperm AR *in vitro* and this blockage is eluded by exogenous lysophospholipids (LPLs) (J Exp Zool 1993; 267-269). In addition, it has been shown that dilauroylphosphatidylcholine induces the AR of human spermatozoa (J Androl. 1992; 13: 260). However this increase was accompanied by a substantial decrease in sperm motility. In the present work we have evaluated the effect of different LPLs on the human sperm AR.

MATERIALS AND METHODS:
Motile spermatozoa selected by a Percoll gradient, were resuspended in modified Tyrode's medium supplemented with 2.6% BSA at 10.10^6 cells/ml. The sperm were incubated at 37 °C and 5% CO2. After 5 or 20 hr, the spermatozoa were treated with 100 or 200 µg/ml of lysophosphatidylcholine (LPC), lysophosphatidylethanolamine (LPE), lysophosphatidylserine (LPS) or lysophosphatidylinositol (LPI) for 15 min. In some experiments, the BSA concentration in the sperm suspension was decreased by washing and resuspending the spermatozoa in medium supplemented with either 0.5 or 0.7% BSA. The different LPLs were then added as above. The AR in living spermatozoa was detected using FITC-PSA and Hoechst 33258. At least 200 spermatozoa were scored in each experiment.

RESULTS:
When added to spermatozoa capacitated for 20 hr (in medium with 2.6% BSA), none of the LPLs tested induced the AR. This was true at both doses of LPLs (100 and 200 µg/ml). In addition, at 2.6% BSA none of the LPLs affected the motility of spermatozoa. When the cells were suspended in 0.5% BSA before adding the LPLs, both LPC and LPI induced the spermatozoa to undergo the AR (control = 12.4±2; LPC = 33.3±7; LPI = 34.6±8). the treatment with these LPLs, however, significantly decreased sperm motility. In other experiments, spermatozoa incubated for 5 hr in

medium supplemented with 2.6% BSA were washed and suspended in medium with either 0.5% or 0.7% BSA. Then, different concentrations of LPC were added. There was a significant relationship between the dose of LPC used and the ability of the spermatozoa to undergo the AR ($p<0.001$); This was true at both BSA concentrations. Moreover, there was no detrimental effect on sperm motility at all doses of LPC tested, except at 200 µg/ml. At this highest concentration of LPC the percentage of motile spermatozoa was significantly decreased only in those cells suspended in 0.5% BSA. The LPC-induced AR were morphologically normal as evidenced by transmission electron microscopy.

CONCLUSION:
The present results suggest that massive production of an endogenous lysophospholipid may be the trigger for the membrane events on the human, sperm AR.

Financed by Fondecyt 688/93 and European Economic Community N° CI1-CT92-0022.

Evidence suggesting that reacted human spermatozoa express a L-selectin

Lucas H.*[§], Harb J. [§], Le Pendu J. [§], Mirrallie S. *, Bercegeay S. *, Jean M.* , Barriere P.*

* Unité de Biologie de la Reproduction, [§] INSERM U 419, CHU de Nantes, France

OBJECTIVES:
The aim of this study was to examine the presence of a leukocyte selectin (L-Selectin) on human spermatozoa correlatively to acrosomal status by cytofluorimetry. L-Selectin was a cell adhesion molecule expressed on leukocyte which plays a role in endothelium-leukocyte interactions during inflammation and lymphocytes homing to high endothelial venules. We have previously observed an immunoreactivity with antibody directed against this adhesion molecule on the head of methanol-fixed human spermatozoa and identified two of its potential ligands, sialyl-lewis-a and sialyl-lewis-x oligosaccharides on zonae pellucidae, under immunocytochemical condition. Otherwise, anti-L-selectin monoclonal antibody (anti-LECAM-1 mAb) inhibits sperm zona pellucida binding under hemizona assay conditions.

MATERIALS AND METHODS:
Sperm was obtained from one volunteer of proven fertility who had fathered a child in the last two years. The sperm concentration was $> 50 \; 10^6$ /ml and the progressive motility $> 50\%$. Spermatozoa used in immunocytochemistry were prepared by a swim-up procedure in Menezo B2 medium then methanol fixed on slides. The sperm used in cytofluorimetric analysis was separated into two aliquots, the first was capacitated by a single swim-up procedure, and the second was capacitated in presence of 20 µm calcium ionophore A 23187.
Methanol-fixed spermatozoa for immunochemistry, and calcium ionophore A 23187 treated or not spermatozoa studied by cytofluorimetry, were incubated with anti-LECAM-1 mAb overnight at room temperature, then with secondary FITC-conjugated mAb. Negative controls were performed by omission of the primary mAb. $5 \; 10^3$ cells were analyzed for each aliquots on a Becton Dickinson FACScan cytofluorimeter. χ^2 test was used for statistical analysis.

RESULTS:
100 % spermatozoa treated with ani-LECAM-1 mAb presented an intense fluorescence on the half anterior part of the head and a lower on the midpiece,

whereas the negative controls did not present any fluorescence on methanol-fixed spermatozoa by immunocytochemical procedure.

Sperm capacitated without calcium ionophore A 23187 then treated with anti-LECAM-1 mAb revealed a 29.2% subpopulation of spermatozoa with a mean fluorescence intensity of 44 and a 70.8% subpopulation with a mean fluorescence of 4.5, whereas control sperm incubated with the single secondary FITC conjugated antibody revealed two cell subpopulations with a mean autofluorescence intensity of 3 (94.3% spermatozoa) and 33.1 (5.7% spermatozoa).

Sperm capacitated without calcium ionophore A 23187 then treated with anti-LECAM-1 mAb revealed a 10.7% subpopulation a with a mean fluorescence intensity of 55 and a 89.3% subpopulation with a mean fluorescence of 2.8, whereas control sperm incubated with the single secondary FITC conjugated antibody revealed two cell subpopulations with a mean autofluorescence intensity of 2 (97.8% spermatozoa) and 35.4 (2.2% spermatozoa). Spermatozoa subpopulations labeled with anti-LECAM-1 mAb show a significant difference when treated or not with calcium ionophore A 23187 ($p=0.001$).

CONCLUSION:

Immunochemistry was applied on a methanol-fixed spermatozoa and 100% of them were able to bind anti-LECAM-1 mAb after permeabilization with methanol. Cytofluorimetric analysis suggest that calcium ionophore induced acrosomal reaction permits to anti-LECAM-1 mAb to bind to the sperm. We could speculate that L-selectin was an inner acrosomal membrane protein exposed with acrosomal region and participated in secondary sperm-zona pellucida binding.

Localization and characterization of protein 4.1 in human spermatozoa

Rousseaux Prevost R.[1], Dalla Venezia N.[2], Saint Pol P.[3], Delaunay J., Rousseaux J.

[1] EA 1719 IRCL Lille, [2] URA CNRS 1171, Institut Pasteur, Lyon, [3] CECOS-Nord, CHRU Lille, France

OBJECTIVES:
We have previously shown that human spermatogenic cells contain proteins antigenically related to protein 4.1, a protein of the membrane cytoskeleton initially described in red cells but also present in various cell types. An abnormal expression of protein 4.1 has been found in some cases of teratospermia (Rousseaux-Prevost et al, 1994, Lancet 343, 764- 765). The aim of this study was: (1) To investigate more precisely the intracellular localization of the protein 4.1-like material present in spermatozoa; (2) to define whether sperm protein 4.1 is a spectrin-actin binding protein as the isoform of red cell membranes.

MATERIALS AND METHODS:
Spermatozoa from fertile donors were analyzed by indirect immunofluorescence either directly or after the following treatments: (1) extraction of sperm cells with MgCl2 1M or Triton X-100, or SDS 1%; (2) Induction of acrosome reaction with ionophore A 23187. Proteins released from spermatozoa were studied by immunoblotting. Antibodies used were : polyclonal anti-protein 4.1 and anti-spectrin antibodies; antibodies specific for the spectrin-actin binding domain (anti-10 kDa domain); monoclonal antibodies to beta-actin (Sigma) and to acrosin (Biomérieux).

RESULTS:
Protein 4.1 was found predominantly located in the sperm acrosome region while actin and spectrin have variable localizations, mostly the equatorial segment and the tail. Protein 4.1 like material of 86 kDa was released by extraction with either MgCl2, Triton X-100 or SDS treatments, while acrosin was mainly found in Triton X 100 or SDS. Immunofluorescent labeling of acrosome reacted sperm with anti-Protein 4.1 antibodies was poor or absent. Protein 4.1-like material of sperm cells was not recognized by antibodies specific for the 10 kDa domain of erythrocyte protein 4.1.

CONCLUSION:
A protein antigenically related to protein 4.1 is present near the plasma membrane in the human acrosome. However, absence of the spectrin-actin binding domain and distinct localizations of spectrin, actin and protein 4.1 indicate that protein 4.1- like material does not contribute to the constitution of a membrane cytoskeleton similar to the one present in red cells. Further studies will show whether sperm protein 4.1, is a specific isoform produced by alternative splicing of protein 4.1 mRNA transcripts or whether it is a member of the protein 4.1 superfamily, composed of various molecules (ezrin, moesin, PTPD1.....) which share a domain homologous to the 30 kDa domain of protein 4.1.

P34H: an epididymal protein associated with the acrosome of human spermatozoa

Sullivan R.*, Blais J.*, Boue F.[#]

*Département d'Obstétrique et Gynécologie, Université Laval, Québec, Canada,
[#] INSERM U33, 94276 Le Kremlin-Bicêtre, France

OBJECTIVES:
During epididymal transit, spermatozoa undergo a series of modifications collectively involved in the acquisition of their fertilizing ability. Using the hamster as a model, we have previously identified a protein, P26h, that is involved in the binding of the male gamete to the zona pellucida. This protein is added to spermatozoa during their epididymal transit. More recently, we have shown that human ejaculated spermatozoa are characterized by a protein, P34H, showing antigenic and functional homologies with hamster P26h. The aim of this study was to determine the localization of P34H on human epididymal spermatozoa and to establish whether capacitation and the acrosome reaction affect the distribution of this sperm antigen.

MATERIALS AND METHODS:
Human testicular and epididymal tissues were obtained through our local organ transplantation program. These tissues were collected from donors of 20 to 33 years of age, following accidental death with no medical antecedent that could affect reproductive function. The tissues were rapidly frozen, cryosections where made and processed for immunohistological detection of P34H using a specific antiserum. Ejaculated spermatozoa were separated on a discontinuous Percoll gradient, washed, used immediately or capacitated for different period of time in B2 medium. After capacitation, the acrosome reaction was induced by the Ca++ ionophore, ~23187. Following these treatments. the percentage of spermatozoa with the acrosomal cap coated with P34H was determined by immunohistological staining using anti-P34H and correlated with the percentage of acrosome-reacted spermatozoa as evaluated by staining with fluorescein-coupled Pisum sativum.

RESULTS:
Our results have shown that spermatozoa within the seminiferous tubules as well as within the vasa efferentia did not stain following incubation with the anti-P34H antiserum. Labeling restricted to the acrosomal cap first appeared in the lumen of the caput epididymal tubules and its intensity increased during epididymal transit.

P34H detection appeared to be optimal on cauda epididymal spermatozoa. Ejaculated spermatozoa obtained from fertile donors showed the same pattern of P34H distribution e.g. on the acrosomal cap, but the intensity of labeling was much lower than that characterizing cauda epididymal spermatozoa. The ability of the anti-P34H antiserum to bind to the surface of the spermatozoa was reestablished during incubation in B2 medium and culminated in an intense labeling of the acrosomal cap after capacitation. Following acrosomal exocytosis induced by Ca^{2+} ionophore, the percentage of anti-P34H labeled spermatozoa decreased proportionally to the acrosomal reacted spermatozoa as determined by P. sativum labeling.

CONCLUSION:
We have previously proposed that P34H is involved in the interactions of spermatozoa with zona pellucida in humans. The sequence of appearance and accumulation of this sperm antigen during epididymal transit, followed by its unaccessibility associated with ejaculation and its reappearance during capacitation are in agreement with the proposed function of P34H.

(Supported by "Medical Research Council of Canada" and "Fonds de la Recherches en Sante du Quebec")

Human sperm acrosome reaction. Eds P. Fénichel, J. Parinaud.
Colloque INSERM/John Libbey Eurotext Ltd © 1995. Vol. 236, pp. 418

Relationship between timing of the acrosome reaction induction and the fusiogenic capacity of human spermatozoa

Cozzi J, Chevret E, Rousseaux S, Pelletier R, Sele B.

Laboratoire Dyogen, Unité de Biologie de la Reproduction, Institut Albert Bonniot, La Tronche 38706, France

OBJECTIVES:

The aim of this study was to assess the influence of the timing of acrosome reaction induction on the fusiogenic capacity of human spermatozoa.

MATERIALS AND METHODS:

The fusiogenic capacity of spermatozoa from four men presenting normal semen parameters was assessed using subzonal sperm insemination (SUZI) into hamster oocytes. Acrosome reaction was induced before SUZI by exposing sperm to calcium ionophore A23187 (10µM, 30 min) or after SUZI by incubating oocytes, already injected, in medium containing A23187 (10~M, 30 min).

RESULTS:

A total of 843 hamster oocytes were analysed. When acrosome reaction was induced before SUZI, rates of fertilizing spermatozoa among those injected were respectively 0.9%, 0.8%, 2.8% and 3.5% for donors A, B, C and D. When acrosome reaction was induced after SUZI, these rates were significantly increased to 4.5%, 10.3%, 11.9% and 8.2%. A control showed that such increase was not due to activation of oocytes by calcium

CONCLUSION:

The fusiogenic ability of acrosome reacted spermatozoa is time limited. Sperm treatment by A23187 after SUZI synchronize the acrosome reaction with the meeting of gametes and allowed more spermatozoa to fuse with the vitelline membrane of oocytes. Therefore, timing of acrosome reaction induction is of great importance when assessing the fusiogenic capacity of human spermatozoa.

Induction of human sperm capacitation and acrosome reaction in the reproductive tract of hamster cultured *in vitro*

Dhindsa J.S., Sidhu K.S., Guraya S.S.

Andrology Laboratory, Department of Zoology, Punjab Agricultural University, Lhudiana, India

OBJECTIVES:
To study the xenogenic site for inducing sperm hyperactive motility, capacitation and acrosome reaction in human in the reproductive tract of female hamster cultured *in vitro*.

MATERIALS AND METHODS:
Hamster reproductive tract at estrous and diestrous stages of the estrous cycle cultured *in vitro* and human semen samples incubated in cultured reproductive tract. Hamsters uterus alone and uterus with intact oviduct at estrous and diestrous stages were cultured *in vitro*. Washed human spermatozoa were injected into the reproductive tract of hamster cultured *in vitro* and sperm hyperactive motility, capacitation and acrosome reaction were assessed during incubation.

RESULTS:
The occurrence of maximum sperm hyperactive motility, capacitation and acrosome reaction were significantly ($P<0.01$) higher when the human spermatozoa were incubated in uterus with intact oviduct of estrogen-dominated hamster.

CONCLUSION:
The endocrine status of the female hamster and the intactness of the oviduct with uterus affect the onset of sperm hyperactive motility, capacitation and acrosome reaction in human. The estrogen-dominated uterus with intact oviduct of hamster cultured *in vitro* induced the maximum sperm hyperactive motility, capacitation and acrosome reaction in human.

Mechanisms underlying ANP-induced acrosomal exocytosis in bovine sperm

Zamir N.[1], Barkan D.[1], Keynan N.[1], Naor Z.[2], Breibart H.[3]

1: Department of Physiology and Pharmacology, Sackler School of Medecine Tel Aviv University
2: Department of Biochemistry, Faculty of Life Sciences, Tel Aviv University, 69978 Tel Aviv
3. Department of Life Sciences, Bar Ilan University, Ramat Gan 52900 Israel

OBJECTIVES:

The signal transduction mechanisms underlying ANP-induced acrosomal exocytosis in capacitated bull spermatozoa were studied *in vitro*. Typically, ANP exerts its action via activation of ANPR-A receptor (a particulate guanylyl cyclase receptor and/or ANPR-C receptor (also termed clearance receptor). ANPR-C receptor is coupled to the adenyl-cyclase/cAMP system in several cells types.

MATERIALS AND METHODS:

We have recently demonstrated that ANP induced the acrosome reaction via activation of ANPR-A receptors and enhanced formation of cGMP in capacitated bull spermatozoa.

RESULTS:

We hypothesized that ANP-induced acrosome reaction is also mediated by activation of ANPR-C receptor. Using cANP $_{4\text{-}23}$, as specific ligand that binds exclusively to these receptors, we found that cANP $_{4\text{-}23}$ induced acrosome reaction in a dose dependent manner. The activation of ANPR-C receptors by cANP $_{4\text{-}23}$ was associated with reduced cAMP formation. This effect is apparently mediated by activation of a pertussis toxin-sensitive G_i protein. In addition, staurosporine, an inhibitor of protein kinase C partially inhibited cANP $_{4\text{-}23}$-induced acrosomal exocytosis.

CONCLUSION:

We suggest that ANP-induced acrosome reaction in capacitated bull spermatozoa, is mediated via activation of ANPR-A and/or ANPR-C receptors.

Role of reactive oxygen species (ROS) on human sperm acrosome reaction

Fernandez PJ[+], Doncel GF[*], Acosta AA[*], Romeu A[+].

[+]*Hospital Universitario La Fe. Servicio de Reproducción. Valencia, SPAIN.* [*]*Jones Institute for Reproductive Medicine. Department of OB/GYN. Eastern Virginia Medical School, Norfolk, VA 23507 USA.*

OBJECTIVES:

The aims of the present work have been 1) to evaluate the levels of ROS generation and AR during *in vitro* incubation; and 2) to investigate the effect of catalase (CAT), superoxide dismutase (SOD) and pentoxifylline (PTX) on the percentage of spontaneously and induced acrosome-reacted sperm.

MATERIALS AND METHODS:

Normal semen samples (n=20) (count ³ 60 x 10^6 spermatozoa/ml, motility ³ 50%, <1 x 10^6 round cells/ml) were used in the study. Motile spermatozoa were collected by the swim-up procedure and incubated 48 hours in Biggers, Whitten and Wittingham [BWW] medium + 0.3% of human serum albumin (room temperature, 20-22°C) supplemented with 0.06 mM PTX; or 100 U/ml CAT; or 100 U/ml SOD. Spontaneous and 10 mM A23187 induced acrosome reaction was evaluated after swim-up (T_0), and after 4 h (T_4), 24 h (T_{24}) and 48 h (T_{48}) of incubation using fluorescein isothiocyanate conjugated-*pisum sativum* agglutinin. Spontaneous reactive oxygen species (ROS) generation during the incubation were measured on a Berthold LB9505C luminometer in the presence of luminol and horseradish peroxidase (or lucigenine for the superoxide anion).

RESULTS:

The presence of CAT or PTX reduced significantly ($p<0.05$) ROS detection (using luminol and peroxidase) during 48 hours of *in vitro* incubation. On the other hand, PTX and SOD reduced significantly ($p<0.001$) superoxide anion generation during the same period.

At T_0, T_4, T_{24} and T_{48} the percentages of spontaneous acrosome reaction were not significantly different among medium BWW alone or with PTX, SOD or CAT. However, spontaneous and induced acrosome reaction were always lower (not significantly) in presence of SOD than with BWW alone or supplemented with PTX or CAT. At T_{24} and T_{48} the presence of SOD gives a percentage of induced acrosome reaction significantly lower ($p<0.05$) than in medium BWW supplemented with PTX.

CONCLUSION:

Superoxide anion, more than hydrogen peroxide, could play a positive role during capacitation and acrosome reaction process.

Superoxide anion production by human spermatozoa as a part of the ionophore induced acrosome reaction process

Griveau J.F., Renard P., Le Lannou D.

*CECOS de l' OUEST, 1 bis rue de la cochardiere, 35000 Rennes, France

OBJECTIVES:
The involvement of superoxide anion ($O_2^{\circ-}$) in human sperm capacitation and/or acrosome reaction was investigated.

MATERIALS AND METHODS:
Sperm motility was analyzed using the ATS 40 motility analyzer.
Evaluation of acrosome reaction was realized with the monoclonal antibody GB24.
Superoxide anion production was measured by the reduction of ferricytochrome C.
Sperm fatty acids were analyzed by gas liquid chromatography.

RESULTS:
Addition of superoxide dismutase (SOD) in the medium at the beginning of the capacitation process or 15 min. before the induction of acrosome reaction decreased the level of ionophore-induced acrosome reaction. Hyperactivation was not affected by the presence of SOD during the capacitation process. Treatment of sperm suspension by calcium ionophore increased the production of $O_2^{\circ-}$ by the spermatozoa by 4-5 fold and induced the acrosome reaction. In the presence of SOD, superoxide anion could not be detected in the medium and the rate of induced-acrosome reaction was greatly decreased. The presence of an inhibitor of protein kinase C inhibited the production of $O_2^{\circ-}$ in the medium and reduced the induced-acrosome reaction. The production of $O_2^{\circ-}$ and the acrosome reaction were also increased by treatment of spermatozoa by 12-myristate 13-acetate phorbol ester, a specific activator of protein kinase C. While the level of spontaneous acrosome reaction was not increased by the direct addition in the medium of $O_2^{\circ-}$, its presence induced the release of unesterified fatty acids from the membrane phospholipids.

CONCLUSION:
These findings suggest that the production of $O_2^{\circ-}$ by the spermatozoa could be implied in the ionophore-induced acrosome reaction, possibly through the deesterification of membrane phospholipids. However this superoxide anion production is not sufficient to induce by itself the exocytotic process.

Participation of protein-kinases in calcium-ionophore induced human acrosome reaction

Asin S., Doncel G.F., Acosta A.A.

Eastern Virginia Medical School, Norfolk, VA., USA and Clinica e Centro de Pesquisa em Reproducao Humana Roger Abdelmassih, Sao Paulo, SP., Brazil

OBJECTIVES:
Zona pellucida proteins appear to elicit the acrosome reaction (AR) in human spermatozoa through multiple pathways including tyrosine (PTK), A (PKA), and C (PKC) protein-kinase activation as well as extracellular calcium (Ca_e) influx. A mechanism of crosstalk has been postulated for these pathways and demonstrated for some of them. The objective of this work was to ascertain whether PTK, PKA, or PKC activation was critically involved in Ca_e-dependent induction of AR.

MATERIALS AND METHODS:
Motile spermatozoa were separated from semen collected by normal healthy volunteers (n=11) using the swim-up procedure. The sperm were then incubated at 37°C for 3 hours in Ham's F10 + 3.5% human serum albumin (HSA) + 1.0 mM $CaCl_2$ or in medium containing 400 uM Genistein, 80 uM Tyrphostin (PTK inhibitors), 500 uM H-8 (PKA inhibitor), or 500 uM H-7 (PKC inhibitor). The inhibitor concentrations used were the highest ones that did not affect motility and sperm membrane integrity (measured through a hypoosmotic swelling test). Inclusion of 2.5 or 10 uM calcium-ionophore A23187 in medium supplemented with 0.3% HSA and 1 mM was followed by an additional 2 hour incubation. Motility percentage and motion parameters were measured with a Hamilton Thorne motion analyzer (IVOS v.10). Sperm acrosomal status was assessed using the fluorescent probes *Pisum sativum* agglutinin and Hoechst 33258.

RESULTS:
The baseline percentage of acrosome-reacted sperm incubated in medium alone was 3.5 ± 0.7% (x±SEM). As expected, 2.5 and 10 uM A23187 significantly increased this value (20.4 ± 2.7 and 41.8 ± 2.9%). Since non-maximal stimulation was more adequate for inhibition experiments, we chose the lowest dose of A23187. Despite the prolonged contact with the sperm, none of the inhibitors, Genistein (25.4 ± 2.5%), Tyrphostin (30.0 ± 3.9%), H-8 (27.1 ± 2.8%), or H-7 (27.5 ± 3.2%) was able to inhibit A23187-induced AR. Motion parameters were not significantly changed by the inhibitors.

CONCLUSION:
An extracellular influx of calcium was solely sufficient to induce the human acrosome reaction, and if any, interactions or "crosstalks" between this calcium-dependent via and the pathways involving PTK, PKA, or PKC were not indispensable for the completion of the reaction.

Progesterone induces Ca^{++} dependent cAMP increase in human spermatozoa

Milhet P., Parinaud J.

Laboratoire de Fécondation In vitro, CHU La Grave, 31052 Toulouse, France

OBJECTIVES:
Progesterone (P) has been reported to modulate numerous sperm functions through the binding to plasma membrane. One of the effects is an increase in sperm hyperactivation, which is known to be cAMP-dependent. The aim of the present study was thus to evaluate the effect of P on cAMP levels.

MATERIALS AND METHODS:
Spermatozoa, obtained from healthy volonteers, were incubated in presence of increasing concentrations of P. cAMP levels were measured after ethanol extraction by radio-immuno-assay. The percentage of hyperactivated spermatozoa was evaluated using Hamilton-Thorn motility analyser.

RESULTS:
P significantly induced cAMP increase in a dose dependent manner, reaching a 3 fold increase at 100µM ($P < 0.01$). When studying the kinetic of P effect, two cAMP peaks were observed: one occuring after a 30 minute incubation, with a 1.5 fold increase ($P < 0.05$) and the second after a 120 minute incubation with a 2.5 fold increase ($P < 0.01$). These effects of P on cAMP levels were correlated with significant rises in the percentage of hyperactivated spermatozoa, occuring at the same times than those of cAMP. In order to evaluate the Ca^{++}-dependence of these P effects, the experiments were performed in presence and in absence of Ca^{++} in the incubation medium. The effects of P, at the 30th minute and the 120th minute, were completely abolished in the absence of Ca^{++}. Moreover, calcium ionophore A23187 induced, after a 30 minute incubation, an increase in cAMP levels identical to that obtained with P. The effect of P was partially reproduced by GABA and inhibited by GABA antagonist picrotoxin. It was also inhibited by tyrosine kinase inhibitor genistein but not by RU486.

CONCLUSION:
Based on these findings, we conclude that P induces Ca^{++}-dependent cAMP increase in human sperm and that this effect is likely due to the influx of Ca^{++} previously reported and partially involves $GABA_A$ like receptors.

The signal transduction pathway of the acrosome reaction in human spermatozoa in response to purified recombinant human ZP3

Brewis I.A.[1,2], Chapman N.R.[1,2], Barratt C.L.R.[2], Hornby D.P.[1], Moore H.D.M.[1,2]

[1]*Departments of Molecular Biology & Biotechnology and Obstetrics & Gynaecology. The University of Sheffield. Sheffield. S10 2UH. UK*

OBJECTIVES:

The purpose of this study was to investigate signal transduction mechanisms involved in the initial interactions between human spermatozoa and zona pellucida proteins. Due to the paucity of native human zona we have used purified recombinant human zona pellucida protein (rhuZP3). The extent of phosphotyrosine kinase activity, levels of intracellular calcium and the acrosomal status of capacitated spermatozoa in response to rhuZP3 have been examined.

MATERIALS AND METHODS:

RhuZP3 was overexpressed in E. coli as a fusion protein with glutathione-S-transferase (GST) and purified by affinity chromatography (see abstract by Chapman et al.,.1995). Tyrosine phosphorylation of sperm proteins in response to incubation with rhuZP3 was determined with an *in vitro* kinase assay using ^{32}P labeling of whole capacitated spermatozoa and also using Western blotting with anti-phosphotyrosine antibodies. Influx of calcium into spermatozoa in response to rhuZP3 was measured and quantified using fura-2/AM and fluorescence spectrometry. The acrosome reaction of capacitated spermatozoa was assessed by immunofluorescence with an acrosomal membrane-specific monoclonal antibody (mab. 18.6).

RESULTS:

There was a marked increase in the phosphorylation of a 95 kDa membrane protein on the spermatozoa in the presence of rhuZP3 compared to the controls as assessed by the *in vitro* kinase assay. This was shown to be tyrosine phosphorylation using Western blotting techniques and anti-phosphotyrosine monoclonal antibodies (both PY20 and Ab-2). To date we have not been able to show any significant changes to the basal levels of intracellular calcium (65-100 nM) in spermatozoa following the addition of rhuZP3 at levels sufficient to cause tyrosine phosphorylation of the 95 kDa protein. No significant changes in the number of acrosome reacted spermatozoa were found in the presence of rhuZP3.

CONCLUSION :
Although in the presence of purified rhuZP3 there was a marked increase in the tyrosine phosphorylation of a 95 kDa protein this was not sufficient to cause changes in the levels of intracellular calcium nor to induce the acrosome reaction. In contrast to native ZP3 the rhuZP3 is unglycosylated and it is possible that this is reason why this form of rhuZP3 failed to affect either the levels of intracellular calcium or to cause the acrosome reaction. In conclusion these results support the premise that the signal transduction mechanism subsequent to spermatozoa-ZP3 interaction involves tyrosine phosphorylation of a 95 kDa protein which is caused by the peptide domain of ZP3.

This work is supported by the MRC and Serono. UK.

Comparison of two cryopreservative media on acrosomal status

Barthelemy C., Saussereau M.H., Fricot G., Hamamah S., Royere D., Tharanne M.J.

CECOS, Unité de Biologie de la Reproduction, CHU Bretonneau, 37044 Tours Cedex France

OBJECTIVES:
Semen cryopreservation is widely used for sperm banking before chemo and/or radiotherapy treatments, vasectomy, or artificial insemination with sperm donors. But freezing-thawing-process induce severe injuries on sperm structure and functions. The aim of our study was to test two different cryopreservative media to evaluate the best for optimal preservation of structure and fertilizing capacity.

MATERIALS AND METHODS:
21 semen samples with normal semen parameters (according Who standard) were divided in 2 aliquots: the first was freezed using Ackerman medium, the second with TEST-Yolk medium (Irvine scientific CA). Glycerol was used as cryoprotective agent (6% final concentration). Cryopreservation was done in 0.25ml straws (IMV F), after 30mn incubation in the medium, using a programmable freezer Minicool LC40 (Air liquide F.. The straws were warmed in a 37°C waterbath 10mn before use.
On each aliquot were evaluated, before and after cryopreservation, the following parameters: motility, alive forms (Eosin-nigrosin and Hoechst stainings), sperm membrane integrity by hypoosmotic test, FITC ConA staining and acrosomal status using PSA-FITC. Results were expressed in means ± sem and compared with non parametrics tests (Wilcoxon).

RESULTS:
These results confirm sperm injuries during freezing-taawing process: semen parameters were significantly different before and after cryopreservation whatever the medium used ($p<0.0001$). Correlation were found between PSA and ConA staining with alive forms before and after freezing ($p<0.01$). A significant difference appears for vitality and acrosomal status between TEST-Yolk and Ackerman medium: the acrosome seems better preserved with TEST medium. The advantage of TEST medium for post thaw motility was previously described but motility is not the only parameter to evaluate fertilizing capacity. A better acrosomal status appears more important for the fertilization process. These results must be confirmed by comparing the fertilizing capacity of these two media in artificial insemination.

Results
COMPARISON OF VALUES BEFORE AND AFTER CRYOPRESERVATION

	BEFORE	AFTER	
		ACKERMAN	TEST-Yolk
% MOTILITY	42.4 ± 1.4	18.7 ± 1.9	17.6 ± 1.9
% VITALITY Eosin	84.2 ± 1.4	37.4 ± 1.8^a	42.7 ± 2.9^a
% VITALITY Hoechst	86.5 ± 0.9	40.2 ± 2.5	44.7 ± 3
% HYPOOSMOTIC TEST	85.7 ± 0.9	67.5 ± 1.6	70.1 ± 2
% PSA-FITC	66.5 ± 2	22.8 ± 2.4^b	27.2 ± 2.6
Con A-FITC	61.7 ± 2.5	28.6 ± 2.3	30.1 ± 2

a $p<0.03$, **b** $p<0.04$, before/after $p<0.0001$ for all parameters.

CONCLUSION:
These results confirm sperm injuries during freezing-thawing process: semen parameters were significantly different before and after cryopreservation whatever the medium used ($p<0.0001$). Correlation were found between PSA and ConA staining with alive forms before and after freezing ($p<0.01$). A significant difference appears for vitality and acrosomal status between TEST-Yolk and Ackerman medium: the acrosome seems better preserved with TEST medium. The advantage of TEST medium for post thay motility was previously described but motility is not the only parameter to evaluate fertilizing capacity. A better acromosal status appears more important for the fertilization process. These results must be confirmed by comparing the fertilization capacity of these two media in artificial insemination.

Effect of caffeine citrate and heparin on post-thawed motility and on acrosomal cap of buffalo bull spermatozoa frozen in different diluents: assay for *in vitro* fertilization technique

Barnabe, V.H., Barnabe R.C.

Department of Animal Reproduction, Faculty of Veterinary Medicine and Zootechny, University of São Paulo, Brazil

OBJECTIVES:
To test three kinds of diluents for buffalo semen and the effect on postthawed progressive motility and on acrosomal cap, of caffeine citrate and heparin. Semen so treated will be utilized for "*in vitro*" capacitation and "*in vitro*" fertilization of buffalo oocytes.

MATERIALS AND METHODS:
30 semen samples from one healthy buffalo bull were diluted in: 1) TRIS ;2) TES-TRIS and GLYCINE. After centrifugation, semen samples were submitted to caffeine citrate 6mM or to heparin 0.8% during 10 minutes. Effects on postthawed progressive motility were recorded, both prior and after treatments. Integrity of the acrosomal cap after treatments was evaluated under interference phase contrast microscopy (1250 X).

RESULTS:
Progressive motility increased 18% in average, in samples treated by caffeine citrate, while those submitted to heparin 0.8%, resulted in an average increase of 20%. Best results of motility were obtained with TES-TRIS diluent. Immediate post-thawed motility was markedly increased in semen diluted in Glycine, as compared to TRIS and TES-TRIS. In general, progressive motility increased in the 3 diluents, either treated by caffeine citrate or heparin. Acrosomal cap was more affected in semen diluted in TRIS and treated by caffeine citrate or heparin.

CONCLUSION:
Sperm progressive motility increases in post thawed frozen semen diluted with TRIS, TES-TRIS and GLYCINE. Sperm showing low progressive motility are better improved by addition of caffeine citrate or heparin to the diluent. Better results regarding sperm progressive motility were obtained with diluent TES-TRIS treated by caffeine or heparin. Diluent TRIS, either added by caffeine or heparin damaged more the acrosomal cap of spermatozoa, than did TES-TRIS or GLYCINE.

Human sperm acrosome reaction. Eds P. Fénichel, J. Parinaud.
Colloque INSERM/John Libbey Eurotext Ltd © 1995. Vol. 236, pp. 431

Effects of lipids in cryoprotective diluants on motility and fertilization potential of post-thaw human spermatozoa

Grizard G., Sion B., Renard P.*, Artonne C., Boucher D.

Service de Biologie Dévoppement et Reproduction, Hôtel Dieu, Clermont-Ferrand, France
*Cecos ouest, Hôtel Dieu, rue de la Cochardière, Rennes, France

OBJECTIVE:
It was suggested that cholesterol (chol) and phospholipids prevent damages of the membrane of spermatozoa during freeze-thaw process. To test this hypothesis, we studied the cryoprotective effects of different phospholipids singly or in combination with chol and compare these effects with those of egg yolk (EY).

MATERIALS AND METHODS:
To investigate the effects exerted by lipids, liposomes have been made from bovine brain phosphatidylserine (PS), EY phosphatidylcholine (PC-EY) bovine brain-PC (PC-BB), distearolyl-PC (PC18) and a mixture (mole/mole) of PC-BB/chol.
Study was performed on semen samples with a sperm concentration $>20.10^6$ spermatozoa/ml and a motility >50%. They were divided into aliquots which were diluted (V/V) with basal medium (BM: 80 mM glutamine, 0.35% fructose, 0.66% sodium citrate, 14% glycerol, 400 mg steptomycin/100ml) and with either BM containing EY or BM containing liposomes. The semen-medium mixtures were equilibrated for 15 min at room temperature, then cooled in liquid nitrogen according to a specific program.

RESULTS:
PS induces a large decrease in post-thaw (PT) progressive motility; this damage occurs principally during equilibration period rather than during freeze-thaws process. Addition of EY or liposomes of PC or PC/chol in BM did not significantly modified PT viability and motility of spermatozoa. But some PT velocity parameters (VCL, ALH) are higher in presence of EY than in BM alone or in BM supplemented with liposomes.
In contrast, using hamster egg penetration test, the percentage of zona-free hamster eggs that was penetrated was significantly greater with spermatozoa frozen/thawed in BM containing PC-BB/chol than in BM alone or in BM supplemented with EY.

CONCLUSION:
It is concluded that diluants containing liposomes of PC/chol may be beneficial to cryopreservation of human spermatozoa.

A simple method for assessment of the human acrosome reaction (AR) of spermatozoa bound to the zona pellucida (ZP): lack of relationship with ionophore A23187 induced AR

Liu D.Y. , Baker H.G.W.

University of Melbourne Department of Obstetrics and Gynaecology and Reproductive Biology Unit, Royal Women's Hospital, Victoria 3035, Australia

OBJECTIVES:
The aims of this study were (1) to develop a simple method for assessment of the human AR of sperm bound to the ZP and (2) to compare the results with of those of the calcium ionophore, A23187 and solubilized human ZP.

MATERIALS AND METHODS:
Sperm samples were obtained from fertile men or men with normal semen analysis and normal sperm-ZP binding. Oocytes were obtained from patients with failure of fertilization after 48h to 60h *in vitro*. Synthetic human tubal fluid (HTF) medium supplemented with 10% human serum was used. Motile sperm selected by swim-up technique were incubated with 10 mM A23187 for 1 h or 4 oocytes for 2 h or solubilized ZP (4ZP/ml) for 2 h. Sperm bound to the ZP were dislodged and collected in a small volume of phosphate buffered saline by aspirating the oocytes with a glass pipette with an inner diameter of 120 mm, which is slightly smaller than the diameter of the oocyte. Acrosome status of sperm was determined using fluorescein labeled Pisum Sativum agglutinin.

RESULTS:
The proportion of sperm undergoing the AR on the ZP at 2h varied over a wide range (5-99%) but the agreement between results for the same semen sample exposed to different groups of oocytes was good: the standard deviations of the differences being 7% for oocytes from the same patients and 13% for oocytes from different patients. Pre-incubation of sperm for 2h did not increase the ZP induced AR. Reincubation of ZP with the same sperm suspension for 2 h after removing ZP-bound sperm from the first 2h incubation produced significantly lower ZP induced acrosome reaction in the second incubation ($22 \pm 16\%$) than in the first incubation ($30\pm14\%$, $P< 0.001$, n=20). There was no significant difference in ZP induced AR with oocytes with ZP which had or had not been penetrated by sperm from the IVF insemination. Pre-incubation of sperm with solubilized ZP blocked sperm-ZP binding. However, the AR induced by solubilized ZP (4ZP/ml) was significantly lower than AR induced by intact ZP

($10\pm5\%$ and $30\pm13\%$, n=11, P<0.001) but there was a high correlation (Spearman r=0.822, P<0.01) between the AR induced by the intact and solubilized ZP. On the other hand, although the average of AR was similar for A23187 (42%) and for ZP (43%), there was no significant correlation between the results for the two stimuli (n=60, P>0.05).

CONCLUSION:

In conclusion, a useful method for assessing the ZP induced AR has been developed using oocytes which failed to fertilize *in vitro*. The lack of relationship between the results of the chemical (A23187) and physiological (ZP) stimuli for the AR in the same subjects questions the biological basis of using A23187 for tests of sperm function. Solubilized human ZP in concentration that blocks sperm-ZP binding but is a less efficient inducer of the AR than is intact ZP. It is possible that the three dimensional structure of the ZP is important for induction of the AR or sperm which bind to the ZP are more likely to AR. Assessment of the physiological AR for diagnosis of sperm defects which interfere with the fertilization process should be concentrated on the sperm which are capable of binding to the ZP.

Clinical characteristics of disordered zona pellucida induced acrosome reaction: a newly described cause of infertility

Baker HWG, Liu D.Y., Bourne H.

University of Melbourne Department of Obstetrics and Gynaecology and Reproductive Biology Unit, Royal Women's Hospital, Victoria 3035, Australia

OBJECTIVES:
We have recently discovered a specific abnormality of the fertilization process: disordered zona pellucida (ZP) induced acrosome reaction (AR) which causes failure of sperm penetration of the ZP and persistent failure of fertilization *in vitro* (Liu and Baker, Human Reprod, 9: 1694, 1994). The clinical features and results of *in vitro* fertilization and intracytoplasmic sperm injection (ICSI) of 24 patients with this condition are reported.

MATERIALS AND METHODS:
The men were aged 28 to 47, mean 34 and the women 23 to 39, mean 31 years at the time of diagnosis. The couples had a long duration of infertility (Mean 5, range 2.5-13 years). Only one couple had produced a natural pregnancy. Most had idiopathic infertility but a variety of abnormalities were found in some patients including ovulatory disorders in 3, endometriosis in 3 and tubal disease in 1 woman, and varicoceles in 6 and intermittent prostatitis in 1 man. There was no family history of male infertility in the majority of men but we found 3 brothers with this condition. Repeated semen analysis results were normal in half the men. Most of the others mild to moderate reduction in sperm concentration, motility, VSL, or morphology in occasional samples. Four patients had sperm morphology below normal range (normal >15%). Four patients had moderate reductions in sperm-mucus penetration (Kremer test). Twenty couples had standard IVF treatments (average 2 cycles) with low fertilization rates. Twelve patients had consistent failure of fertilization and eight of them had low (<25%) fertilization rates. It was noted that often there were many sperm bound to the ZP of the oocytes which failed to fertilize.

RESULTS:
Sperm zona pellucida interaction tests were performed using the oocytes that failed to fertilize in standard IVF from other patients because of severe sperm defects. Sperm from all the patients had normal ZP-binding but the sperm failed to penetrate the ZP. In contrast most of the ZP were penetrated by control sperm from fertile men. The AR of sperm bound to the ZP was significantly lower for the patients (average 5%) than for fertile men (average 60%).

ICSI was performed in 20 patients and the normal fertilization rate was 77%. Four ongoing and two delivered pregnancies were obtained (30%/ patient).

CONCLUSION:
In conclusion, disordered zona pellucida induced acrosome reaction is a cause of severe infertility which can be diagnosed by sperm ZP interaction tests and treated by ICSI.

Correlation between clinical diagnosis and acrosomal protease assay for the evaluation of male infertility

Chen J.S., *Ma J., #Chang H.S.,*ChangT.S., Sensini C., Collodel G., Piomboni P., Baccetti B., Menesini Chen M.G.

*CSCG del CNR and Ist. Biol. Gen. Univ. Siena, Italy.*Devel. Center for, Taiwan, ROC. # Urol. Dept. Taipei Medical College, Taipei, Taiwan, ROC*

OBJECTIVES:
An italian patent has been requested for a biochemical method for the diagnosis of male infertility (Chen, J.S. et al. It. Pat. Appli. N° RM 94 A 000647). This theory was based on the data obtained from animal experiments (Chen J.S.and al 1993 Zygote 1:309-313) and from human samples (Sensini, C. et al., 1993 The Clinical Biochemist-Reviews 14(iv) p. S41).For human ejaculated sperm, the correlation of R value >1.3, expressed by enzyme activity using BAPNA as substrate, resulting from acrosin-like protease [E]/benzamidine resistant protease [E]x was up to 76.9 % of fitness regarding the normal acrosomal pattern which is believed essential for sperm to bind the zona pellucida (Saling P.M. and Storey B.T. 1979 J. Cell Biol.83: 544).This study evaluates the correlation between infertile subjects and the R value.

MATERIALS AND METHODS:
Ejaculated spermatozoa from 24 patients were collected for conventional clinical assays: sperm count, motility, velocity etc., and for the determination of enzyme activity from two acrosomal protease, namely acrosin-like protease [E] and benzamidin resistant protease [E]x according to the method described by Chen et al (It. Pat. Appli. N° RM 94 A 000647).In this study a synthetic substrate, benzoyl-DL-arginine-p-nitroanilide (BAPNA) was used for enzyme assays. The R was computed from [E]/[E]x.

RESULTS:
According to this description, the R value of infertile subjects should be 0-1.29. Based on the motility, cell counts, and R values, samples were classified into 4 groups as follows: a) Astheno n=12 mean R=0.860 ± 0.387; b) relative Oligo-Astheno n=2 mean R=1.103±0.041; c) relative Astheno n=5 mean R=1.2498± 0.2769 and d) normal but known as infertile n=5 mean R=1.061±0.1634. The correlation between the R value and diagnosed cases for each group were up to 91%, 80%, 100% and 100% respectively for a, b, c, and d. Of 24 samples assayed only two cases have R value above 1.3.

CONCLUSION:
The results fulfilled our prediction that up to 91.66 % of patients have R value < 1.3 therefore without a sufficient normal acrosomal structure to sustain a correct acrosome function/reaction.. This biochemical method, the first in the history of spermatology, which is rapid (< one hour), precise (having reduced technical error to a minimum by using the same extract for enzyme activity assay), and reliable, can be a reference parameter for the diagnosis of male infertility in regard to the acrosome function/reaction. It might also be useful for *in vitro* fertilization technology. It is generally accepted that sperm infertility is dependent on an enormous range of factors, recently assembled in one mathematical formula (Baccetti et al., 1995, J. Androl., in press), therefore it is clear that the R value is probably only one of them.

Detection of patients defective in acrosome reaction

Arts E.G.J.M.[1,2], Van Kooij R.J.[2], Kastrop P.M.M.[2], Hobo A.C.[1]

[1]University Hospital, Oostersingel 59, 9713 EZ Groningen and [2]University Hospital, Heidelberglaan 100, 3584 CX Utrecht, the Netherlands

OBJECTIVES:
Failed *in vitro* fertilization (IVF) may be caused by defective sperm functions in the interaction with the oocyte. Assays that test zona pellucida (ZP) binding capacity of spermatozoa cannot explain all failed fertilizations. In this study we combined a ZP binding assay with a new method to detect both acrosomal status and fusogenic activity, and we examined whether possible causes of unexplained fertilization failure could be further defined. The method uses fluorescent liposomes that interact only with the equatorial segment (ES) of acrosome-reacted spermatozoa.

MATERIALS AND METHODS:
Eight normospermic patients who had failed to fertilize oocytes at least two times were admitted to the study. The control group consisted of 5 healthy, normal sperm donors. Incubation of capacitated spermatozoa with human zonae pellucidae and subsequently with phosphatidylserine liposomes was as described (Arts et al., Biochem. J. 304:211, 1994). Spermatozoa were considered acrosome-reacted when fluorescence was confined to the ES; only when this ES-restricted fluorescence was clearly diffuse, the spermatozoa were considered fusogenic.

RESULTS:
The sperm preparations of all 8 patients showed reduced ZP binding capacity: for two patients the number of bound sperm per ZP was less than 40% of the donor value, the spermatozoa of the other 6 patients showed a binding capacity of 40-80% relative to the control value. After binding to the ZP, the spermatozoa of three patients failed to undergo AR. The other 5 patients responded poorly to AR induction: the number of acrosome-reacted spermatozoa per ZP was always less than 5% of the control value. The acrosome-reacted spermatozoa of three patients had acquired fusogenic activity. For the other two patients, liposomes only bound to the ES, but did not fuse.

CONCLUSION:
For only two patients the inability of the spermatozoa to fertilize could be explained by a low ZP binding capacity (Oehninger et al., Fertil. Steril. 51:665, 1989). The liposome test revealed that all other patients were either unable to undergo ZP-induced AR or responded poorly. In addition, some preparations did not acquire fusogenic activity. Inclusion of the liposome test may therefore reduce the false-positive score of a ZP binding test.

Sperm function tests and fertilization failure following IVF

Kalantar S.M.[1], Lenton E.A., Barratt C.L.R[2]

[1]Sheffield Fertility Centre and [2]Department of Obstetrics and Gynaecology, University of Sheffield, U.K.

OBJECTIVES:
Eleven men with abnormal semen parameters and total fertilization failure were recruited as part of an ongoing study to assess the predictive value of sperm function tests in the selection of couples for IVF + ICSI or IVF alone. The men were asked to produce a further semen sample which was then subjected to four recognized tests of sperm function. Control semen was obtained under identical conditions from fertile semen donors.

MATERIALS AND METHODS:
In addition to a comprehensive semen analysis, each sample was assessed for (i) spontaneous live acrosome reaction(AR)(ii) AR after A23187 challenge (iii) DNA maturation by acridine orange (AO)(iv)zona pellucida binding (ZPB). This last test was performed using salt-stored unfertilized oocytes. Sperm-zona binding was assessed following simultaneous incubation with both test and control sperm separately labeled with two different fluorescein dyes and the number of sperm which were tightly bound was counted. Results have been compared using ANOVA statistics.

RESULTS:

Variable	AR % live acrosome reacted		AO % sperm with mature DNA	ZPB N° sperm bound
	Spontaneous	A23187		
Patient	2.09 ± 2.5	24 ± 10.8	23.9 ± 6.4	2.6 ± 3.9
Control	0.9 ± 0.83	58 ± 6.5	53.9 ± 5.9	65.7 ± 33.1

* (Expressed as percentage of AR induced - spontaneous).
The results are shown as mean±SD. For each test the difference was highly significant($p<0.0001$,ANOVA). However the only sperm function test where there was no overlap in the results obtained between the failed fertilization men and the normal controls was the zona binding test (range of test and control results 2-13 and 21-148, respectively).

CONCLUSION:
Although the zona binding test as performed here, has shown a clear difference between the normal controls and the men selected for their previous total failed fertilization at IVF, it is too early to say whether this simple test will be effective in predicting those men who should be managed by ICSI as the primary treatment procedure. Further investigations examine the biochemical/molecular defects in sperm zona binding e. g phosphorylation of ^{32}P are in progress (see Brewis. *et al.,* in this meeting).

(This research is supported by the Iranian MHME)

The effect of testosterone enanthate (TE) administration on the acrosome reaction to ionophore challenge (ARIC) test

Troup, S.A, Bellis, A., WU, F.C.W , Lieberman, B.A.

Manchester Fertility Services, BUPA Hospital, Russel road, Manchester UK

OBJECTIVES:

The aim of the present investigation was to examine the ARIC values of semen samples provided by subjects receiving TE for contraceptive purposes to assess any effect of this agent on acrosomal function.

MATERIALS AND METHODS:

Normospermic subject were given weekly i. m. injections of 200mg TE. Commencing one month after the first injection, subjects provided semen samples at monthly intervals. In addition to a routine semen analysis, spermatozoa were prepared using a Percoll gradient and exposed to 10µM A23187 for 60 minutes, followed by exposure to hypoosmotic solution as a test of spermatozoa viability. The acrosome was visualized using FITC conjugated 18.6 monoclonal antibody and epifluorescence. The proportion of viable spermatozoa which had acrosome reacted in response to A23187 was calculated (the ARIC value).

RESULTS:

The performance of each ARIC test was verified using aliquots of cryopreserved semen. The median spermatozoal concentration pre-treatment was 70.0 million/ml. A significant reduction ($P<0.05$) was observed in spermatozoal concentration following 4 weeks TE (32 million/ml) with a further significant reduction ($p<0.05$) following 8 weeks TE (14.5 million/ml). The median pre-treatment ARIC value was 47.5%. A highly significant reduction ($p<0.005$) was observed in ARIC values following 4 weeks TE (16.0%), although no further reduction was observed following 8 weeks TE (17.3%).

CONCLUSION:

The results of the present investigation demonstrate that spermatozoa produced by subjects taking TE have a significantly reduced ability to acrosome react in response to A 23187. This result would suggest that in addition to its well documented inhibitory spermatogenic effect, TE administration may affect spermatozoal function at the level of the acrosome reaction. The mechanism of such an effect remains unclear, and the effects of male contraceptive agents on the AR are worthy of further investigation.

Use of acrosome reaction for predicting *in vitro* fertilization results

Richoilley G., Moutaffian H., Vieitez G., Milhet P., Labal B., Parinaud J.

Laboratoire de Fécondation In vitro, CHU La Grave, Toulouse, France

OBJECTIVES:
Acrosome plays an essential role in fertilization process and some IVF failures has been related to acrosome dysfunctions. Nevertheless, the place of acrosome function in assessing fertilizing ability remained to be evaluated. This study aimed to determine whether or not acrosome evaluation can enhance the prediction of IVF results when associated to conventional semen parameters.

MATERIALS AND METHODS:
Spontaneous and induced acrosome reactions as well as sperm concentration, viability, motility and morphology were recorded in 210 semen samples from patients undergoing an IVF attempt. Fertilization occurred in 172 cases (82%). According to WHO criteria, 104 sperms (50%) were abnormal. Acrosome reaction was measured by cytofluorimetry (Coultronics) using GB24 monoclonal antibody (Théramex). Spontaneous acrosome loss was assessed after a 6 hour and a 24 hour incubation in B2 medium (Δ 24h). Acrosome reaction was also induced a phorbol ester (Δ TPA). Motility was measured by Hamilton computerized system analysis.

RESULTS:

Z values	Serie 1 (n=131)	Serie 2 (n=79)	Overall results (n=210)
< -100	95%	98%	95%
-100 to 100	76%*	86%	81%*
> 100	46%**	30%***	42%***

Table 1: Fertilization rates according to the Z score values
* $P < 0.05$ versus group with Z < -100 in the same series
** $P < 0.01$ versus group with Z < -100 in the same series;
*** $P < 0.001$ versus group with Z < -100 in the same series

On a first series of 131 samples we established a score predicting IVF results calculated as follows: Z = 1198.70 - (2.97 x % of normal forms) - (1.99 x % rapid motility) + (5.73 x Δ 24h) - (63.64 x % of enlarged heads) + (78.34 x % multiflagellar forms) - (9.94 x linear motility) - (5.84 x viability) - (6.42 x Δ TPA).

This score was then validated on a separate series of 79 samples and the discriminating ability of the score was identical in both series.

CONCLUSION:

The study of acrosome function, through spontaneous acrosome loss and response to TPA, is of great interest in clinical practice, when associated to some parameters of motility and morphology. The calculated score allowed to predict fertilization failures with a 56% sensitivity, a 91% specificity, a 56% positive predictive value and a 91% negative predictive value. Therefore, it can be used in routine to choice between conventional IVF and ICSI.

Use of acrosome reaction for predicting *in vitro* fertilization results

Richoilley G., Moutaffian H., Vieitez G., Milhet P., Labal B., Parinaud J.

Laboratoire de Fécondation In vitro, CHU La Grave, Toulouse, France

OBJECTIVES:
Acrosome plays an essential role in fertilization process and some IVF failures has been related to acrosome dysfunctions. Nevertheless, the place of acrosome function in assessing fertilizing ability remained to be evaluated. This study aimed to determine whether or not acrosome evaluation can enhance the prediction of IVF results when associated to conventional semen parameters.

MATERIALS AND METHODS:
Spontaneous and induced acrosome reactions as well as sperm concentration, viability, motility and morphology were recorded in 210 semen samples from patients undergoing an IVF attempt. Fertilization occurred in 172 cases (82%). According to WHO criteria, 104 sperms (50%) were abnormal. Acrosome reaction was measured by cytofluorimetry (Coultronics) using GB24 monoclonal antibody (Théramex). Spontaneous acrosome loss was assessed after a 6 hour and a 24 hour incubation in B2 medium (Δ 24h). Acrosome reaction was also induced a phorbol ester (Δ TPA). Motility was measured by Hamilton computerized system analysis.

RESULTS:

Z values	Serie 1 (n=131)	Serie 2 (n=79)	Overall results (n=210)
< -100	95%	98%	95%
-100 to 100	76%*	86%	81%*
> 100	46%**	30%***	42%***

Table 1: Fertilization rates according to the Z score values
 * $P < 0.05$ versus group with $Z < -100$ in the same series
 ** $P < 0.01$ versus group with $Z < -100$ in the same series;
 *** $P < 0.001$ versus group with $Z < -100$ in the same series

On a first series of 131 samples we established a score predicting IVF results calculated as follows: Z = 1198.70 - (2.97 x % of normal forms) - (1.99 x % rapid motility) + (5.73 x Δ 24h) - (63.64 x % of enlarged heads) + (78.34 x % multiflagellar forms) - (9.94 x linear motility) - (5.84 x viability) - (6.42 x Δ TPA).

This score was then validated on a separate series of 79 samples and the discriminating ability of the score was identical in both series.

CONCLUSION:
The study of acrosome function, through spontaneous acrosome loss and response to TPA, is of great interest in clinical practice, when associated to some parameters of motility and morphology. The calculated score allowed to predict fertilization failures with a 56% sensitivity, a 91% specificity, a 56% positive predictive value and a 91% negative predictive value. Therefore, it can be used in routine to choice between conventional IVF and ICSI.

Prognostic value of hamster test with Ca-ionophore A 23187

Van Kooy R.J., Arts E.G.J.M, Kastrop P.M.M., Velde E.R.

University Hospital Utrecht, Heidelberglan 100, 3584 CX Utrecht, The Netherlands

OBJECTIVES:
To evaluate the prognostic value of the hamster oocyte test with and without pretreatment of the spermatozoa by Ca-ionophore A 23187.

MATERIALS AND METHODS:
Spermatozoa from two groups of IVF patients were tested with hamster oocyte tests with and without pretreatment of the spermatozoa with A 23187. Group I were patients who had total fertilization failure in their first IVF treatment. Group II were patients who did fertilize at least some ova in their first IVF-treatment.
Hamster tests were performed according to WHO-guidelines.

RESULTS:
Upto now 41 patients have been tested with both hamster test systems. The test system with A 23187 produced much higher penetration rates. In group I (IVF negative patients) 24 patients were tested upto now. The hamster test according to the classical protocol was negative in 14 cases. The test with A 23187 was negative in only four cases. In group II (IVF positive controls) 17 patients were tested upto now. In the A 23187 protocol 16 were positive and 1 negative. In the classical protocol 2 were negative, 15 positive. The study is still ongoing for both groups.

CONCLUSION:
Spermatozoa seem to be forced to undergo an acrosome reaction and get fusogenic properties by the action of A 23187. Provisional results show that A 23187 does not improve the prognostic value.

A novel method for evaluating the acromosal status of mammalian spermatozoa

Margalit I., Rubinstein S., Breitbart H.

Department of Life Sciences, Bar-Ilan University, Ramat-Gan, Israël

OBJECTIVES:
To develop a simple, objective, low cost assay to evaluate the acrosome reaction in ram, bull and human sperm for clinical and research purposes.

MATERIALS AND METHODS
The acrosome reaction (AR) was induced in ram, bull and human spermatozoa by known inducers of the AR (e.g., A23187, ionomycin, progesterone etc.). The acrosomal status was monitored by the new method and was compared to conventional methods such as staining with Pisum sativum agglutinin and also with fertilization rates in IVF (human only). Working conditions were optimized for the new method..

RESULTS
A novel method was developed to evaluate the acrosomal status of mammalian spermatozoa. The new method correlates well with conventional methods results and has advantage such as simplicity, objectiveness, rapidity, low cost, only standard laboratory is needed, there is no need for tedious slide reading by microscopes and many samples can be processed in parallel. I can be applied in hospitals and centers for artificial insemination of farm animals.

CONCLUSION:
Testing of this aspect -acrosomal status- of sperm function is an important diagnostic tool in sperm analysis that is not widely used today, perhaps because of the lack of a convenient method. The method presented here can overcome this problem.

Changes in lectin receptors in ejaculated, capacitated and acrosome reacted rhesus monkey spermatozoa

Sivashanmugam P., Navaneetham D., Rajalakshmi M.

All India Institute of Medical Sciences, New Delhi, India.

OBJECTIVES:
In this study changes in sperm surface glycoconjugates were analyzed in ejaculated spermatozoa incubated in capacitation medium *in vitro*, using lectin probes. The results were evaluated by lectin fluorescence and lectin immunoassay. The occurrence of acrosome reaction in capacitated spermatozoa and the changes in sperm surface glycoconjugates during this reaction were also studied.

MATERIALS AND METHODS:
Spermatozoa were collected from six adult male rhesus monkeys by penile electroejaculation. Capacitation was induced experimentally by incubating sperm in Tyrode's medium for five hours in a CO_2 incubator at 37° C. Lectin labeling (PNA, WGA, Con A) was done using FITC labeled lectins. To quantitate lectin receptors, a cellular lectin enzymeimmunoassay (CLEIA) was established; the validity of CLEIA was done using different concentrations of lectins, antilectin antibodies and cell number. Appropriate inhibitor saccharide sugars were used as controls.

RESULTS:
Approximately 30% of sperm underwent the acrosome reaction when incubated in capacitation medium. Ejaculated spermatozoa showed intense labeling of lectins in the acrosome while the postacrosomal area did not bind lectins and showed a quantitative increase in lectin binding compared to caudal spermatozoa. In capacitated acrosome reacted spermatozoa, the localization of lectins was restricted to mainly the equatorial segment while sperm that did not undergo the acrosome reaction showed a pattern similar to ejaculated uncapacitated spermatozoa. The restriction of lectin labeling to the equatorial region of spermatozoa which had undergone acrosome reaction indicates the important role the equatorial segment plays during fertilization since fusion with ovum takes place at the equatorial segment.

CONCLUSION:
Lectins thus provide a suitable marker to monitor the acrosome reaction.

Human sperm acrosome reaction. Eds P. Fénichel, J. Parinaud.
Colloque INSERM/John Libbey Eurotext Ltd © 1995. Vol. 236, pp. 449

Expression of sperm binding-receptors in different groups of human spermatozoa

Friedrich K.J., Haidl G., Deiss B., Kreysel H.W.

Department of Dermatology, University of Bonn, Sigmund-Freud Str. 25, 53105 Bonn/GERMANY

OBJECTIVES:
The aim of our study was to investigate the binding capacity of 1) immature epididymal and 2) morphologically disturbed spermatozoa.

MATERIALS AND METHODS:
Therefore, samples of epididymal spermatozoa from patients who underwent orchidectomy because of prostatic cancer were collected and divided into samples from caput, corpus and cauda epididymidis. In addition semen samples from andrological patients were collected containing either high amounts of acrosome-defect or hyperelongated spermatozoa. Binding capacity was analysed by determination of mannose binding receptors after capacitation *in vitro* (Benoff, 1993). Spermatozoa were incubated with mannose labeled FITC-neoglycoproteinligands and expression of receptors was assessed by fluorescence microscopy.

RESULTS:
The results revealed a significantly increasing amount of spermatozoa expressing the receptors during epididymal transit from 6 % in caput to 20 % in cauda epididydimidis. Analysis of morphologically disturbed samples showed that only normal formed spermatozoa and slightly hyperelongated cells (also known as "tapers") are able to express binding receptors in contrast to acrosome-defect or totally amorphous forms.

CONCLUSION:
The results are indicative of changes in the ability of sperm binding during epididymal maturation of spermatozoa and can explain poor fertilization rates using epididymal spermatozoa from the caput for assisted reproduction. On the other side a markedly reduced binding capacity of severely disturbed spermatozoa is confirmed while the role of the so-called "taperforms" in classification of pathological morphology should be discussed again.

Modifications of lectin binding sites on the surface of human sperm during acrosome reaction: analysis in flow cytometry and electron microscopy

Fierro R.C., Daniel M., Foliguet B., Bene M.C., Barbarino P., Faure G., Grignon G.

Laboratoire d' Histologie Embryologie, Faculté de Médecine, BP 184, 54505 NANCY Laboratoire d' Immunologie, Faculté de Médecine de NANCY Laboratoire de Biologie Sexuelle, Maternité Régionale NANCY Depto. Ciencias Salud. Univ. Autonoma Metropolitana Iztapalapa, MEXICO

OBJECTIVES:
Biochemical surface modifications occur during the capacitation and acrosome reaction of human sperm (among those, variations in the expression of carbohydrate moieties).
We report a dynamic study where the binding of wheat germ agglutinin (WGA), concanavalin A (ConA), peanut agglutinin (PNA), and Ulex-1 was assessed on normal human sperm samples during *in vitro* induction of the acrosome reaction with calcium ionophore A 23 187.

MATERIALS AND METHODS:
Thirty samples of human sperm were centrifuged over a Percoll gradient. Aliquots of each sperm sample were collected before and respectively 30, 60 and 120 minutes after initiation of the acrosome reaction by addition of 10 mMol/L calcium ionophore. Each aliquot was studied in flow cytometry and electron microscopy (CM12 Philips), after incubation respectively with fluorescein-, ferritin- or gold-conjugated lectins. The samples used for flow cytometry were also labeled indirectly with GB24 (THERAMEX) and phycoerythrin-conjugated anti-mouse antiserum in order to appreciate the amount of sperm having undergone the acrosome reaction.
For each sample, the percentage of labeled sperm and their fluorescence intensity, recorded using EPICS-XL flow cytometer (Coultronics Company, Hialeah, FL), were used to calculate a labeling index taking both these parameters into account.

RESULTS:
WGA was shown to bind strongly the whole surface of sperm before induction of the acrosome reaction, and in a lesser amounts after incubation with calcium ionophore. This resulted in a significant decrease of the labeling index during the

first 30 minutes of incubation, persisting at later times. GB24 binding increased proportionally to this decrease.

PNA and mostly Con-A binding evolved in an opposite pattern, with an increase of the labeling index parallel to that of GB24 binding. Electron microscopy allowed to demonstrate that this was the result of the increasing labeling of the acrosomes inner membrane, significant 60 minutes after induction of the acrosome reaction.

Ulex-1 was found to bind faintly on unstimulated sperm, but a significant labeling was observed after incubation with calcium ionophore, concomitant with access of the lectin to the acrosomes inner membrane.

In vitro induction of the acrosome reaction, which has been shown to induce an increase in GB24 binding, also results in a increased labeling of human sperm with ConA, PNA and Ulex-1, and a decreased binding of WGA. Electron microscopy confirmed that the fluorescence patterns observed correlated with increased access to the inner membrane of the acrosome.

CONCLUSION:
This suggests that the modifications of both protein detection and glycosylation patterns occur during the acrosome reaction, which can be assessed in flow cytometry.

Response of human spermatozoa to five different acrosome reaction inducers

Kohn F.M.[1], El-Mulla K.F.[1,2], El-Beheiry A.H.[2], Schill W.B.[1]

[1] Dept. Derm Androl., Justus Liebig Univ., Giessen, Germany, [2] Dept. Derm. Androl., Alexandria Univ., Egypt

OBJECTIVES:
The aim of the study was to compare five different protocols for human sperm acrosome reaction. The AR can be induced by artificial increase of intracellular calcium levels (ionophore A 23187, progesterone), direct activation of protein kinase A (dbcAMP) or C (phorboldiesters, PMA), inhibition of phosphodiesterase (pentoxifylline, Ptx) and moderate cold treatment activation.

MATERIALS AND METHODS:
Semen samples from 50 patients attending an andrological outpatient department were filtered through glass woll and washed twice in human tubular fluid (HTFM) containing 1 % human serum albumin. Each semen sample (5×10^6/ml) was divided into 8 aliquots and treated for the induction of AR. Four aliquots were capacitated for 18 hours at 37°C; subsequently they were incubated with 1 mM dbcAMP (in phosphate buffered saline, PBS), 10 µM ionophore (in 0.1% DMSO), 10 µM PMA (in 0.1% DMSO) and 10 µM progesterone (in 0.1% DMSO) for 1 hour at 37°C, respectively. Two other aliquots were first kept at 4°C for 15 hours and then incubated at 37°C for 3 hours in the presence of 1 mg/ml Ptx (cold treatment + Ptx) or without any treatment (cold treatment). The corresponding controls were two specimens capacitated for 18 hours at 37°C and treated with PBS or 0.1% DMSO for 1 hour at 37°C. Living acrosome reacted spermatozoa were detected by triple staining.

RESULTS:
The numbers (mean±SEM) of acrosome reacted spermatozoa in PBS- and DMSO-treated controls were similar (13.2±1.0% vs. 12.8±0.9%). Treatment with ionophore (28.1±1.3%, $p<0.001$), progesterone (21.0±1.3%, $p<0.001$), PMA (21.7±1.4%, $p<0.001$), Ptx (25.0±1.2%, $p<0.001$), dbcAMP (21.1±1.3%, $p<0.001$) and cold (24.9±1.2%, $p<0.001$) increased the percentages of acrosome reacted spermatozoa significantly. Significant positive correlations were found between all the numbers of acrosome reacted spermatozoa as detected by the various protocols. The highest correlations were found between progesterone and ionophore ($r=0.67$), progesterone and PMA ($r=0.70$), Progesterone and db cAMP ($r=0.63$), dbcAMP and PMA

(r=0.72), dbcAMP and ionophore (r=0.69), Ptx and cold-treatment (r=0.85), Ptx and PMA (r=0.62). However, only 18 of 50 patients (36%) responded to all inducers with an increase of acrosome reaction of at least 5%. The best responses were found after treatment with ionophore and cold treatment. The most non-responders were found after treatment with progesterone (14/50=28%), dbcAMP (16/50=32%) and PMA (9/50=18%).

CONCLUSION:
Individual semen samples do not respond uniformly to various AR inducers. Therefore, correlations between the inducibility of AR and the fertilizing capacity are dependent on the stimulus used. Since the various inducers represent different second messenger systems, the pattern of response may provide information about their function.

Human sperm acrosome reaction. Eds P. Fénichel, J. Parinaud.
Colloque INSERM/John Libbey Eurotext Ltd © 1995. Vol. 236, pp.454-455

Studies on the kinetics of human sperm acrosome reaction. A mathematical model for assessment.

Henkel R.[1], Franken D.R.[2], Maritz J.S.[3], Schill W.B.[1], Habenicht U.F.[4]

[1]*Dept. Dermatol. Androl., JLU Giessen, Germany,* [2]*Dept. Obstet. Gynaecol., Univ. Stellenbosch, Tygerberg, RSA,* [3]*Dept. of Statistics, Univ. Stellenbosch, Stellenbosch, RSA and* [4]*Ernst Schering Research Foundation, Berlin, Germany*

OBJECTIVES:
To evaluate the influence of solubilized human zona pellucida proteins on acrosomal status and to calculate kinetics of human sperm acrosome reaction.

MATERIAL AND METHODS:
Sperm samples from fertile donors were prepared by double-wash and swim-up. Post mortem derived immature human oocytes were used for solubilization. Zona pellucida solutions were prepared by dissolving zonae pellucidae in NaH_2PO_4 (pH 2.5) to obtain solutions 0.1, 0.15, 0.3, 0.5 and 1.0 zonae pellucidae/µl. The zona solvent containing no zona proteins plus a modified HTF medium was taken for control. Following treatment of zona solutions with modified HTF medium to adjust pH sperm were added (final conc.: 4×10^6 cells/ml) and the samples were incubated at 37°C. For evaluation of acrosomal status of sperm aliquots were taken after 20, 40 and 60 minutes of incubation, respectively. Samples were stained with Bismarck Brown and Rosé Bengal and evaluated in a bright field microscope at 1000x. Time dependence of acrosome reaction was then calculated by a 'logistic regression' model. Using the fitted model it was possible to obtain estimates of the rate of change in Y with t at t=0 for different concentrations of zona pellucida.

RESULTS:
The results showed a distinct time- and dose dependence of acrosome reaction induced by means of solubilized human zona pellucida proteins. After 20 minutes of incubation in 0.1 zonae/µl already about 40% of the sperm showed signs of acrosome reaction. After 60 minutes of incubation in 1.0 zonae/µl 82% of the sperm showed signs of acrosomal loss. The percentage of completely acrosome-reacted sperm, however, were 9% and 36%, respectively. Using the mathematical model we could calculate V_0 and constants of equilibrium of both sperm that were completely acrosome-reacted and those that show signs of acrosome reaction. Calculated V_0 had the same levels of approximately 2%/min. for both completely acrosome-reacted sperm and all those sperm showing signs of acrosome reaction. Constants of

equilibrium differed by factor 10; 2.0 zonae/µl and 0.2 zonae/µl for completely reacted sperm and all those sperm showing signs of acrosome reaction, respectively.

CONCLUSION:
Following induction by means of human zona pellucida moieties human sperm acrosome reaction shows a distinct time- and dose dependence. V_0 and constants of equilibrium of human sperm acrosome reaction could be calculated in a mathematical model.

This study was supported by the 'Stifterverband für die Deutsche Wissenschaft' grant number TS 017/23.

The application of scanning probe microscopy to the visualization of the human sperm acrosome reaction

Sweeney A., Tomkins P.T.

Toxicology Unit, Regional College, Athlone, Ireland

OBJECTIVES:
A primary objective of this study was to establish optimal operating conditions and experimental configuration for the application of scanning tunneling microscopy (STM) and atomic force microscopy (AFM) to the visualization of the human sperm acrosome and ascription of acrosomal status with reference to scanning electron microscopy (SEM) and localization of fluorescent lectin probes.

MATERIALS AND METHODS:
Sperm from clinical samples were motile selected on discontinuous Percoll gradients or Sephadex columns and prepared at a density of 5×10^6 ml^{-1} in culture medium. The acrosome reaction was induced by exposure to calcium ionophores A23187 and ETH-129 at concentrations of 1 - 20 mM and by electropermeabilization in the presence of 3.4 mM $CaCl_2$ using a square wave generator in high viability non-contact mode. For AFM of 'preserved' cells, sperm were fixed in 4% glutaraldehyde, anchored to treated glass substrates, dehydrated and critical point dried prior to examination on a Burleigh SPM. For AFM of live cells, cleaved sperm heads were anchored to poly-l-lysine coated polished glass substrates in a 5 - 10 ml drop of medium containing ionophore. For STM, fixed cells were uniformly coated with gold prior to examination. SEM and lectin studies were performed according to established procedures in this laboratory.

RESULTS:
Low resolution AFM images of fixed cells were readily obtained by AFM provided cells were dried by a CPD method and density was restricted to prevent overlapping. Despite minimization of cell movement, vibration damping and application of image processing, obtaining high resolution AFM images of fixed and live cells proved difficult and gold depth for effective STM was found to be critical (1 nm). AFM permitted visualization of sequential intermembranous fusions and surface geometry during the acrosome reaction which tentatively supports the notion of an atypical reaction for human cells. The configuration for visualizing live cells demanded that the AFM probe be manually approached to the cell surface. Initial analysis indicates a significant positive correlation between AFM, SEM and fluorescent probe based classification of acrosomal status. The kinetics of non-viable acrosome reactions induced by ETH-129 were >5x faster than those induced by A23187.

CONCLUSION:
Visualization of the human sperm acrosome is routinely possible using scanning probe microscopy and in the long term, AFM offers the tantalizing prospect of clearly visualizing the conduct of the acrosome reaction at surface and whole cell resolution in living cells.

Using flow cytometry for acrosome status evaluation in human sperm

Nikolaeva M.A., Goukasian I.A., Philippova R.D., Sukhikh G.T.

Scientific Center for Obstetrics, Gynaecology and Perinatology, Oparin 4, 117815, Moscow. Russia.

OBJECTIVES:
Acrosome status in human spermatozoa was evaluated by flow cytometry (FCM) analyzer FACSCAN (Becton Dickinson, USA). Dual fluorescence staining of methanol fixed spermatozoa was performed with the probes targeting the outer acrosomal membrane (OAM) (rodamine-conjugated Arachis hypogea lectin) or constituents of the acrosomal vesicle (fluorescein isothiocyanate-conjugated Pisum sativum lectin).

MATERIALS AND METHODS:
Sperm samples were obtained from 10 men with normal semen analysis. Motile spermatozoa selected by swim up technique were subsequently incubated for 1 hour with: Medium 199 with 0,5% bovine serum albumin (Medium A), Medium A with the ionophore A23187 (10 μM) and Medium A with rabbit antiserum against human spermatozoa (1:8 dilution).

RESULTS:
FCM-analysis revealed distinct subpopulations of spermatozoa: 1) with high level of green and red fluorescence (acrosome-intact spermatozoa); 2) with high level of green and reduced level or absence of red fluorescence (probably, spermatozoa with intact acrosomal matrix and dispersed or absent OAM); 3) with reduced level of green and red fluorescence (probably, spermatozoa with dispersed both acrosomal matrix and OAM); 4) without red and green fluorescence (probably, spermatozoa without OAM and acrosomal matrix); 5) spermatozoa with very high level of green fluorescence and different level of red fluorescence (probably, spermatozoa with enhanced content of acrosomal matrix and intact, dispersed or absent OAM). Induction of acrosome reaction with the ionophore A23187 resulted in reliable enhancement of the number of spermatozoa in subpopulation with reduced level of green and red fluorescence from 6,7% to 19,2% ($p<0,02$) and in subpopulation with very high level of green fluorescence from 10,1% to 16,1% ($p<0,01$). Incubation of spermatozoa with rabbit antiserum resulted in the dramatically enhanced number of spermatozoa with very high level of green fluorescence from 10,3% to 41,2% ($p<0,001$). It is possible that ionophore A23187 and antisperm antibodies can stimulate synthesis of acrosomal matrix.

CONCLUSION:
Thus, a possibility of quantitative estimation of heterogeneity of spermatozoa has been demonstrated during acrosomal reaction. The evaluation of acrosome reaction by FCM seemed to be more objective and sensitive than those methods using fluorescent microscopy.

The extrusion of doublet-ODF$_S$ (outer dense fibers) 5-6 associating with fibrous sheath sliding in mouse sperm flagella

Si Y. , Okuno M.

Department of biology, College of Arts & Sciences, the University of Tokyo, Tokyo 153, Japan.

OBJECTIVES:
A previous study (Si & Okuno, 1993. exp. Cell Res. 208: 170-174) provided evidence the fibrous sheath (FS) slid headward to middle piece in the activated mouse sperm flagella when doublet microtubules together with their ODFs extruded from the axoneme. The aim of the present study was to investigate which one, of the extruded doublet-ODFs, was responsible for the FS sliding.

MATERIALS AND METHODS:
It was observed that the sliding of FS was always associated with the first doublet-ODF extruding from the axoneme. When the preferential extrusion of doublet-ODF associating with FS sliding was performed, vanadate sodium, a dynein ATPase inhibitor, was added to inhibit other doublet-ODFs to extrude. Electron microscopy was employed to examine the configurations of the cross section of the microtubule-extruded spermatozoa. It was expected that the doublet-ODF' extruding preferentially would be missing in these flagellar cross sections.

RESULTS:
Under the condition of mild trypsinization, only doublet ODFs 4, 5-6 and 7 extruded from the axoneme. Furthermore, it was found that 81 % and 91% of spermatozoa ejected their doublet ODFs 5-6 in their principal and middle pieces, respectively, while only 9% and 2% of spermatozoa ejected their doublet -ODF 4 in their principal and middle pieces, respectively. Thus the extrusion of doublet-ODFs 5 and 6 was identified to precede doublet-ODFs 4 and 7, and was considered the candidate responsible for FS sliding. In contrast high concentration trypsinization led to the extrusion of doublets-ODFs 1,2 and 9 following doublet-ODFs 4, 5-6 and 7. FS sliding, however, did not occur.

CONCLUSION:
The results demonstrated that the nine doublet microtubules is demembranated mouse sperm flagella had a difference in their sliding disintegration activity, which might be involved in the regulatory system for flagellar movement in situ. under the present experimental circumstances, it was found that; the doublet-ODF's 5-6 extruded preferentially from the axoneme and associated with FS sliding, then the doublet-ODF 4 or 7 extruded. Doutlet-ODFs 1, 2 and 9 were the last to be extruded, however, doublet 3-central pair-8 did not extrude.

Colloques INSERM
ISSN 0768-3154

Other *Colloques* published as co-editions by John Libbey Eurotext and INSERM

133 Cardiovascular and Respiratory Physiology in the
Fetus and Neonate. *Physiologie Cardiovasculaire et Respiratoire du Fœtus et du Nouveau-né.*
Scientific Committee : P. Karlberg,
A. Minkowski, W. Oh and L. Stern;
Managing Editor : M. Monset-Couchard.
ISBN : John Libbey Eurotext 0 86196 086 6
INSERM 2 85598 282 0

134 Porphyrins and Porphyrias. *Porphyrines et Porphyries.*
Edited by Y. Nordmann.
ISBN : John Libbey Eurotext 0 86196 087 4
INSERM 2 85598 281 2

137 Neo-Adjuvant Chemotherapy. *Chimiothérapie Néo-Adjuvante.*
Edited by C. Jacquillat, M. Weil and D. Khayat.
ISBN : John Libbey Eurotext 0 86196 077 7
INSERM 2 85598 283 7

139 Hormones and Cell Regulation (10th European Symposium). *Hormones et Régulation Cellulaire (10ᵉ Symposium Européen).*
Edited by J. Nunez, J.E. Dumont and R.J.B. King.
ISBN : John Libbey Eurotext 0 86196 084 X
INSERM 2 85598 284 7

147 Modern Trends in Aging Research. *Nouvelles Perspectives de la Recherche sur le Vieillissement.*
Edited by Y. Courtois, B. Faucheux, B. Forette,
D.L. Knook and J.A. Tréton.
ISBN : John Libbey Eurotext 0 86196 103 X
INSERM 2 85598 309 6

149 Binding Proteins of Steroid Hormones. *Protéines de liaison des Hormones Stéroïdes.*
Edited by M.G. Forest and M. Pugeat.
ISBN : John Libbey Eurotext 0 86196 125 0
INSERM 2 85598 310 X

151 Control and Management of Parturition. *La Maîtrise de la Parturition.*
Edited by C. Sureau, P. Blot, D. Cabrol, F. Cavaillé and G. Germain.
ISBN : John Libbey Eurotext 0 86196 096 3
INSERM 2 85598 311 8

Colloques INSERM
ISSN 0768-3154

153 Hormones and Cell Regulation (11th European Symposium). *Hormones et Régulation Cellulaire (11ᵉ Symposium Européen).*
Edited by J. Nunez and J.E. Dumont.
ISBN : John Libbey Eurotext 0 86196 104 8
 INSERM 2 85598 324 X

158 Biochemistry and Physiopathology of Platelet Membrane. *Biochimie et Physiopathologie de la Membrane Plaquettaire.*
Edited by G. Marguerie and R.F.A. Zwaal.
ISBN : John Libbey Eurotext 0 86196 114 5
 INSERM 2 85598 345 2

162 The Inhibitors of Hematopoiesis. *Les Inhibiteurs de l'Hématopoïèse.*
Edited by A. Najman, M. Guignon, N.C. Gorin and J.Y. Mary.
ISBN : John Libbey Eurotext 0 86196 125 0
 INSERM 2 85598 340 1

164 Liver Cells and Drugs. *Cellules Hépatiques et Médicaments.*
Edited by A. Guillouzo.
ISBN : John Libbey Eurotext 0 86196 128 5
 INSERM 2 85598 341 X

165 Hormones and Cell Regulation (12th European Symposium). *Hormones et Régulation Cellulaire (12ᵉ Symposium Européen).*
Edited by J. Nunez, J.E. Dumont and E. Carafoli.
ISBN : John Libbey Eurotext 0 86196 133 1
 INSERM 2 85598 347 9

167 Sleep Disorders and Respiration. *Les Evénements Respiratoires du Sommeil.*
Edited by P. Lévi-Valensi and D. Duron.
ISBN : John Libbey Eurotext 0 86196 127 7
 INSERM 2 85598 344 4

169 Neo-Adjuvant Chemotherapy. *Chimiothérapie Néo-Adjuvante.*
Edited by C. Jacquillat, M. Weil, D. Khayat.
ISBN : John Libbey Eurotext 0 86196 150 1
 INSERM 2 85598 349 5

171 Structure and Functions of the Cytoskeleton. *La Structure et les Fonctions du Cytosquelette.*
Edited by B.A.F. Rousset.
ISBN : John Libbey Eurotext 0 86196 149 8
 INSERM 2 85598 351 7

Colloques INSERM
ISSN 0768-3154

172 The Langerhans Cell. *La Cellule de Langerhans.*
Edited by J. Thivolet, D. Schmitt.
ISBN : John Libbey Eurotext 0 86196 181 1
INSERM 2 85598 352 5

173 Cellular and Molecular Aspects of Glucuronidation. *Aspects Cellulaires et Moléculaires de la Glucuronoconjugaison.*
Edited by G. Siest, J. Magdalou, B. Burchell
ISBN : John Libbey Eurotext 0 86196 182 X
INSERM 2 85598 353 3

174 Second Forum on Peptides. *Deuxième Forum Peptides.*
Edited by A. Aubry, M. Marraud, B. Vitoux
ISBN : John Libbey Eurotext 0 86196 151 X
INSERM 2 85598 354 1

176 Hormones and Cell Regulation (13th European Symposium). *Hormones et Régulation Cellulaire (13ᵉ Symposium Européen).*
Edited by J. Nunez, J.E. Dumont, R. Denton
ISBN : John Libbey Eurotext 0 86196 183 8
INSERM 2 85598 356 8

179 Lymphokine Receptors Interactions. *Interactions Lymphokines-récepteurs.*
Edited by D. Fradelizi, J. Bertoglio
ISBN : John Libbey Eurotext 0 86196 148 X
INSERM 2 85598 359 2

191 Anticancer Drugs (1st International Interface of Clinical and Laboratory responses to anticancer drugs). *Médicaments anticancéreux (1ʳᵉ Confrontation internationale des réponses cliniques et expérimentales aux médicaments anticancéreux).*
Edited by H. Tapiero, J. Robert, T.J. Lampidis
ISBN : John Libbey Eurotext 0 86196 223 0
INSERM 2 85598 393 2

193 Living in the Cold (2nd International Symposium). *La Vie au Froid (2ᵉ Symposium International).*
Edited by A. Malan, B. Canguilhem
ISBN : John Libbey Eurotext 0 86196 234 9
INSERM 2 85598 395 9

Colloques INSERM
ISSN 0768-3154

194 Progress in Hepatitis B Immunization. *La Vaccination contre l'épatite B.*
Edited by P. Coursaget, M.J. Tong
ISBN : John Libbey Eurotext 0 86196 249 4
    INSERM 2 85598 396 7

196 Treatment Strategy in Hodgkin's Disease. *Stratégie dans la maladie de Hodgkin.*
Edited by P. Sommers, M. Henry-Amar,
J.H. Meezwaldt, P. Carde
ISBN : John Libbey Eurotext 0 86196 226 5
    INSERM 2 85598 398 3

198 Hormones and Cell Regulation (14th European Symposium). *Hormones et Régulation Cellulaire (14ᵉ Symposium Européen).*
Edited by J. Nunez, J.E. Dumont
ISBN : John Libbey Eurotext 0 86196 229 X
    INSERM 2 85598 400 9

199 Placental Communications : Biochemical, Morphological and Cellular Aspects. *Communications placentaires : aspects biochimique, morphologique et cellulaire.*
Edited by L. Cedard, E. Alsat, J.C. Challier,
G. Chaouat, A. Malassiné
ISBN : John Libbey Eurotext 0 86196 227 3
    INSERM 2 85598 401 7

204 Pharmacologie Clinique : Actualités et Perspectives. (6ᵉ Rencontres Nationales de Pharmacologie clinique).
Edited by J.P. Boissel, C. Caulin, M. Teule
ISBN : John Libbey Eurotext 0 86196 225 7
    INSERM 2 85598 454 8

205 Recent Trends in Clinical Pharmacology (6th National Meeting of Clinical Pharmacology).
Edited by J.P. Boissel, C. Caulin, M. Teule
ISBN : John Libbey Eurotext 0 86196 256 7
    INSERM 2 85598 455 6

206 Platelet Immunology : Fundamental and Clinical Aspects. *Immunologie plaquettaire : aspects fondamentaux et cliniques.*
Edited by C. Kaplan-Gouet, N. Schlegel,
Ch. Salmon, J. McGregor
ISBN : John Libbey Eurotext 0 86196 285 0
    INSERM 2 85598 439 4

Colloques INSERM
ISSN 0768-3154

207 Thyroperoxidase and Thyroid Autoimmunity. *Thyroperoxydase et auto-immunité thyroïdienne.*
Edited by P. Carayon, T. Ruf
ISBN : John Libbey Eurotext 0 86196 277 X
INSERM 2 85598 440 8

208 Vasopressin. *Vasopressine.*
Edited by S. Jard, R. Jamison
ISBN : John Libbey Eurotext 0 86196 288 5
INSERM 2 85598 441 6

210 Hormones and Cell Regulation (15th European Symposium). *Hormones et Régulation Cellulaire (15e Symposium Européen).*
Edited by J.E. Dumont, J. Nunez, R.J.B. King
ISBN : John Libbey Eurotext 0 86196 279 6
INSERM 2 85598 443 2

211 Medullary Thyroid Carcinoma. *Cancer Médullaire de la Thyroïde.*
Edited by C. Calmettes, J.M. Guliana
ISBN : John Libbey Eurotext 0 86196 287 7
INSERM 2 85598 440 0

212 Cellular and Molecular Biology of the Materno-Fetal Relationship. *Biologie cellulaire et moléculaire de la relation materno-fœtale.*
Edited by G. Chaouat, J. Mowbray
ISBN : John Libbey Eurotext 0 86196 909 1
INSERM 2 85598 445 9

215 Aldosterone. Fundamental Aspects. *Aspects fondamentaux.*
Edited by J.P. Bonvalet, N. Farman, M. Lombes, M.E. Rafestin-Oblin
ISBN : John Libbey Eurotext 0 86196 302 4
INSERM 2 85598 482 3

216 Cellular and Molecular Aspects of Cirrhosis. *Aspects cellulaires et moléculaires de la cirrhose.*
Edited by B. Clément, A. Guillouzo
ISBN : John Libbey Eurotext 0 86196 342 3
INSERM 2 85598 483 1

217 Sleep and Cardiorespiratory Control. *Sommeil et contrôle cardio-respiratoire.*
Edited by C. Gaultier, P. Escourrou, L. Curzi-Dascalora
ISBN : John Libbey Eurotext 0 86196 307 5
INSERM 2 85598 484 X

Colloques INSERM
ISSN 0768-3154

218 Genetic Hypertension. *Hypertension génétique.*
Edited by J. Sassard
ISBN : John Libbey Eurotext 0 86196 313 X
INSERM 2 85598 485 8

219 Human Gene Transfer. *Transfert de gènes chez l'homme.*
Edited by O. Cohen-Haguenauer, M. Boiron
ISBN : John Libbey Eurotext 0 86196 301 6
INSERM 2 85598 497 1

220 Medicine and Change: Historical and Sociological Studies of Medical Innovation. *L'innovation en médecine : études historiques et sociologiques.*
Edited by Ilana Löwy
ISBN : John Libbey Eurotext 2 7420 0010 0
INSERM 5 85598 508 0

221 Structures and Functions of Retinal Proteins. *Structures et fonctions des rétino-protéines.*
Edited by J.L. Rigaud
ISBN : John Libbey Eurotext 0 86196 355 5
INSERM 2 85598 509 9

222 Cellular and Molecular Biology of the Adrenal Cortex. *Biologie cellulaire et moléculaire du cortex surrénal.*
Edited by J.M. Saez, A.C. Brownie, A. Capponi, E.M. Chambaz, F. Mantero
ISBN : John Libbey Eurotext 0 86196 362 8
INSERM 2 85598 510 2

223 Mechanisms and Control of Emesis. *Mécanismes et contrôle du vomissement.*
Edited by A.L. Bianchi, L. Grélot, A.D. Miller, G.L. King
ISBN : John Libbey Eurotext 0 86196 363 6
INSERM 2 85598 511 0

224 High Pressure and Biotechnology. *Haute pression et biotechnologie.*
Edited by C. Balny, R. Hayashi, K. Heremans, P. Masson
ISBN : John Libbey Eurotext 0 86196 363 6
INSERM 2 85598 512 9

Colloques INSERM
ISSN 0768-3154

228 Non-Visual Human-Computer Interactions. *Communication non visuelle homme-ordinateur.*
Edited by D. Burger, J.C. Sperandio
ISBN : John Libbey Eurotext 2 7420 0014 3
INSERM 2 85598 540 4

229 The negative regulation of hematopoiesis, from fundamental aspects to clinical applications. *Régulation négative de l'hématopoïèse, des aspects fondamentaux à l'application clinique.*
Edited by Y. Beuzard
ISBN : John Libbey Eurotext 2 7420 0015 1
INSERM 2 85598 541 2

230 From Research in Oncology to Therapeutic Innovations. *De la recherche oncologique à l'innovation thérapeutique.*
Edited by P. Tambourin, M. Boiron
ISBN : John Libbey Eurotext 2 7420 0016 X
INSERM 2 85598 542 0

231 Human Ochratoxicosis and its pathologies. *Ochratoxicose humaine et ses pathologies.*
Edited by E.E. Creppy, M. Castegnaro, G. Dirheimer
ISBN : John Libbey Eurotext 2 7420 0017 8
INSERM 2 85598 543 9

232 Anxiety : Neurobiology, Clinic and Therapeutic Perspectives. *Anxiété : Neurobiologie, Clinique et Perspectives Thérapeutiques.*
Edited by M. Hamon, H. Ollat, M.-H. Thiébot
ISBN : John Libbey Eurotext 2 7420 0018 6
INSERM 2 85598 544 7

234 Sickle cell disease and thalassaemias : new trends in therapy. *Drépamocytose et thalassémies : nouvelles tendances thérapeutiques.*
Edited by Y. Beuzard, B. Lubin, J. Rosa
ISBN : John Libbey Eurotext 2 7420 0063 1
INSERM 2 85598 578 1

LOUIS-JEAN
avenue d'Embrun, 05003 GAP cedex
Tél. : 92.53.17.00
Dépôt légal : 651 — Août 1995
Imprimé en France